The Current and Future Impact of Cytopathology on Patient Care

Editor

CHRIS VANDENBUSSCHE

SURGICAL PATHOLOGY CLINICS

www.surgpath.theclinics.com

Consulting Editor
JASON L. HORNICK

September 2024 • Volume 17 • Number 3

ELSEVIER

1600 John F. Kennedy Boulevard • Suite 1800 • Philadelphia, Pennsylvania, 19103-2899

http://www.theclinics.com

SURGICAL PATHOLOGY CLINICS Volume 17, Number 3
September 2024 ISSN 1875-9181, ISBN-13: 978-0-443-13129-5

Editor: Taylor Hayes
Developmental Editor: Saswoti Nath

Surgical Pathology Clinics (ISSN 1875-9181) is published quarterly by Elsevier Inc., 360 Park Avenue South, New York, NY 10010. Months of issue are March, June, September, and December. Business and Editorial Office: Elsevier Inc., 1600 John F. Kennedy Blvd., Ste. 1800, Philadelphia, PA 19103-2899. Accounting and Circulation Offices: Elsevier Inc., 3251 Riverport Lane, Maryland Heights, MO 63043. Periodicals postage paid at New York, NY and at additional mailing offices. Subscription prices are $253.00 per year (US individuals), $100.00 per year (US students/residents), $294.00 per year (Canadian individuals), $307.00 per year (foreign individuals), and $120.00 per year (international students/residents), $100.00 per year (Canadian students/residents). For institutional access pricing please contact Customer Service via the contact information below. Foreign air speed delivery is included in all *Clinics'* subscription prices. All prices are subject to change without notice. Orders, claims, and journal inquiries: Please visit our Support Hub page https://service.elsevier.com for assistance.

Reprints. For copies of 100 or more, of articles in this publication, please contact the Commercial Reprints Department, Elsevier Inc., 360 Park Avenue South, New York, NY 10010-1710. Tel. 212-633-3874; Fax: 212-633-3820; E-mail: reprints@elsevier.com.

Surgical Pathology Clinics of North America is covered in *MEDLINE/PubMed (Index Medicus)*.

Contributors

CONSULTING EDITOR

JASON L. HORNICK, MD, PhD
Director of Surgical Pathology and
Immunohistochemistry, Brigham and Women's
Hospital, Professor of Pathology, Harvard
Medical School, Boston, Massachusetts, USA

EDITOR

CHRIS VANDENBUSSCHE, MD, PhD
Associate Professor of Oncology and
Pathology, Department of Pathology, Johns
Hopkins University School of Medicine,
Baltimore, Maryland, USA

AUTHORS

DEREK B. ALLISON, MD
Associate Professor of Pathology and Urology,
Vice Chair for Research, Department of
Pathology and Laboratory Medicine, University
of Kentucky College of Medicine, Assistant
Director and Quality Officer, Biospecimen
Procurement and Translational Pathology SRF,
Markey Cancer Center, Lexington, Kentucky,
USA

ALESSANDRO CAPUTO, MD
Pathologist, Department of Pathology,
University Hospital "San Giovanni di Dio e
Ruggi d'Aragona", Salerno, Italy

VALERIA CILIBERTI, MD
Pathologist, Department of Advanced
Biomedical Sciences, Pathology Unit,
University of Naples Federico II, Naples, Italy

DANIELLE D'AMBROSIO, MD
Pathologist, Department of Pathology, New
York University Grossman School of Medicine,
New York, New York, USA

ANGELA D'ARDIA, BS
Department of Pathology, University Hospital
"San Giovanni di Dio e Ruggi d'Aragona",
Salerno, Italy

NIYATI DESAI, MD
Pathology Resident, Department of Pathology
and Cell Biology, New York-Presbyterian
Hospital, Columbia University Irving Medical
Center, New York, New York, USA

KATYA S. DOMBROWSKI, MD
Pathology Resident, Department of Pathology,
The Johns Hopkins University School of
Medicine, Baltimore, Maryland, USA

FIONA HANLY, MS
MD/MBA Candidate, University of Miami Miller
School of Medicine, Miami, Florida, USA

JONAS J. HEYMANN, MD
Associate Professor of Clinical Pathology and
Laboratory Medicine, Department of Pathology
and Laboratory Medicine, New York-
Presbyterian Hospital, Weill Cornell Medicine,
New York, New York, USA

ERIC C. HUANG, MD, PhD
Director of Cytopathology, Director of HPV
Molecular Diagnostics Laboratory, Program
Director of Cytopathology Fellowship,
Associate Professor, Department of
Laboratory Medicine and Pathology, University
of Washington School of Medicine, Harborview
Medical Center, Seattle, Washington, USA

PETER B. ILLEI, MD
Associate Professor, Department of Pathology, The Johns Hopkins University School of Medicine, Baltimore, Maryland, USA

VICKIE Y. JO, MD
Associate Professor of Pathology, Brigham and Women's Hospital, Harvard Medical School, Boston, Massachusetts, USA

MERCE JORDA, MD, PhD, MBA
Chair, Department of Pathology and Laboratory Medicine, Desai Sethi Urology Institute, Sylvester Comprehensive Cancer Center, University of Miami Miller School of Medicine, Miami, Florida, USA

DARCY A. KERR, MD
Associate Professor of Pathology, Department of Pathology and Laboratory Medicine, Dartmouth-Hitchcock Medical Center, Lebanon, New Hampshire, USA; Geisel School of Medicine at Dartmouth, Hanover, New Hampshire, USA

OLEKSANDR N. KRYVENKO, MD
Director of Genitourinary Pathology, Department of Pathology and Laboratory Medicine, Desai Sethi Urology Institute, Department of Radiation Oncology, Sylvester Comprehensive Cancer Center, University of Miami Miller School of Medicine, Miami, Florida, USA

MELANIE C. KWAN, MD
Resident, Department of Pathology, Massachusetts General Hospital, Boston, Massachusetts, USA

SIGFRED LAJARA, MD
Assistant Professor, Department of Pathology, UPMC Shadyside Hospital, Cancer Pavilion, Pittsburgh, Pennsylvania, USA

JOSHUA LEVY, PhD
Director of Digital Pathology Research, Department of Pathology and Laboratory Medicine, Dartmouth-Hitchcock Medical Center, Lebanon, New Hampshire, USA; Cedars-Sinai Medical Center, Los Angeles, California, USA

ELISABETTA MAFFEI, MD
Pathologist, Department of Pathology, University Hospital "San Giovanni di Dio e Ruggi d'Aragona", Salerno, Italy

VARSHA MANUCHA, MD
Professor, Director, Division of Cytology, Section Chief, Head and Neck and Urologic Pathology, University of Mississippi Medical Center, Jackson, Mississippi, USA

ANTONINO MULÈ', MD
Pathologist, Division of Anatomic Pathology and Histology, Fondazione Policlinico Universitario "Agostino Gemelli", IRCCS, Rome, Italy

DAVA W. PIECORO, MD
Associate Professor, Department of Pathology and Laboratory Medicine, University of Kentucky College of Medicine, Lexington, Kentucky, USA

FEDERICA POLICARDO, MD
Pathologist, Division of Anatomic Pathology and Histology, Fondazione Policlinico Universitario "Agostino Gemelli", IRCCS, Rome, Italy

CAROL N. RIZKALLA, MB BCh, BAO
Resident, Department of Laboratory Medicine and Pathology, University of Washington School of Medicine, Seattle, Washington, USA

ESTHER DIANA ROSSI, MD, PhD
Associate Professor, Division of Anatomic Pathology and Histology, Fondazione Policlinico Universitario "Agostino Gemelli", IRCCS, Rome, Italy

FRANCESCO SABBATINO, MD
Pathologist, Department of Oncology, University Hospital "San Giovanni di Dio e Ruggi d'Aragona", Salerno, Italy

FERNANDO SCHMITT, MD, PhD, FIAC
IPATIMUP Diagnostics, IPATIMUP – Institute of Molecular Pathology and Immunology of Porto University, Faculty of Medicine of the University of Porto, Porto, Portugal

BIANCA SERIO, MD
Pathologist, Department of Hematology, University Hospital "San Giovanni di Dio e Ruggi d'Aragona", Salerno, Italy

RICELLA SOUZA DA SILVA, MD, PhD
IPATIMUP Diagnostics, IPATIMUP – Institute of
Molecular Pathology and Immunology of Porto
University, Porto, Portugal

LOUIS J. VAICKUS, MD, PhD
Associate Professor of Pathology, Department
of Pathology and Laboratory Medicine,
Dartmouth-Hitchcock Medical Center,
Lebanon, New Hampshire, USA; Geisel School
of Medicine at Dartmouth, Hanover, New
Hampshire, USA

JAYLOU M. VELEZ TORRES, MD
Assistant Professor and Associate Professor of
Pathology, Department of Pathology and
Laboratory Medicine, University of Miami Miller
School of Medicine, Miami, Florida, USA

PIO ZEPPA, MD, PhD
Pathologist, Department of Pathology,
University Hospital "San Giovanni di Dio e
Ruggi d'Aragona", Salerno, Italy

M. LISA ZHANG, MD
Instructor, Department of Pathology, Harvard
Medical School, Massachusetts General
Hospital, Boston, Massachusetts, USA

YIQIN ZUO, MD, PhD
Attending Physician in Cytopathology, Director
of Renal Pathology Service, Department of
Pathology and Laboratory Medicine, Sylvester
Comprehensive Cancer Center, University of
Miami Miller School of Medicine, Miami,
Florida, USA

Contents

Over the last decade, cancer diagnostics has undergone a notable transformation with increasing complexity. Minimally invasive diagnostic tests, driven by advanced imaging and early detection protocols, are redefining patient care and reducing the need for more invasive procedures. Modern cytopathologists now safeguard patient samples for vital biomarker and molecular testing. In this article, we explore ancillary testing modalities and the role of biomarkers in organ-specific contexts, underscoring the transformative impact of precision medicine. Finally, the advent of more than 80 Food and Drug Administration-approved predictive biomarkers signals a new era, guiding cancer care toward personalized and targeted strategies.

Fine-needle aspiration represents a valid tool for the diagnosis/management of salivary gland lesions. The past years assessed the lack of uniform diagnostic reports for salivary cytopathology leading to interpretative issues. In 2015, an international group of cytopathologists developed an evidence-based tiered classification system for reporting salivary gland fine-needle aspiration (FNA) specimens, the "Milan System for Reporting Salivary Gland Cytopathology" (MSRSGC). The present landscape of salivary cytology is represented by the growing adoption of the MSRSGC and the assessment of its diagnostic role. The future landscape is characterized by the increasing role of ancillary techniques for diagnostic and prognostic purposes.

The discovery of multiple novel biomarkers in head and neck tumors has led to an increasing interest in utilizing head and neck cytology material as the primary specimens for testing diagnostic and prognostic biomarkers. Although human papillomavirus and programmed death ligand 1 are the most well-established biomarkers tested in cytology specimens, their utilization in cytology is limited by the absence of standardized protocols for specimen collection and fixation. This has led to a quest for innovative techniques to explore the genomic landscape in head and neck tumors and its application in cytology.

Thyroid cytology is a rapidly evolving field that has seen significant advances in recent years. Its main goal is to accurately diagnose thyroid nodules, differentiate between benign and malignant lesions, and risk stratify nodules when a definitive diagnosis is not possible. The current landscape of thyroid cytology includes the use of fine-needle aspiration for the diagnosis of thyroid nodules with the use of uniform, tiered reporting systems such as the Bethesda System for Reporting Thyroid Cytopathology. In recent years, molecular testing has emerged as a reliable preoperative diagnostic tool that stratifies patients into different risk categories (low, intermediate, or high) with varying probabilities of malignancy and helps guide patient treatment.

Urine cytology is a non-invasive, cost-efficient, and sensitive test to detect high-grade urothelial carcinoma. The Paris System (TPS) for Reporting Urinary Cytology is an evidence-based system that uses the risk of malignancy to guide patient management. Since its inception, TPS has standardized urine cytology reports, facilitating communication among pathologists and between pathologists and clinicians. It is imperative to correlate the urine cytology findings with the concurrent tissue sample to avoid false-negative and false-positive results when possible. Several ancillary tests and artificial intelligence algorithms are being developed to increase the accuracy of urine cytology interpretation.

Small biopsies of lung are routinely obtained by many methods, including several that result in cytologic specimens. Because lung cancer is often diagnosed at a stage for which primary resection is not an option, it is critical that all diagnostic, predictive, and prognostic information be derived from such small biopsy specimens. As the number of available diagnostic and predictive markers expands, cytopathologists must familiarize themselves with current requirements for specimen acquisition, handling, results reporting, and molecular and other ancillary testing, all of which are reviewed here.

With the advancement of tissue procurement techniques, in-depth knowledge of morphology is crucial for cytopathologists to diagnose neoplastic and nonneoplastic lung diseases optimally. Cytopathologists must also be well versed in immunohistochemistry/immunocytochemistry markers and their interpretation for an accurate diagnosis.

Cervical cancer is the fourth most common malignancy in women worldwide. The identification of *human papillomavirus* (HPV) as the main etiologic cause of cervical cancer has led to the development and adaptation of HPV molecular diagnostics as a cervical cancer screening and prevention tool. This article highlights six Food and Drug Administration-approved HPV molecular platforms, each with unique advantages and disadvantages. In addition, HPV vaccination and the emergence of HPV self-collection as an alternative testing strategy are discussed.

Pancreatic lesions can be solid or cystic and comprise a wide range of benign, premalignant, and malignant entities. Endoscopic ultrasound–guided fine needle aspiration (EUS-FNA) is the current primary sampling method for the preoperative diagnosis of pancreatic lesions. Optimal handling of cytology/small tissue specimens is critical to ensure that the often-scant diagnostic material is appropriately utilized for ancillary and/or molecular studies when appropriate. Ultimately, evaluation of EUS-FNA cytology and small biopsy material can provide accurate and timely diagnoses to guide patient management and triage them to surveillance or surgical intervention.

Precision medicine translates through molecular assays and in minimally invasive diagnosis, evident in analyses of effusions that serve therapeutic and diagnostic purposes. This cost-effective and low-risk approach provides advantages, playing a pivotal role in late-stage oncology and frequently standing as the primary resource for cancer diagnosis and treatment pathways. This article outlines the workflow for managing serous fluid and explores how cytology effusion analysis extends beyond immunocytological diagnosis. Combined with current molecular tests it showcases the potential to be a skillful tool in precision cytopathology.

Soft tissue neoplasms pose many diagnostic challenges on fine-needle aspiration (FNA), owing largely to their rarity, large number of entities, and histologic diversity. Advances in ancillary testing now allow detection of the characteristic immunophenotypes and molecular alterations for many neoplasms and include reliable surrogate immunohistochemical markers for underlying molecular events that are highly efficient in small biopsies. A morphology-based framework is recommended to guide appropriate differentials and judicious selection of ancillary tests for small biopsies. The accurate diagnosis of soft tissue tumors is crucial for patient management and prognostication, with many potential implications in this era of precision medicine.

Lymph node (LN) fine-needle aspiration cytology (FNAC) is a common diagnostic procedure for lymphadenopathies. Despite the qualities and potentialities of LN-FNAC, the number of possible pathologies and the variety of clinical contexts represent a challenge and require a continuous upgrading of the procedure according to the emerging clinical requests and new technologies. This study presents an overview of the current and future impact of LN-FNAC on the care of patients with lymphadenopathy.

The practice of cytopathology has been significantly refined in recent years, largely through the creation of consensus rule sets for the diagnosis of particular specimens (Bethesda, Milan, Paris, and so forth). In general, these diagnostic systems have focused on reducing intraobserver variance, removing nebulous/redundant categories, reducing the use of "atypical" diagnoses, and promoting the use of quantitative scoring systems while providing a uniform language to communicate these results. Computational pathology is a natural offshoot of this process in that it promises 100% reproducible diagnoses rendered by quantitative processes that are free from many of the biases of human practitioners.

SURGICAL PATHOLOGY CLINICS

SERIES OF RELATED INTEREST

Clinics in Laboratory Medicine
http://www.labmed.theclinics.com/
Medical Clinics
https://www.medical.theclinics.com/

Preface

The Current and Future Impact of Cytopathology on Patient Care

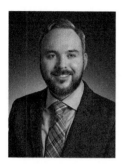

Chris VandenBussche, MD, PhD
Editor

Cytopathology, the microscopic examination of individual cells and fluids, has long served as a cornerstone of medical diagnosis. Its minimally invasive nature and ability to detect abnormalities from various body sites have made it an invaluable tool. However, the field is poised for a transformative leap forward with the emergence of precision cytopathology.

Precision cytopathology ushers in a new paradigm that leverages the power of advanced technologies like molecular analysis and artificial intelligence. By incorporating these tools alongside the expertise of cytopathologists, this refined approach promises significant advancements in diagnostic accuracy, personalized treatment, and the earlier detection of neoplastic processes.

Each article in this issue focuses on a particular specimen type and is written by prominent authors with expertise in each area. These experts not only describe the current state of cytopathology as applied to clinical care but also have been encouraged to imagine how cytopathology will be impacted in the near future by recently published studies.

The journey of precision cytopathology is just beginning. We stand at the threshold of a new era in cytopathologic diagnosis that promises an even brighter outlook for patient care.

Chris VandenBussche, MD, PhD
Department of Pathology
Johns Hopkins University School of Medicine
Pathology Room 406, 600 North Wolfe Street
Baltimore, MD 20850, USA

E-mail address:
cjvand@jhmi.edu

Surgical Pathology 17 (2024) xiii
https://doi.org/10.1016/j.path.2024.04.001
1875-9181/24/© 2024 Published by Elsevier Inc.

Precision Medicine in Cytopathology

Dava W. Piecoro, MD[a], Derek B. Allison, MD[a,b,c],*

KEYWORDS

- Precision medicine • Cytopathology • Ancillary testing • Immunohistochemistry
- Next-generation sequencing • Predictive biomarkers

Key points

- Over the past decade, the field of cancer diagnostics has seen a remarkable surge in complexity, with a multitude of tumor types and subtypes identified through advanced diagnostic modalities.

- Minimally invasive diagnostic testing is increasing, meaning modern cytopathologists, beyond their diagnostic role, now safeguard patient samples for vital biomarker and molecular testing, including prognostic and predictive tumor-specific and tumor-agnostic markers.

- It is crucial for the cytopathologist to have a solid understanding of these ancillary and molecular tests so we can appropriately triage and utilize specimens and adequately and accurately answer clinical care questions.

ABSTRACT

Over the last decade, cancer diagnostics has undergone a notable transformation with increasing complexity. Minimally invasive diagnostic tests, driven by advanced imaging and early detection protocols, are redefining patient care and reducing the need for more invasive procedures. Modern cytopathologists now safeguard patient samples for vital biomarker and molecular testing. In this article, we explore ancillary testing modalities and the role of biomarkers in organ-specific contexts, underscoring the transformative impact of precision medicine. Finally, the advent of more than 80 Food and Drug Administration-approved predictive biomarkers signals a new era, guiding cancer care toward personalized and targeted strategies.

OVERVIEW

Over the past decade, the complexity of cancer diagnostics has rapidly expanded. The number of newly defined tumor types and subtypes that have unique morphology, immunochemical protein expression, and molecular findings has dramatically increased and has led to better risk stratification and treatment options for patients in most primary sites.[1] Simultaneously, there have been a number of advancements regarding protein expression and molecular drivers that have been found to predict response to targeted therapies.[2–4] Despite this increased complexity, we have been progressively able to do more with less tumor sample.[5–7] With the advent of high-resolution computed tomography (CT), multisequence MRI, and early detection cancer screening protocols,

---

[a] Department of Pathology and Laboratory Medicine, 800 Rose Street, MS117, University of Kentucky College of Medicine, Lexington, KY 40536, USA; [b] Markey Cancer Center, Lexington, KY 40536, USA; [c] Department of Urology, University of Kentucky College of Medicine, Lexington, KY 40536, USA
* Corresponding author. Department of Pathology and Laboratory Medicine, 800 Rose Street, MS117, University of Kentucky College of Medicine, Lexington, KY 40536.
E-mail address: Derek.Allison@uky.edu

Surgical Pathology 17 (2024) 329–345
https://doi.org/10.1016/j.path.2024.04.002
1875-9181/24/© 2024 Elsevier Inc. All rights are reserved, including those for text and data mining, AI training, and similar technologies.

patients often rely on minimally invasive diagnostic tests to target previously untargetable lesions, obviating a more invasive or morbid procedure.[8,9] With these samples, we have moved beyond the need to merely provide an accurate diagnosis. The modern cytopathologist must be a good steward of the patient's sample and preserve the specimen for relevant biomarkers and molecular testing when indicated. This role requires the cytopathologist to have a functional understanding of the specimen needs for each accompanying diagnosis and clinical scenario. Fortunately, many of these studies can be performed with relatively low tumor fractions and low minimum nucleic acid quantities.[10]

When discussing biomarkers, a definition of terms is warranted. First, diagnostic markers are used for the purpose of rendering a primary diagnosis. These include immunostains such as p40 or thyroid transcription factor 1 (TTF-1) that help support squamous differentiation or a lung or thyroid primary site of disease, fluorescence in situ hybridization (FISH) studies that detect murine double minute 2 (MDM2) amplification in a well-differentiated liposarcoma, or RNA sequencing that detects a nuclear protein of the testis family member 1 (NUTM1) fusion in a nuclear protein of the testis (NUT) carcinoma, to name a few.[11–14] Next, prognostic markers provide information about the likely course of a disease, regardless of treatment. Essentially, these markers help predict the natural history of the disease or the overall outcome. These include markers such as Ki-67, alpha-thalassemia mental retardation X-linked (ATRX), and death-associated protein 6 (DAXX) in pancreatic neuroendocrine tumors, DNA polymerase ε (POLE) and p53 in endometrioid carcinomas, and microsatellite instability (MSI) in colon cancer, to name a few.[15–18] Finally, predictive markers essentially forecast the likelihood of benefit for a particular therapy. Examples include estrogen receptor (ER)/progesterone receptor (PR) and human epidermal growth factor receptor 2 (HER2) expression in breast cancer, anaplastic lymphoma kinase (ALK) gene fusions in lung adenocarcinoma, and programmed death-ligand 1 (PD-L1) expression and tumor mutational burden (TMB) in many solid tumor types.[4,19–22] These predictive biomarkers can be further subdivided into tumor-specific markers, meaning the correlation of therapy depends on the specific tumor type, and tumor-agnostic markers, meaning response to therapy is independent of the specific diagnosis. For example, an epidermal growth factor receptor (EGFR) mutation in lung adenocarcinoma would be tumor specific while a neurotrophic tropomyosin-receptor kinase (NTRK) gene fusion

in any solid tumor would be tumor agnostic and considered actionable in the proper clinical setting.[23,24] Due to the interdisciplinary complexity in integrating all of this information, some centers are developing molecular tumor boards to improve clinical care.[10,25]

As laboratory physicians, it is crucial for the cytopathologist to have a solid understanding of these ancillary and molecular tests so we can adequately and accurately answer clinical care questions for our clinicians. This understanding further affects how we handle rapid onsite evaluation cases, triage specimens, and make procedural recommendations to clinicians. In this review, we will provide an overview of the current major ancillary testing modalities, the role of molecular diagnostic testing for clinical decision-making in cytopathology, and precision medicine biomarkers that can be performed in exfoliative, aspiration, and small core needle biopsy samples.

DISCUSSION

ANCILLARY TESTING MODALITIES

There a several important methodologies that are utilized for detecting biomarkers in cytopathology samples. These include immunochemistry, FISH, chromogenic in situ hybridization (CISH), MSI, DNA sequencing, and RNA sequencing, in addition to polymerase chain reaction (PCR) testing for human papillomavirus (HPV) testing in gynecologic cytology samples. Test selection depends on the specimen type, the specific biomarker, and the specimen requirements.

Immunochemistry

Briefly, immunochemistry relies on the use of antibodies to detect the presence, abundance, and localization of specific proteins in the sample and can be performed on both alcohol-fixed smears, liquid-based preparations, and cytospins, as well as more commonly on formalin-fixed paraffin embedded (FFPE) cell blocks and core needle biopsies. However, several of the predictive biomarkers have specific preanalytical variable requirements that are important to be aware of. For example, breast biomarkers require 10% neutral buffered formalin fixation for 6 to 72 hours because both underfixation and overfixation can result in false negatives.[26,27] In addition, some drugs require a specific clone of antibody for predictive purposes (Fig. 1A–D). For example, the PD-L1 clone 22C3 is a Food and Drug Administration (FDA)-approved companion diagnostic test for pembrolizumab in certain clinical settings for patients with non-small cell lung carcinoma (NSCLC),

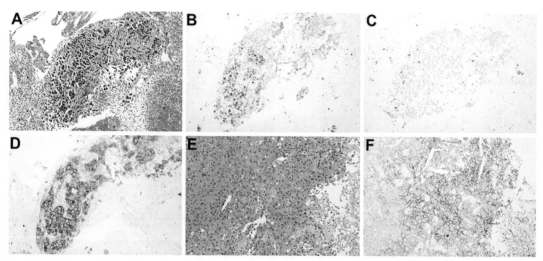

Fig. 1. (*A*) Metastatic ductal carcinoma of breast, hematoxylin and eosin stain (H&E) 20×; cell block section from station 7 lymph node endobronchial ultrasound-guided fine needle aspiration biopsy. (*B*) Metastatic ductal carcinoma of breast, ER immunostain 20×, interpreted as moderate intensity staining in 61% to 70% of tumor cells. (*C*) Metastatic ductal carcinoma of breast, PR immunostain 20×, interpreted as moderate intensity staining in 1% to 10% of tumor cells. (*D*) Metastatic ductal carcinoma of breast, HER-2/neu immunostain 20×, interpreted as positive (score 3+). (*E*) Adenocarcinoma of lung, H&E 20×, CT-guided core needle biopsy from right upper lobe of lung. (*F*) Adenocarcinoma of lung, PD-L1 IHC 22C3 pharmDx 20×, interpreted as 60% tumor proportion score.

cervical squamous cell carcinoma (SqCC), endocervical adenocarcinoma, urothelial carcinoma, head and neck and esophageal SqCC, and triple-negative breast cancer; however, the scoring method and the threshold for positivity is tumor specific (**Fig.** 1E, F).[28–33] In contrast, the PD-L1 SP142 clone is an FDA-approved companion diagnostic test for atezolizumab only in patients with urothelial carcinoma and advanced NSCLC.[34,35] Due to these differences, each clone and each primary site has to be separately validated. As a result, it is important to be aware of which clone or clones your laboratory has inhouse and to be aware of which specific primary tumor types have been validated. Wasting tissue on an improperly ordered PD-L1 stain for which your laboratory is not validated may deplete the tumor cellularity and require the patient to undergo a repeat procedure. In other settings, immunochemistry can be used as a quick triage technique. For example, immunochemistry for ALK and ROS proto-oncogene 1 (ROS1) in non-small cell lung cancer can be performed to identify cases that can subsequently be confirmed to have a gene rearrangement by FISH, PCR, or sequencing studies, making the patient eligible for a tyrosine kinase inhibitor.

Fluorescence In Situ Hybridization

FISH studies use fluorescent probes to visualize the present and location of a specific DNA sequence and can be performed on cytologic slide preparations as well as FFPE cell blocks and core biopsies for diagnostic and predictive purposes. As examples, FISH can be used to detect *HER2*, *c-MYC*, and *MDM2* gene amplifications, deletions such as 1p/19q codeletions, and fusions involving *ALK*, *ROS1*, *RET*, *SS18::SSX*, and many more.[13,20,23,36–40] There are several different ways to perform a FISH assay depending on the type of aberration that you need to detect. The most frequently utilized types of assays for solid tumors include break-apart, dual fusion, and centromere enumeration probe FISH. Briefly, break-apart FISH detects chromosomal rearrangements by labeling and hybridizing to 2 separate regions of a target gene. The test is considered to be positive for a fusion if the distance between the probe signals is far apart, correlating with a break and rearrangement of a gene, irrespective of the fusion partner (**Fig. 2**A, B). Dual fusion FISH, on the other hand, utilizes 2 differently colored probes that each hybridize to the 2 genes involved in the fusion. The test is considered positive if the 2 separate genes appear close together in signal, but the fusion partner must be known, noting that noncanonical variant fusions may be missed. Amplification can be detected with centromeric enumeration probes, like is done for HER2. By using a probe that targets the centromere of a specific chromosome, you can get information on the chromosomal copy number. Each FISH assay has its own minimum cellularity requirement but, unlike sequencing techniques,

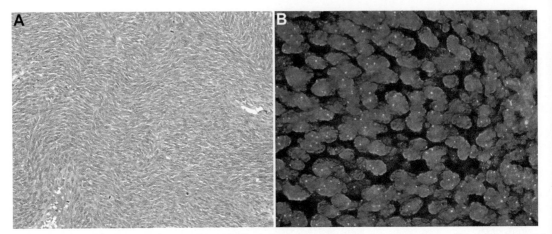

Fig. 2. (*A*) Synovial sarcoma, H&E 20×, CT-guided core needle biopsy from left upper lobe of lung. (*B*) Synovial sarcoma; positive SS18 (SYT) paraffin FISH analysis using break apart probes (note numerous isolated *red* and *green* signals).

the overall percent tumor nuclei in the sample is less of a concern, as long as the tumor nuclei can be easily distinguished from the background normal cellularity. In addition, cytologic slide preparations, such as direct smears, touch imprints, cytospins, and liquid-based preparations allow for examination of the entire nucleus, unlike FFPE sections that transect nuclei and can result in nuclear truncation artifact. As a result, performing FISH on a touch prep slide and preserving the cell block for PD-L1 may make a lot of sense in some situations.

Chromogenic In Situ Hybridization

CISH combines elements of both immunochemistry and FISH. Like FISH, it allows the visualization of specific nucleic acid sequencing in tissue by using a probe; however, like immunochemistry, that probe is visually detected with a chromogen. The epstein-barr virus (EBV)-encoded RNA (EBER) test is a common CISH used to detect the presence of EBV in tumor cells of patients with

nasopharyngeal carcinoma, sinonasal natural killer (NK) cell lymphomas, plasmablastic lymphoma, and some high-grade B-cell lymphomas (**Fig. 3**A, B).[41,42] In addition, high-risk (HR)-mRNA in situ hybridization (ISH) is another CISH used most commonly to detect transcriptionally active high-risk HPV in oropharyngeal SqCC tumor cells by hybridizing high-risk specific *E6* and *E7* mRNA.[43,44] CISH assays for *HER2* are performed instead of FISH in some laboratories due to ease of interpretation with a traditional brightfield microscope, precluding a second workflow.[45]

Microsatellite Instability

MSI testing is a method used to assess the stability of microsatellite repeats in the DNA, which are short (2–10 nucleotides in length), repetitive sequences scattered throughout the genome. MSI testing is often employed to identify tumors with deficiencies in DNA mismatch repair (MMR) mechanisms, which can lead to the accumulation of errors in microsatellite regions that cannot be

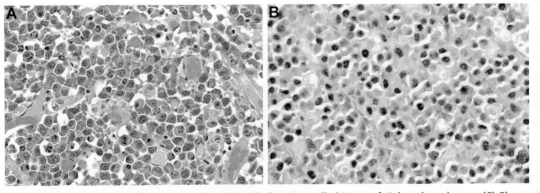

Fig. 3. (*A*) Plasmablastic lymphoma, H&E 50×, CT-guided core needle biopsy of right adnexal mass. (*B*) Plasmablastic lymphoma, Epstein-Barr virus in situ hybridization stain.

repaired during DNA synthesis. Two common methodologies for MSI testing are MMR protein immunochemistry and PCR analysis, though next generation sequencing (NGS) assays are also being increasingly utilized.[18,46] Four key proteins are typically evaluated to assess the integrity of the MMR complex by immunochemistry. These proteins are mutl homolog 1 (MLH1), postmeiotic segregation increased 2 (PMS2), muts homolog 2 (MSH2), and muts homolog 6 (MSH6) (**Fig. 4**). Each protein plays a specific role in the MMR pathway, and their expression levels are examined to identify potential deficiencies in MMR function that may be related to either mutation or promoter methylation. Loss of function in one of these proteins can be identified by a complete lack of nuclear staining by immunochemistry. Based on the findings, additional studies may be warranted to determine if the patient has Lynch syndrome or a sporadic case of MMR deficiency.

PCR is performed by extracting DNA from the tumor sample and typically adjacent normal tissue. Primers are designed to amplify specific microsatellite loci, and the PCR products are then analyzed for size differences. MSI is then identified by the presence of additional or fewer repeats in the tumor compared to the normal sample. A tumor is considered to be MSI-high if there is significant instability in 2 or more markers, MSI-low if instability in 1 marker, or microsatellite stable if no instability markers are identified. In summary, MSI testing can be used to help identify individuals at risk for hereditary cancer syndromes and to guide therapeutic strategies, such as selection for immunotherapy, in certain cancer types.

DNA and RNA Sequencing

Although several sequencing methods have been developed over the years, NGS is a versatile, high-throughput, unbiased, parallel technology that can be applied to both DNA and RNA sequencing workflows. As shown in **Fig. 5**, DNA-based NGS assays can detect single nucleotide variants, small insertions and deletions (<~50 bp), copy number alterations, and karyotypes, as well as various genomic signatures, such as MSI status, TMB, genomic loss of heterozygosity (LOH), and homologous recombination deficiency. In contrast, RNA-Seq is the preferred method for detecting gene fusions, largely due to its unique capabilities in directly examining transcripts produced by genes, resulting in increased sensitivity, increased efficiency, and a functionally definitive assessment of gene fusions compared

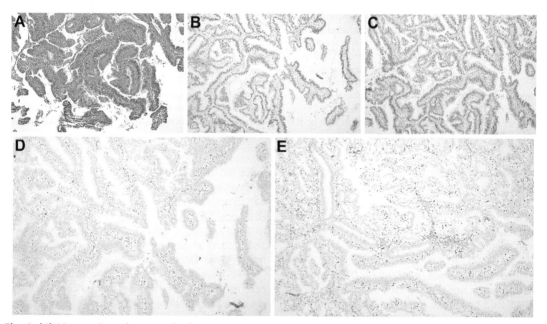

Fig. 4. (A) Metastatic endometrioid adenocarcinoma of endometrium, H&E 10×, CT-guided core needle biopsy from right lower lobe of lung. (B) Metastatic endometrioid adenocarcinoma, MLH1 with intact nuclear expression in tumor cells and background benign cells, 10×. (C) Metastatic endometrioid adenocarcinoma, PMS2 with intact nuclear staining in tumor cells and background benign cells, 10×. (D) Metastatic endometrioid adenocarcinoma, MSH2 with loss of nuclear staining in tumor cells and positive nuclear staining in background benign cells, 10×. (E) Metastatic endometrioid adenocarcinoma, MSH6 with loss of nuclear staining in tumor cells and positive nuclear staining in background benign cells, 10×. Loss of MSH2 and MSH6 in tumor cells corresponds to a deficiency in DNA mismatch repair.

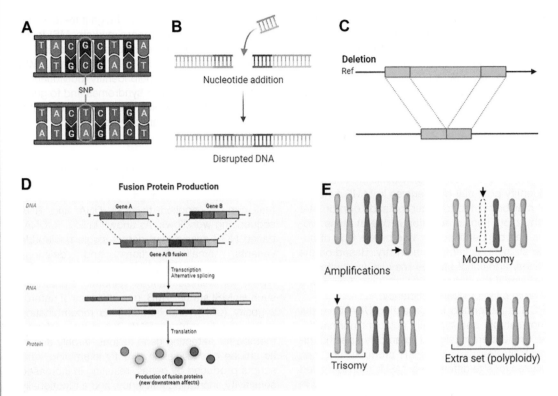

Fig. 5. Selected alterations detected by DNA and RNA NGS. (*A*) Single nucleotide polymorphisms, which correspond to variations in a single position of a DNA sequence. These can be silent and result in no change in the amino acid sequence or can result in a missense mutation (a change in the encoded amino acid) or a nonsense mutation (resulting in a premature stop codon). The pathogenicity depends on additional variables, such as whether or not the change occurs in a noncoding versus coding region, or whether or not the amino acid that is encoded is very biologically different than the wild type amino acid. (*B*) Nucleotide addition, or insertion, is where one or more nucleotides are added to the DNA sequence, thus resulting in a shift in the reading frame or the addition of extraneous codons. (*C*) Internal deletions can also cause a shift in the reading frame, as well as loss of important codons, depending on where in the gene the alteration occurs. (*D*) Gene fusions occur when a segment of DNA moves from one location to another, either within the same chromosome or between chromosomes. This change can lead to loss of function of the genes involved or can result in novel fusion products. (*E*) Larger amplifications and deletions can result in partial or complete aneuploidy or polyploidy.

to DNA-based methods.[47,48] For example, a recent study including 2522 NSCLC cases were sequenced with DNA-based methods, and 76.7% were shown to have at least one oncogenic driver alteration.[47] In a group of 232 cases without driver mutations identified, RNA-Seq was performed and 36 (15.5%) oncogenic fusions were identified that were not detected by DNA-Seq, 33 of which were actionable. One notable strength of RNA-Seq lies in its ability to capture the variability in gene fusion breakpoints at the DNA level. Even when the same fusion arises, different breakpoints within a gene can be identified, providing a more nuanced understanding of genomic alterations. Crucially, RNA-Seq directly identifies fusion transcripts generated by tumor cells only, which improves the limits of detection in cases with low tumor fractions.[49] Moreover, RNA-Seq's

focus on transcripts helps circumvent the need to interpret DNA variants that do not translate into changes at the RNA level. This emphasis on RNA adds a layer of direct functional relevance to the analysis, ensuring a more comprehensive and accurate assessment of gene fusions and the ability to target them.

FFPE-based NGS can be performed on small core needle biopsies and cell blocks from fine-needle aspiration (FNA) and effusion cytology samples that have been fixed in 10% neutral-buffered formalin for between 6 and 72 hours without the use of a strong acid for decalcification, which degrades nucleic acids. Fortunately, biopsies containing bone that have been softened using ethylenediaminetetraacetic acid (EDTA) chelation agents are typically successful for sequencing.[50] Specimen requirements are fairly variable depending on the platform and workflow but generally require a tumor volume of 1 mm^3 with a tumor nuclei fraction of 20%. When looking at a slide, a 5 mm × 5 mm area equates to 25 mm^2 of tissue. As long as approximately 10 slides can be cut at 4 μm levels, there should be sufficient tumor volume (1 mm^3) to perform most NGS assays. It is important to note that some workflows include tumor microdissection, which can allow for the enrichment of tumor nuclei and drastically improve the nucleic acid extraction process, making previously insufficient samples adequate for sequencing.[51,52]

Sequencing can be also be performed on non-FFPE tissue, including from scrapes from FNA smears.[51] The lower limits of detection are dependent on the assay design and platform. For example, the Ion Torrent NGS platform typically requires at least 10 ng of DNA while the Illumina NGS platforms requires a higher input of DNA ranging from 30 to 270 ng. To put this into context, a single intact diploid cell will yield approximately 6 to 7 pg of DNA, meaning that a molecular assay that requires 1 ng of DNA would require approximately 1500 intact tumor cells.[53–56]

MOLECULAR DIAGNOSTIC TESTING IN PATIENT MANAGEMENT DECISIONS

Molecular diagnostic testing on cytology samples plays a crucial role in clinical decision-making across various organ systems, including the cervix, thyroid, urine, biliary tract, and pancreatic cyst fluid. Although detailed discussions regarding these site-specific management questions will be addressed in other articles in this series, it is helpful to provide a brief overview here.

HPV Testing in Gynecologic Specimens

The most classic example is the performance of HPV testing, most commonly via PCR, in residual liquid-based Pap preservation media.[57] The presence of HR-HPV helps determine screening intervals and guide clinical management in cases of indeterminate cytology. In fact, there is a growing push for primary HPV screening, resulting in a reflex cytology evaluation for patients that are shown to be positive for HR-HPV.

Molecular Testing in Thyroid FNA Samples

Next, there are several platforms that assist clinicians in managing patients with indeterminate diagnoses following thyroid FNA. For example, the ThyroSeq Genomic Classifier utilizes DNA and RNA NGS to interrogate 112 relevant genes that can parse thyroid lesions into 4 main classes of molecular alterations.[58] Although the exact details of the panel are proprietary, the panel can detect

mutations in genes such as *BRAF*, *RAS*, and *TERT;* gene fusions such as *RET*, *NTRK*, and *ALK;* copy number alterations like those seen in oncocytic nodules and follicular carcinomas; and gene expression alterations like those seen in medullary thyroid carcinoma or parathyroid nodules. Results are reported as positive or negative with the associated mutations findings, risk of recurrence, and personalized management recommendation. Although the negative predictive value (NPV) is excellent at greater than 95%, which can help patients avoid an unnecessary surgery, the positive predictive value is only 66%, due to a high rate of false positives from *RAS* and *RAS*-like alterations in nodules that end up being benign.[59–63] On the other hand, Veracyte's Afirma Genomic Sequencing Classifier only utilizes RNA-Seq to analyze expression of 10,196 nuclear and mitochondrial genes, which are used to identify or group nodules into parathyroid tissue, medullary thyroid carcinoma, *BRAF V600 E* mutation, *RET::PTC1/PTC3* fusion, follicular cell content index, oncocytic cell index, and oncocytic cell neoplasm index.[64,65] Results are reported out as benign (low risk of malignancy, ≤ 4%) or suspicious (high risk of malignancy, ≥50%). If the result is suspicious, additional but limited molecular data are reported. In comparison to the ThyroSeq panel, Afirma has a similarly high NPV of greater than 95%, but similarly low-positive predictive value of approximately 65%.[64,66] Additional panels, such as the ThyGeNEXT and ThyraMIRv2, utilizing microRNA expression, exist but with limited clinical applications to date.[67]

Molecular Testing in Urine Samples

Ancillary tests for urinary tract specimens typically aim to achieve 1 of 2 objectives. First, ensuring patients under surveillance have no residual or recurrent disease by emphasizing a high NPV. Second, accurately identifying high-grade lesions in situations where biopsy options are limited, requiring a high positive predictive value. Commercial tests often prioritize maximizing NPV, as it impacts a larger patient population.[68] Ancillary tests for urinary tract specimens come in 2 types: slide-based and slide-free. Slide-based tests involve a separate slide preparation, potentially impacting laboratory workflow, while slide-free tests eliminate the need for an additional slide, allowing centralized or on-site testing. Both urinary tract cytology (UTC) and ancillary tests can produce "false false positive" results, where a positive finding occurs without detectable lesions on cystoscopy or biopsy. This scenario can be particularly relevant for

Table 1
Summary of selected ancillary tests for the detection of urothelial carcinoma in urine specimens

Test	Specimen Type	Clinical Utility	Methodology	Sensitivity	Specificity	Additional Comments
UroVysion	Slide-based	Primary screening and surveillance	Fluorescence in situ hybridization using chromosomal enumeration probes to detect copy number increases in chromosomes 3, 7, and 17 and band assessment of 9p21 to detect homozygous deletion	All cases • 72%[70] Noninvasive pTa tumors • 65%–73%[71,72] Invasive pT1-T4 tumors • 95%–100%[71,72] Upper tract tumors • 35%–87.5%[71,72]	All cases • 83%[70]	• Issue of anticipatory positive: 2/3 of surveillance patients with a positive result and negative cytology and cystoscopy develop recurrence within 29 mo[73] • Logistical issues with reflex testing, cost, and questionable utility in equivocal cases
uCyt+/ImmunoCyt	Slide-based	Surveillance	Utilizes 3 fluorescent antibodies to detect abnormally glycosylated carcinoembryonic antigens	78%–90%[74,75]	77%–87%[74,75]	• Protein-based test that may result in false positives in setting of urinary tract infections, stones, and so forth • Good sensitivity, especially in detecting low-grade disease
Anti-hTERT	Slide-based	Limited data	Immunochemical stain utilizing an antibody to the catalytic subunit of telomerase	52%–60%[76]	70%–91%[76]	• Not all tumors have alterations in telomerase activity • Nonurothelial cells may stain positive, resulting in challenges with interpretation
ProEx C	Slide-based	Limited data	Immunochemical stain utilizing an antibody cocktail to topoisomerase IIα and MMP-2	78%[77]	96%[77]	• Likely has low sensitivity with populations with larger numbers of low-grade tumors

Name	Type	Use	Description	Sensitivity	Specificity	Comments
NMP22 BladderChek	Slide-free	Primary screening and surveillance	Enzyme-linked immunosorbent assay (ELISA) that detects nuclear mitotic apparatus proteins	62%–75%[75]	70%–83%[75]	• Point of care option that results in 30 min • Only requires 4 drops of urine
BTA stat, BTA TRAK	Slide-free	Surveillance	ELISA that detects complement factor H and complement factor H-related protein	54%–75%[75,78]	64%–82%[75,78]	• Point of care option that results in 5 min • Only requires 5 drops of urine
UroSEEK	Slide-free	Primary screening and surveillance	NGS panel analyzing TERT promoter mutations in addition to a 10 gene panel and aneuploidy analysis	71%–95%[79]	80%–93%[79]	• Theoretic improved performance with multigene and aneuploidy analysis • Decreased sensitivity probably due to increased "false false positives" • Expensive and technically complex

Table 2
Summary of selected ancillary tests on pancreatic cyst fluid specimens

Diagnosis	Amylase	CEA	DNA-Seq	Malignant Potential	Treatment
Pseudocyst	High	Low	None	None	Medical management
Serous cystadenoma	Low	Low	VHL mutation is specific for the diagnosis[85]	None	Surgery if symptomatic
Mucinous cystic neoplasm	Low	High	KRAS mutation is specific (>90%) but not specific (<50%)[86–88] PIK3CA, PTEN, and TP53 may be seen in cases that have transformed to malignancy[89–91]	Moderate	Surgery
Intraductal papillary mucinous neoplasm	High	High	KRAS and GNAS mutations are specific (>90%) but are not sensitive (<50%)[86–88] PIK3CA, PTEN, and TP53 may be seen in cases that have transformed to malignancy[89–91]	High	Surgery and postresection surveillance
Solid pseudopapillary mucinous neoplasm	Low	Low	CTNNB1 mutations are specific[85]	Moderate to high	Resection

Table 3
Selected Food and Drug Administration-approved and emerging tumor-specific and tumor-agnostic biomarkers

Examples of FDA-Approved Tumor-Specific Biomarkers	Testing Methodology	Example Tumor Types	Examples of Therapy
ER/PR	IHC	Breast	Tamoxifen, fulvestrant, anastrozole, and leuprorelin
HER2	IHC/CISH/FISH	Breast, gastric/gastroesophageal junction	Trastuzumab
PD-L1	IHC	NSCLC, cervical, esophageal, and head and neck SqCC, endocervical adenocarcinoma, urothelial carcinoma, and triple-negative breast cancer	Nivolumab, pembrolizumab, atezolizumab, and durvalumab
EGFR	DNA-Seq	NSCLC and pancreatic cancer	Erlotinib, osimertinib, gefitinib, and afatinib
BRCA	DNA-Seq	Breast, ovarian, fallopian tube, and primary peritoneal cancer	Olaparib, rucaparib, niraparib, and talazoparib
ALK fusion	FISH/RNA-Seq (IHC screen)	NSCLC	Crizotinib, entrectinib, ceritinib, alectinib, brigatinib, and lorlatinib
ROS1 fusion	FISH/RNA-Seq (IHC screen)	NSCLC	Crizotinib, entrectinib, ceritinib, and lorlatinib
FOLR1	IHC	Ovarian cancer	Mirvetuximab soravtansine
Examples of FDA-approved tumor-agnostic biomarkers			
MSI-H	PCR/DNA-Seq	Metastatic solid cancers	Pembrolizumab, nivolumab, and nivolumab–ipilimumab combination
dMMR	IHC	Metastatic solid cancers	Pembrolizumab, nivolumab, and nivolumab–ipilimumab combination
TMB	DNA-Seq	Adult and pediatric patients with unresectable or metastatic solid tumors	Pembrolizumab
BRAF V600 E	IHC/DNA-Seq	Adult and pediatric unresectable or metastatic solid tumors who have progressed or have no alternative therapies	Dabrafenib with trametinib

(continued on next page)

Table 3
(continued)

Examples of FDA-Approved Tumor-Specific Biomarkers	Testing Methodology	Example Tumor Types	Examples of Therapy
RET gene fusion	RNA-Seq	Any solid tumor	Selpercatinib
NTRK fusion	RNA-Seq	Adults and pediatric patients with a solid tumor	Entrectinib and larotrectinib
Examples of emerging biomarkers			
METex14 skipping	DNA-Seq/RNA-Seq	NSCLC	Capmatinib and tepotinib
FGFR alterations	DNA-Seq/RNA-Seq	Urothelial carcinoma and cholangiocarcinoma	Erdafitinib and pemigatinib
NRG1 fusion	RNA-Seq	NSCLC	Afatinib

certain lesions, like flat urothelial carcinoma in situ (CIS), and may prompt a more aggressive clinical investigation, potentially enabling earlier detection despite the challenges in assessing new tumors.[69] Ancillary tests may also uncover dysplastic changes not easily visible with light microscopy. In many circumstances, however, it is difficult to know how to manage a patient with a positive ancillary test and negative cytology/cystoscopy, even knowing with the understanding of the concept of a "false false positive." Furthermore, these tests are more expensive than urine cytology, labor intensive, and technically difficult. As a result, many of these tests are not widely utilized. See **Table 1** for a summary of selected urine ancillary diagnostic tests.

Molecular Testing in Biliary Tract Samples

Biliary tract samples may undergo FISH testing utilizing chromosomal enumeration probes to identify copy number gains in chromosomes 3, 7, and 17, similar to the UroVysion test performed in UTC. Other laboratories utilize a FISH panel with probes specific to 1q21, 7q12, 8q24, and 9p21 for polysomy. Depending on the particular FISH assay, sensitivity ranges from 45% to 55% with a specificity of greater than 95%.[80] Compared to cytology assessment, which has a sensitivity of around 35% and specificity of 99%, this test offers only a modest improvement in sensitivity.[80] This test can be performed inhouse or sent to one of several reference laboratories. Samples must be from FNA or biliary brushings submitted in nongynecologic ThinPrep media or in CytoLyt solution. As an adjunct to conventional cytology assessment, this test may be useful in some settings to increase confidence in a reactive stricture versus a malignant stricture.

Ancillary Testing in FNA Samples of Pancreatic Cyst Fluid

Pancreatic cysts can be challenging to diagnose by FNA.[81–83] The procedure often results in paucicellular cyst fluid contents only without a definitive epithelial component to evaluate. Furthermore, the differential includes a variety of lesions, including reactive pseudocysts, lymphoepithelial cysts, serous cystadenomas, mucinous cystic neoplasms, intraductal papillary mucinous neoplasms, and solid pseudopapillary neoplasm, the last 3 of which may have dysplasia and may transform to malignancy.[84] As a result, cell-free ancillary testing can be useful to select patients for surveillance versus surgery. Cyst fluid ancillary testing includes chemistry tests for amylase and carcinoembryonic antigen (CEA) analysis, as well as DNA-Seq for

KRAS, GNAS, TP53, PIK3CA, PTEN, VHL, and *CTNNB1.* See **Table 2** for how this testing can be used to suggest a diagnosis and manage patients.

PRECISION MEDICINE RELIES ON PREDICTIVE MARKERS

There are over 80 FDA-approved predictive biomarkers with therapy associations. As previously mentioned, these include both tumor-specific biomarkers and tumor-agnostic biomarkers. The incidence of an actionable alteration is largely dependent on the tumor type. Obtaining the biomarker status of a tumor is recommended for a number of tumor types depending on the clinical scenario, including primary versus metastatic, resectable versus nonresectable, second-line or third-line therapy assessment, or no other treatment options available. In addition to these scenarios, however, nearly 20% of solid tumors will be positive for one or more tissue-agnostic biomarker, which means preserving tissue for potential future molecular considerations is paramount.[10,92,93] **Table 3** includes a selection of tumor-specific and tumor-agnostic biomarkers, as well as some emerging biomarkers that are likely to be FDA-approved in the near future. It is important to realize that this list is just a portion of a larger group of biomarkers that are only going to increase as our understanding of tumor biology continues and as therapeutic options with proven efficacy continue to be tested.

SUMMARY

Over the past decade, the field of cancer diagnostics has seen a remarkable surge in complexity, with a multitude of tumor types and subtypes identified through advanced diagnostic modalities. This evolution has enabled improved risk stratification and treatment options for patients. Notably, the shift toward minimally invasive diagnostic tests, aided by high-resolution imaging and early detection protocols, has allowed for more extensive analysis with smaller tumor samples. Modern cytopathologists, in this intricate landscape, play a pivotal role not just in accurate diagnosis but also as custodians of patient samples, preserving them for relevant biomarker and molecular testing.

Various ancillary testing modalities are utilized for precision medicine in the modern era, including immunochemistry, FISH, CISH, MSI testing, and DNA and RNA sequencing. These techniques, each with specific applications and considerations, contribute to the identification of diagnostic, prognostic, and predictive markers critical for clinical decision-making. It is crucial to have a comprehensive understanding of the testing methodology and specimen requirements to navigate the intricacies of sample handling and processing. Already, we have seen the role molecular diagnostic testing impact patient management decisions in areas such as gynecologic, thyroid, urinary tract, biliary tract, and pancreatic cyst fluid samples. Furthermore, small samples from solid tumors from all sites are being increasingly utilized for precision medicine testing. Notably, there are over 80 FDA-approved markers influencing therapy decisions, both tumor-specific and tumor-agnostic, marking a crucial paradigm shift in cancer care. Therefore, it is up to the modern cytopathologist to be a great steward in triaging, diagnosing, and handling these specimens.

CLINICS CARE POINTS

- Cytopathologists are tasked with utilizing a number of ancillary testing methods for primary diagnostic, prognostic, and predictive testing, which means specimens must be handled and processed appropriately for a wide range of potential testing.

- Cytopathology samples are commonly used to perform immunochemistry, FISH, chromogenic in situ hybridization, MSI testing, DNA sequencing, RNA sequencing, and PCR testing, each of which has workflow and technical weaknesses and benefits.

- It is important to understand the different molecular diagnostic testing platforms that may be used to inform patient management decisions, including in the gynecologic tract, thyroid, urinary tract, biliary tract, and pancreatic cyst fluid and how to interpret those findings.

- With over 80 FDA-approved predictive biomarkers with therapy, there are increasing indications for ancillary testing beyond making a diagnosis.

- Due to the interdisciplinary complexity in integrating all of this information, some centers are developing molecular tumor boards to improve clinical care.

ACKNOWLEDGMENTS

Author DBA and this manuscript were supported by the Biospecimen Procurement & Translational Pathology Shared Resource Facility of the University of Kentucky Markey Cancer Center (P30CA177558).

DISCLOSURE

The other authors have no relevant conflicts of interest to disclose.

REFERENCES

1. Angerilli V, Galuppini F, Pagni F, et al. the role of the pathologist in the next-generation era of tumor molecular characterization. Diagnostics 2021;11(2).
2. Vogelstein B, Papadopoulos N, Velculescu VE, et al. Cancer genome landscapes. Science 2013; 339(6127):1546–58.
3. Harris TJ, McCormick F. The molecular pathology of cancer. Nat Rev Clin Oncol 2010;7(5):251–65.
4. Lindeman NI, Cagle PT, Aisner DL, et al. Updated molecular testing guideline for the selection of lung cancer patients for treatment with targeted tyrosine kinase inhibitors: Guideline From the College of American Pathologists, the International Association for the Study of Lung Cancer, and the Association for Molecular Pathology. J Mol Diagn 2018;20(2):129–59.
5. Sanchez A, Bocklage T. Precision cytopathology: expanding opportunities for biomarker testing in cytopathology. J Am Soc Cytopathol 2019;8(2):95–115.
6. Lilo MT, Allison DB, Younes BK, et al. The critical role of EBUS-TBNA cytology in the staging of mediastinal lymph nodes in lung cancer patients: A correlation study with positron emission tomography findings. Cancer Cytopathol 2017;125(9):717–25.
7. Souza da Silva R, Pinto R, Cirnes L, et al. Tissue management in precision medicine: What the pathologist needs to know in the molecular era. Front Mol Biosci 2022;9:983102.
8. Medical imaging in personalised medicine: a white paper of the research committee of the European Society of Radiology (ESR). Insights Imaging 2015; 6(2):141–55.
9. Jassim TK, Ferreira JE, Murphy MB, et al. The use of diagnostic patterns for interventional cytopathology during rapid on-site evaluation and final classification. Semin Diagn Pathol 2022;39(6):394–404.
10. Harbin LM, Gallion HH, Allison DB, et al. Next generation sequencing and molecular biomarkers in ovarian cancer-an opportunity for targeted therapy. Diagnostics 2022;12(4).
11. Lilo MT, Allison D, Wang Y, et al. Expression of P40 and P63 in lung cancers using fine needle aspiration cases. Understanding clinical pitfalls and limitations. J Am Soc Cytopathol 2016;5(3):123–32.
12. Vidarsdottir H, Tran L, Nodin B, et al. Comparison of three different TTF-1 clones in resected primary lung cancer and epithelial pulmonary metastases. Am J Clin Pathol 2018;150(6):533–44.
13. Coindre JM, Pédeutour F, Aurias A. Well-differentiated and dedifferentiated liposarcomas. Virchows Arch 2010;456(2):167–79.

14. Allison DB, Rueckert J, Cornea V, et al. Thyroid Carcinoma with NSD3::NUTM1 Fusion: a Case with Thyrocyte Differentiation and Colloid Production. Endocr Pathol 2022;33(2):315–26.

15. Yachida S, Vakiani E, White CM, et al. Small cell and large cell neuroendocrine carcinomas of the pancreas are genetically similar and distinct from well-differentiated pancreatic neuroendocrine tumors. Am J Surg Pathol 2012;36(2):173–84.

16. VandenBussche CJ, Allison DB, Graham MK, et al. Alternative lengthening of telomeres and ATRX/DAXX loss can be reliably detected in FNAs of pancreatic neuroendocrine tumors. Cancer Cytopathol 2017;125(7):544–51.

17. Casey L, Singh N, POLE MMR. MSI Testing in Endometrial Cancer: Proceedings of the ISGyP Companion Society Session at the USCAP 2020 Annual Meeting. Int J Gynecol Pathol 2021;40(1):5–16.

18. Sinicrope FA, Sargent DJ. Molecular pathways: microsatellite instability in colorectal cancer: prognostic, predictive, and therapeutic implications. Clin Cancer Res 2012;18(6):1506–12.

19. Najjar S, Allison KH. Updates on breast biomarkers. Virchows Arch 2022;480(1):163–76.

20. Conde E, Rojo F, Gómez J, et al. Molecular diagnosis in non-small-cell lung cancer: expert opinion on ALK and ROS1 testing. J Clin Pathol 2022; 75(3):145–53.

21. Dong A, Zhao Y, Li Z, et al. PD-L1 versus tumor mutation burden: Which is the better immunotherapy biomarker in advanced non-small cell lung cancer? J Gene Med 2021;23(2):e3294.

22. Sha D, Jin Z, Budczies J, et al. Tumor mutational burden as a predictive biomarker in solid tumors. Cancer Discov 2020;10(12):1808–25.

23. Dong J, Li B, Lin D, et al. Advances in targeted therapy and immunotherapy for non-small cell lung cancer based on accurate molecular typing. Front Pharmacol 2019;10:230.

24. Drilon A, Laetsch TW, Kummar S, et al. Efficacy of Larotrectinib in TRK Fusion-Positive Cancers in Adults and Children. N Engl J Med 2018;378(8): 731–9.

25. Huang B, Chen Q, Allison D, et al. molecular tumor board review and improved overall survival in non-small-cell lung cancer. JCO Precis Oncol 2021. https://doi.org/10.1200/po.21.00210.

26. Allison KH, Hammond MEH, Dowsett M, et al. Estrogen and progesterone receptor testing in breast cancer: ASCO/CAP Guideline Update. J Clin Oncol 2020;38(12):1346–66.

27. Arber DA. Effect of prolonged formalin fixation on the immunohistochemical reactivity of breast markers. Appl Immunohistochem Mol Morphol 2002;10(2):183–6.

28. Reck M, Rodríguez-Abreu D, Robinson AG, et al. Pembrolizumab versus Chemotherapy for PD-L1-Positive Non-Small-Cell Lung Cancer. N Engl J Med 2016;375(19):1823–33.

29. Chung HC, Ros W, Delord JP, et al. Efficacy and safety of pembrolizumab in previously treated advanced cervical cancer: results from the phase II KEYNOTE-158 Study. J Clin Oncol 2019;37(17):1470–8.

30. Balar AV, Castellano D, O'Donnell PH, et al. First-line pembrolizumab in cisplatin-ineligible patients with locally advanced and unresectable or metastatic urothelial cancer (KEYNOTE-052): a multicentre, single-arm, phase 2 study. Lancet Oncol 2017; 18(11):1483–92.

31. Burtness B, Harrington KJ, Greil R, et al. Pembrolizumab alone or with chemotherapy versus cetuximab with chemotherapy for recurrent or metastatic squamous cell carcinoma of the head and neck (KEYNOTE-048): a randomised, open-label, phase 3 study. Lancet 2019;394(10212):1915–28.

32. Cortes J, Cescon DW, Rugo HS, et al. Pembrolizumab plus chemotherapy versus placebo plus chemotherapy for previously untreated locally recurrent inoperable or metastatic triple-negative breast cancer (KEYNOTE-355): a randomised, placebo-controlled, double-blind, phase 3 clinical trial. Lancet 2020;396(10265):1817–28.

33. Kojima T, Shah MA, Muro K, et al. Randomized Phase III KEYNOTE-181 Study of Pembrolizumab Versus Chemotherapy in Advanced Esophageal Cancer. J Clin Oncol 2020;38(35):4138–48.

34. Balar AV, Galsky MD, Rosenberg JE, et al. Atezolizumab as first-line treatment in cisplatin-ineligible patients with locally advanced and metastatic urothelial carcinoma: a single-arm, multicentre, phase 2 trial. Lancet 2017;389(10064):67–76.

35. Lantuejoul S, Damotte D, Hofman V, et al. Programmed death ligand 1 immunohistochemistry in non-small cell lung carcinoma. J Thorac Dis 2019; 11(Suppl 1):S89–s101.

36. Bartley AN, Washington MK, Ventura CB, et al. HER2 Testing and Clinical Decision Making in Gastroesophageal Adenocarcinoma: Guideline From the College of American Pathologists, American Society for Clinical Pathology, and American Society of Clinical Oncology. Arch Pathol Lab Med 2016;140(12): 1345–63.

37. Li S, Seegmiller AC, Lin P, et al. B-cell lymphomas with concurrent MYC and BCL2 abnormalities other than translocations behave similarly to MYC/BCL2 double-hit lymphomas. Mod Pathol 2015;28(2): 208–17.

38. Brandner S, McAleenan A, Jones HE, et al. Diagnostic accuracy of 1p/19q codeletion tests in oligodendroglioma: A comprehensive meta-analysis based on a Cochrane systematic review. Neuropathol Appl Neurobiol 2022;48(4):e12790.

39. Baker JA, Sireci AN, Marella N, et al. Analytical Accuracy of RET Fusion Detection by Break-Apart

Fluorescence In Situ Hybridization. Arch Pathol Lab Med 2021;146(3):351–9.

40. Tay TKY, Sukma NB, Lim TH, et al. Correlating SS18-SSX immunohistochemistry (IHC) with SS18 fluorescent in situ hybridization (FISH) in synovial sarcomas: a study of 36 cases. Virchows Arch 2021;479(4):785–93.

41. Gulley ML, Glaser SL, Craig FE, et al. Guidelines for interpreting EBER in situ hybridization and LMP1 immunohistochemical tests for detecting Epstein-Barr virus in Hodgkin lymphoma. Am J Clin Pathol 2002;117(2):259–67.

42. Chan JK. Virus-associated neoplasms of the nasopharynx and sinonasal tract: diagnostic problems. Mod Pathol 2017;30(s1): S68–s83.

43. Mills AM, Dirks DC, Poulter MD, et al. HR-HPV E6/E7 mRNA In Situ Hybridization: Validation Against PCR, DNA In Situ Hybridization, and p16 Immunohistochemistry in 102 Samples of Cervical, Vulvar, Anal, and Head and Neck Neoplasia. Am J Surg Pathol 2017;41(5):607–15.

44. Allison DB, Miller JA, Coquia SF, et al. Ultrasonography-guided fine-needle aspiration with concurrent small core biopsy of neck masses and lymph nodes yields adequate material for HPV testing in head and neck squamous cell carcinomas. J Am Soc Cytopathol 2016;5(1):22–30.

45. Bartlett JM, Campbell FM, Ibrahim M, et al. Chromogenic in situ hybridization: a multicenter study comparing silver in situ hybridization with FISH. Am J Clin Pathol 2009;132(4):514–20.

46. McCarthy AJ, Capo-Chichi JM, Spence T, et al. Heterogenous loss of mismatch repair (MMR) protein expression: a challenge for immunohistochemical interpretation and microsatellite instability (MSI) evaluation. J Pathol Clin Res 2019;5(2):115–29.

47. Benayed R, Offin M, Mullaney K, et al. High Yield of RNA Sequencing for Targetable Kinase Fusions in Lung Adenocarcinomas with No Mitogenic Driver Alteration Detected by DNA Sequencing and Low Tumor Mutation Burden. Clin Cancer Res 2019; 25(15):4712–22.

48. Kumar S, Vo AD, Qin F, et al. Comparative assessment of methods for the fusion transcripts detection from RNA-Seq data. Sci Rep 2016;6:21597.

49. Uhrig S, Ellermann J, Walther T, et al. Accurate and efficient detection of gene fusions from RNA sequencing data. Genome Res 2021;31(3):448–60.

50. Miquelestorena-Standley E, Jourdan ML, Collin C, et al. Effect of decalcification protocols on immunohistochemistry and molecular analyses of bone samples. Mod Pathol 2020;33(8):1505–17.

51. da Cunha Santos G, Saieg MA. Preanalytic specimen triage: Smears, cell blocks, cytospin preparations, transport media, and cytobanking. Cancer Cytopathol 2017;125(S6):455–64.

52. Jain D, Roy-Chowdhuri S. Molecular Pathology of Lung Cancer Cytology Specimens: A Concise Review. Arch Pathol Lab Med 2018;142(9):1127–33.

53. Dejmek A, Zendehrokh N, Tomaszewska M, et al. Preparation of DNA from cytological material: effects of fixation, staining, and mounting medium on DNA yield and quality. Cancer Cytopathol 2013;121(7):344–53.

54. Ranek L. Cytophotometric studies of the DNA, nucleic acid and protein content of human liver cell nuclei. Acta Cytol Mar-Apr 1976;20(2):151–7.

55. Vigliar E, Malapelle U, de Luca C, et al. Challenges and opportunities of next-generation sequencing: a cytopathologist's perspective. Cytopathology 2015; 26(5):271–83.

56. Roh MH. The utilization of cytologic and small biopsy samples for ancillary molecular testing. Mod Pathol 2019/01/01/2019;32:77–85.

57. Williams J, Kostiuk M, Biron VL. Molecular Detection Methods in HPV-Related Cancers. Front Oncol 2022; 12:864820.

58. Nikiforova MN, Mercurio S, Wald AI, et al. Analytical performance of the ThyroSeq v3 genomic classifier for cancer diagnosis in thyroid nodules. Cancer 2018;124(8):1682–90.

59. Steward DL, Carty SE, Sippel RS, et al. Performance of a Multigene Genomic Classifier in Thyroid Nodules With Indeterminate Cytology: A Prospective Blinded Multicenter Study. JAMA Oncol 2019;5(2):204–12.

60. Chin PD, Zhu CY, Sajed DP, et al. Correlation of ThyroSeq Results with Surgical Histopathology in Cytologically Indeterminate Thyroid Nodules. Endocr Pathol 2020;31(4):377–84.

61. Guan H, Toraldo G, Cerda S, et al. Utilities of RAS Mutations in Preoperative Fine Needle Biopsies for Decision Making for Thyroid Nodule Management: Results from a Single-Center Prospective Cohort. Thyroid 2020;30(4):536–47.

62. Schatz-Siemers N, Brandler TC, Oweity T, et al. Hürthle cell lesions on thyroid fine needle aspiration cytology: Molecular and histologic correlation. Diagn Cytopathol 2019;47(10):977–85.

63. Desai D, Lepe M, Baloch ZW, et al. ThyroSeq v3 for Bethesda III and IV: An institutional experience. Cancer Cytopathol 2021;129(2):164–70.

64. Velez Torres JM, Tjendra Y, Kerr DA. A triumvirate:: correlating thyroid cytopathology, molecular testing, and histopathology. Surg Pathol Clin 2023;16(1):1–14.

65. Whitmer D, Phay JE, Holt S, et al. Risk of malignancy in cytologically indeterminate thyroid nodules harboring thyroid stimulating hormone receptor mutations. Front Endocrinol 2022;13:1073592.

66. Nasr CE, Andrioli M, Endo M, et al. Real-World Performance of the Afirma Genomic Sequencing Classifier (GSC)-A Meta-analysis. J Clin Endocrinol Metab 2023;108(6):1526–32.

67. Finkelstein SD, Sistrunk JW, Malchoff C, et al. A retrospective evaluation of the diagnostic performance of an interdependent pairwise microrna expression analysis with a mutation panel in indeterminate thyroid nodules. Thyroid 2022;32(11):1362–71.

68. Allison DB, VandenBussche CJ. A review of urine ancillary tests in the era of the Paris System. Acta Cytol 2020;64(1–2):182–92.

69. van der Aa MN, Steyerberg EW, Bangma C, et al. Cystoscopy revisited as the gold standard for detecting bladder cancer recurrence: diagnostic review bias in the randomized, prospective CEFUB trial. J Urol 2010;183(1):76–80.

70. Hajdinjak T. UroVysion FISH test for detecting urothelial cancers: meta-analysis of diagnostic accuracy and comparison with urinary cytology testing. Urol Oncol 2008;26(6):646–51.

71. Halling KC, King W, Sokolova IA, et al. A comparison of BTA stat, hemoglobin dipstick, telomerase and Vysis UroVysion assays for the detection of urothelial carcinoma in urine. J Urol 2002;167(5):2001–6.

72. Bubendorf L, Grilli B, Sauter G, et al. Multiprobe FISH for enhanced detection of bladder cancer in voided urine specimens and bladder washings. Am J Clin Pathol 2001;116(1):79–86.

73. Yoder BJ, Skacel M, Hedgepeth R, et al. Reflex UroVysion testing of bladder cancer surveillance patients with equivocal or negative urine cytology: a prospective study with focus on the natural history of anticipatory positive findings. Am J Clin Pathol 2007;127(2):295–301.

74. Greene KL, Berry A, Konety BR. Diagnostic Utility of the ImmunoCyt/uCyt+ Test in Bladder Cancer. Rev Urol. Fall 2006;8(4):190–7.

75. Chou R, Gore JL, Buckley D, et al. Urinary Biomarkers for Diagnosis of Bladder Cancer: A Systematic Review and Meta-analysis. Ann Intern Med 2015;163(12):922–31.

76. Allison DB, Sharma R, Cowan ML, et al. Evaluation of Sienna Cancer Diagnostics hTERT Antibody on 500 Consecutive Urinary Tract Specimens. Acta Cytol 2018;62(4):302–10.

77. Moatamed NA, Rao JY, Alexanian S, et al. ProEx C as an adjunct marker to improve cytological detection of urothelial carcinoma in urinary specimens. Cancer Cytopathol 2013;121(6):320–8.

78. Guo A, Wang X, Gao L, et al. Bladder tumour antigen (BTA stat) test compared to the urine cytology in the diagnosis of bladder cancer: A meta-analysis. Can Urol Assoc J 2014;8(5–6):E347–52.

79. Eich ML, Rodriguez Pena MDC, Springer SU, et al. Incidence and distribution of UroSEEK gene panel in a multi-institutional cohort of bladder urothelial carcinoma. Mod Pathol 2019;32(10):1544–50.

80. Adler DG, Witt B. Cytologic diagnosis of biliary strictures: FISH or cut the sensitivity rate? Dig Dis Sci 2018;63(3):549–50.

81. Lilo MT, VandenBussche CJ, Allison DB, et al. Serous cystadenoma of the pancreas: potentials and pitfalls of a preoperative cytopathologic diagnosis. Acta Cytol 2017;61(1):27–33.

82. Abdelkader A, Hunt B, Hartley CP, et al. cystic lesions of the pancreas: differential diagnosis and cytologic-histologic correlation. Arch Pathol Lab Med 2020;144(1):47–61.

83. Jhala N, Jhala D. Approach to FNA of Pancreatic Cysts. Adv Anat Pathol 2022;29(6):349–57.

84. Pusateri AJ, Krishna SG. Pancreatic cystic lesions: pathogenesis and malignant potential. Diseases 2018;6(2).

85. Springer S, Wang Y, Dal Molin M, et al. A combination of molecular markers and clinical features improve the classification of pancreatic cysts. Gastroenterology 2015;149(6):1501–10.

86. Khalid A, Zahid M, Finkelstein SD, et al. Pancreatic cyst fluid DNA analysis in evaluating pancreatic cysts: a report of the PANDA study. Gastrointest Endosc 2009;69(6):1095–102.

87. Nikiforova MN, Khalid A, Fasanella KE, et al. Integration of KRAS testing in the diagnosis of pancreatic cystic lesions: a clinical experience of 618 pancreatic cysts. Mod Pathol 2013;26(11):1478–87.

88. Singhi AD, Nikiforova MN, Fasanella KE, et al. Preoperative GNAS and KRAS testing in the diagnosis of pancreatic mucinous cysts. Clin Cancer Res 2014;20(16):4381–9.

89. Schönleben F, Qiu W, Ciau NT, et al. PIK3CA mutations in intraductal papillary mucinous neoplasm/carcinoma of the pancreas. Clin Cancer Res 2006;12(12):3851–5.

90. Garcia-Carracedo D, Turk AT, Fine SA, et al. Loss of PTEN expression is associated with poor prognosis in patients with intraductal papillary mucinous neoplasms of the pancreas. Clin Cancer Res 2013;19(24):6830–41.

91. Singhi AD, McGrath K, Brand RE, et al. Preoperative next-generation sequencing of pancreatic cyst fluid is highly accurate in cyst classification and detection of advanced neoplasia. Gut 2018;67(12):2131–41.

92. Schlauch D, Fu X, Jones SF, et al. Tumor-specific and tumor-agnostic molecular signatures associated with response to immune checkpoint inhibitors. JCO Precision Oncology 2021;(5):1625–38.

93. Tan AC. Tumor-agnostic biomarkers: heed caution, and why cell of origin still matters. Onco 2021;1(2):95–100.

Salivary Gland Fine-Needle Aspiration
The Current and Future Landscape

Federica Policardo, MD, Antonino Mule', MD,
Esther Diana Rossi, MD, PhD*

KEYWORDS

• Fine needle-aspiration cytology • Salivary lesions • Immunocytochemistry • Molecular testing
• Personalized medicine

Key points

- The role of cytology in the evaluation of salivary gland lesions

- The comparison between the descriptive report versus the use of a classification system

- Overview and details from the Milan System I and II editions

- The future of salivary cytology and the role of ancillary techniques, especially molecular testing

---

ABSTRACT

Fine-needle aspiration represents a valid tool for the diagnosis/management of salivary gland lesions. The past years assessed the lack of uniform diagnostic reports for salivary cytopathology leading to interpretative issues. In 2015, an international group of cytopathologists developed an evidence-based tiered classification system for reporting salivary gland fine-needle aspiration (FNA) specimens, the "Milan System for Reporting Salivary Gland Cytopathology" (MSRSGC). The present landscape of salivary cytology is represented by the growing adoption of the MSRSGC and the assessment of its diagnostic role. The future landscape is characterized by the increasing role of ancillary techniques for diagnostic and prognostic purposes.

THE PAST AND PRESENT OF SALIVARY CYTOLOGY

According to the literature, neoplasms of salivary glands account for between 2% and 6.5% of all head and neck tumors and up to 80% of these originate in the parotid gland.[1] However, due to the evidence that the majority of these tumors are benign, it is crucial to exclude malignancy preoperatively for proper management. In this regard, FNA represents a valid diagnostic procedure for salivary gland lesions. Its value is mostly associated to the fact that it is a rapid and easy method, minimally invasive, safe, and inexpensive.[1–18] The role of FNA is always combined with the evaluation of the clinical and radiologic findings in order to have a global definition of the lesions before any surgical intervention. The possibility to perform an FNA, especially under ultrasound guidance, is possible in almost every salivary gland, especially for the major salivary glands. Some additional difficulties might be encountered for the minor salivary glands of the oral cavity, for which the adoption of small biopsies is likely to help for the diagnostic evaluation.

The role of FNA has been extensively defined by the ability to differentiate between neoplastic and non-neoplastic salivary gland lesions, to diagnose commonly occurring benign tumors and in most cases to distinguish low-grade from high-grade

---

Division of Anatomic Pathology and Histology, Fondazione Policlinico Universitario "Agostino Gemelli", IRCCS, Rome, Italy
* Corresponding author.
E-mail address: esther.rossi@policlinicogemelli.it

Surgical Pathology 17 (2024) 347–358
https://doi.org/10.1016/j.path.2024.04.003
1875-9181/24/

carcinomas. In fact, FNA (SG-FNA) is critical in providing useful information for planning of surgical treatment of patients with a neoplasm and can obviate the need for surgery in up to one-third of patients with non-neoplastic diseases. Several salivary gland tumors (SGTs) are likely to be treated with surgery which is defined by the results of FNA in terms of the nature (primary vs secondary) and grade (low grade vs high grade) of the neoplasm. Furthermore, FNA is also crucial in determining the facial nerve preservation and neck dissection depending on the specific diagnosis. Although benign SGTs such as pleomorphic adenoma (PA) and Warthin tumor (WT) are very frequently treated with a conservative surgery, they might be managed nonsurgically by clinical and radiologic follow-up, depending upon patient age, preferences, and comorbidities.

Numerous studies and textbooks assessed that the cytomorphologic features of salivary gland lesions in FNA specimens have been well-documented in the literature.[1–22] Nonetheless, salivary gland lesions represent one of the most challenging diagnostic areas in cytopathology. The difficulties are the result of different aspects as (1) diversity of both benign and malignant SGTs, with more than 40 distinct epithelial tumor subtypes recognized by the World Health Organization (WHO) in 2022[23]; (2) the morphologic similarities and overlaps between many benign and low-grade malignant SGTs; (3) the wide spectrum and morphologic heterogeneity of cellular elements within the same SGT (ie, PA); and (4) the rarity of many SGTs making it difficult for the practicing cytopathologist to become familiar with their cytologic features.

Different investigators, in their comprehensive systematic review and meta-analyses of the literature, have reported that the sensitivity and specificity of FNA in differentiating benign and malignant SGTs in the parotid gland is high and of 80% and 97%, respectively. Furthermore, several studies documented a 25% prevalence of malignancy, 90% positive predictive value (PPV) and 94% negative predictive value (NPV). If we consider the prevalence of neoplastic conditions, which is at around 85%, the PPV was 100% and the NPV was 81%. These figures are mostly due to the fact that PA, WT, and metastatic carcinomas to intraparotid lymph nodes are among the most commonly encountered salivary gland (SG) lesions, representing approximately 70% to 80% of tumors and easily recognized on cytologic samples. According to a large review of 6249 SG-FNAs from 1999 to 2003[15] as part of the inter-laboratory comparison program in nongynecologic cytology, spearheaded by the College of American

Pathologists, the highest false-negative (FN) rates were associated to lymphoma (57%), acinic cell carcinoma (49%), low-grade mucoepidermoid carcinoma (MEC; 43%), and adenoid cystic carcinoma (AdCC, 33%), while benign cases with the highest false-positive rates were mostly monomorphic adenoma (53%), intraparotid lymph nodes (36%), and oncocytoma (18%).

To note, there are several preanalytical and postanalytical factors that can influence the diagnostic accuracy of salivary FNA as for instance: the prevalence and distribution of SGT in a given population; FNA techniques such as manual/palpation versus ultrasound (u/s) guided; FNA operator's experience; use of rapid on-site evaluation; cytologic preparation; diagnostic experience of the cytopathologist; reporting terminology; characteristics of the SGT; and the use of ancillary studies. An important point is to reduce the number of inadequate and indeterminate results which might have an impact on the diagnosis. Furthermore, for some uncommon low-grade SGTs, FNA lacks specificity in being able to precisely classify the tumor subtype based on cytomorphology alone.[1,19] Hence, although most of the high-grade carcinomas are easily recognized as malignant,[1,18] the distinction between salivary duct carcinoma, high-grade MEC, and high-grade adenocarcinoma can be problematic and it needs the support of ancillary techniques in several cases.[19–29]

Data from literature reported that the prevalence of malignancy varies depending upon the size and the location of the SGT, being inversely proportional to the size of the salivary gland.[1] It increases from 15% to 32% in the parotid gland, to 35% to 50% in the submandibular gland, and to 50% to 90% in the sublingual and minor salivary glands.[1] However, parotid gland cytology represents more than 70% of salivary gland FNAs.

THE NEED FOR A CLASSIFICATION SYSTEM

Before 2018, several attempts of reporting terminologies for salivary gland cytology had been proposed from different institutions throughout the world or in the same country and even by individual cytopathologists within the same institution. The effect has been the evidence of a wide range of diagnostic categories, descriptive diagnoses, and even the use of surgical pathology terminology for SG-FNA specimens creating confusion among pathologists and treating clinicians as well as patients, who may have access to their pathology reports. Further problems, associated with the diversity in the reports and terminology, are represented by the confusion in the direct correlation with a risk of malignancy (ROM; ie, risk stratification) and management as well as sharing of data for quality control and clinicopathologic studies is problematic. All this confusion led to the general agreement in the cytopathology community that a defined set of diagnostic categories for salivary gland FNA has been necessary.[1,2,30–34] The Bethesda system for cervical cytology,[35] launched in 1988, has been a model for the development of several subsequent standardized cytopathology reporting systems for thyroid, pancreas, urine, and lung[36–39] in which each diagnostic category is associated with a ROM and recommendations for clinical management. One of the first proposed reporting system for SG-FNA specimens was initially shared as part of guidelines developed by the Japanese Society of Clinical Cytology,[40] but it had little impact in Western countries. In these last years, some proposal of classification schemes has been suggested from institutions in different countries.[2,28,30–32,40] Each of the classification schemes shares the following: they are tiered and consist of clinically relevant diagnostic categories, and most provide a framework for reporting indeterminate FNA specimens. Together with these institutional efforts, in 2015, an international group of cytopathologists decided to develop a reporting system for salivary gland FNA specimens using a framework consisting of 6 diagnostic categories. The reporting system was named the "Milan System for Reporting Salivary Cytopathology", because of the first meeting of the core group during the 2015 annual meeting of the European Cytology Congress held in Milan, Italy. The MSRSGC is sponsored by both the American Society of Cytopathology (ASC) and the International Academy of Cytology, and the working group consisted of over 47 participants from 15 countries, including mostly experienced cytopathologists but also surgical pathologists and head and neck surgeons. The MSRSGC was structured as an evidence-based system (based on literature review) which aims to correlate each diagnostic category with a ROM and clinical managements. The MSRSGC working group consensus was developed over 2 years, with also the support of two large online surveys of the cytopathology community were performed to gather data, assess experience, and identify problematic areas and unresolved issues.[34] Several clinicopathological studies were also initiated in order to gather more evidence-based data, leading to a number of over 200 since its publication in 2018 to 2023.[41–47] The format is in the "Bethesda style" including 10 chapters with definitions, criteria, and explanatory notes along with numerous images and tables for each diagnostic category. There are also separate chapters on FNA technique, indications, ancillary studies,

histologic correlation, and management. Furthermore, a web-based atlas was linked to the atlas including many supplemental images available electronically through the ASC. The main objective of the MSRSGC is to improve communication among clinicians and between different institutions and to ultimately improve patient care by providing a practical and uniform reporting system that is user-friendly and internationally accepted. Since its publication in 2018, numerous FNA studies, including meta-analyses have been published using the MSRSGC diagnostic criteria and confirming the value and role of the Milan system as a practical and useful classification system including more than 200 studies from North America, Europe, Africa, Australia, and several Asian countries. The majority of these studies were in line with the mean ROM for each category within the recommended range published by the MSRSGC and they were useful for the recent update of the Milan system. In fact, in July 2023, the second edition of the MSRSGC has been published. Specifically, the second edition shows some refined ROMs for each diagnostic category, a new chapter on imaging studies for salivary glands, updates on the application of ancillary studies to salivary gland FNA, as well as updated nomenclature and entities in keeping with the latest 2022 WHO classification. Furthermore, additional pictures substituting half of the original ones have been added as well as a complete revision of the diagnostic chapters with an emphasis for the neoplastic chapter and its subclassification. The atlas maintained the identical diagnostic categories which were classified as: nondiagnostic, non-neoplastic, atypia of undetermined significance and neoplastic category subclassified as neoplastic—benign and salivary gland neoplasm of uncertain malignant potential (SUMP), suspicious for malignancy, and malignant.

THE FUTURE OF SALIVARY CYTOLOGY

While the present of salivary cytology is defined by the adoption of a classification system for diagnosing salivary lesions, the future seems to be characterized by the growing enthusiasm toward the application of ancillary techniques, with diagnostic and prognostic purposes. In fact, the major role of salivary FNA is to contribute to the definition of the most tailored clinical management of any salivary lesion. Despite the valid aid of morphology for the diagnosis of the majority of salivary lumps, in few cases it is not able to make a definitive conclusion. Despite the fact that morphology is able to recognize the majority of lesions, in a minority of cases immunohistochemistry (IHC) can represent an additional diagnostic tool. Therefore, as for other cytologic fields, ancillary studies should be considered primarily for aspirates in which the results would modify clinical management or clinical risk within the MSRSGC.[52] The added value of ancillary depends on the specific diagnostic concerns and potential impact and clinical management. As for the thyroid FNAs, ancillary studies are most useful for some aspirates in the indeterminate categories of SUMP or SFM, as they can help to refine the differential diagnosis and potentially place the specimen in a more definitive diagnostic category with implications for management. More than 50% of some malignant entities such as AdCC, acinic cell carcinoma (AciCC), SC, and MEC are diagnosed as malignant by cytomorphology alone, but the remaining 50% are diagnosed as SUMP (43%) or suspicious for malignancy (SFM) (11%).[47] In these last decades, the new emerging genetic alterations associated with specific salivary entities have been playing an important role in improving the diagnostic accuracy of salivary gland FNAC, especially within the framework of the MSRSGC. In fact, the majority of SGT is characterized by specific genetic alterations that can be used for diagnostic purposes and that can be evaluated on cytologic material.[2] The characteristic immunophenotypic and cytogenetic features of various SGTs are well described in the literature and now have significant diagnostic (and sometimes therapeutic) implications.[2,3] The most common molecular alterations were included in the latest WHO definitions of several SGTs including MEC, AdCC, SC, polymorphous adenocarcinoma, and hyalinizing clear cell carcinoma.[2] For example, the 2021 American Society of Clinical Oncology (ASCO) guidelines recommend that pathologists may perform ancillary testing (IHC or molecular studies) on FNAs and core needle biopsy (CNBs) to support diagnosis and ROM.[3] Several new immunomarkers have been developed and can be very useful to refine the differential diagnostic list or to favor a specific entity when cytomorphology alone is not sufficient.[48–52]

Fluorescence in situ hybridization (FISH), in particular, can be used to improve the diagnostic accuracy of cytologic samples, as well as other methods such as RT-PCR and next-generation sequencing (NGS).[53] NGS is often used in clinical practice to diagnose salivary gland tumors due to its capacity to test several genes at the same time and find partner genes in chromosomal rearrangements. In salivary gland neoplasms, a pattern-based method can help us decide which ancillary test to apply. An initial distinction between salivary gland neoplasms is frequently based on the observation of peculiar pattern related with the morphology or the many types of cells that comprise the tumor, such as basaloid, oncocytic, clear cell, and biphasic tumors, or the presence of extracellular matrix.[53,54]

BASALOID LESIONS

One of the most difficult patterns to diagnose with aspiration cytology is basaloid salivary gland neoplasms since the differential diagnosis encompasses tumors with a wide range of biologic behavior, from benign neoplasms to aggressive carcinomas. The stromal features are extremely useful in differential diagnosis. A limited proportion of fibrillar stroma is related with neoplasms with low ROM, notably PA. A stroma with more hyaline characteristics (streaks or spherules) indicates basal cell neoplasms or AdCC. In the absence of stroma, identification can be especially difficult because most basaloid neoplasms are composed of monomorphic and bland tumor cells, and cytologic samples only rarely exhibit clearly malignant characteristics (nuclear pleomorphism, significant mitotic activity, or apoptosis/necrosis).[53]

Pleomorphic Adenoma

The most common salivary gland tumor, PA, has mixed myoepithelial and epithelial cells with substantial chondromyxoid fibrillar matrix, to which myoepithelial cells are frequently connected. The architectural and cytologic organization may be heterogeneous and individual parts may vary in presence both within and between tumors.

Over 70% of PAs have known genetic changes. The most common ones are

- Rearrangement of the PLAG1 gene (50%–60% of all PAs).
- Rearrangement of the HMGA2 gene (10%–20%).
- Amplification of the MDM2 gene (less common).[54]

PLAG1 and HMGA2 rearrangements can be detected using both FISH and sequencing methods. However, the availability of immunohistochemistry stains that detect PLAG1 (with intense nuclear reactivity) and HMGA2 overexpression makes them more useful because they are more convenient and efficient to conduct than molecular studies.[53,54] On immunohistochemical tests, it shows positivity for pancytokeratin, CK7, CAM5.2 (epithelial cell component) and SMA, calponin, muscle-specific actin, SMMHC, P63, CK14, GFAP, S100 (myoepithelial cells component).[55]

Carcinoma ex Pleomorphic Adenoma

Carcinoma ex PA accounts for roughly 12% of salivary gland malignant neoplasms and, unlike

Fig. 1. (*A–C*) Epithelial and myoepithelial cells intermixed with the chondromyxoid stromal component of a pleomorphic adenoma (Pap stain 200x).

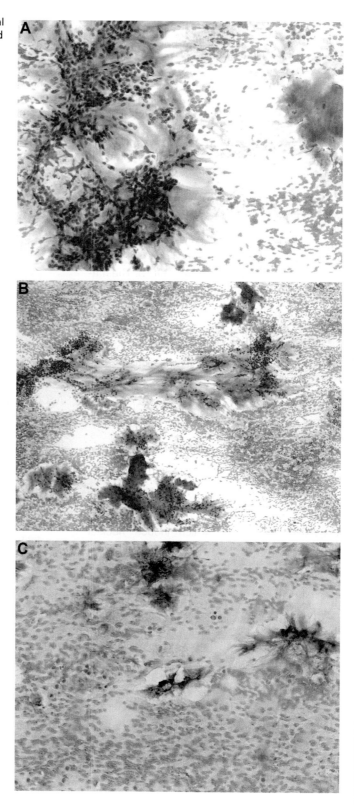

PA, has a monophasic appearance due to the existence of only the epithelial cellular component with an intercalated ductlike phenotype.[54] It frequently develops on top of pre-existing PA and, when it does, it retains the PA-specific gene rearrangements (PLAG1 and HMGA2), the overexpression of which is easily detected by immunohistochemistry.[53]

Furthermore, *HER2* amplification was found in 39% of carcinoma ex PA, and *TP53* mutations were detected in 37% of intracapsular carcinoma ex PA[56,57] (Fig. 1A–C).

Immunohistochemical stains vary based on the type of malignant component present: CK7, EMA, HER2, AR, *P53*(salivary duct carcinoma), calponin, *P63*, *P40*, SMMHC (myoepithelial carcinoma), CK7, CK5/6 (squamoidlike cells), *P63* (squamous cells), mucin stains (mucous cells; MEC). The malignant component has a very high Ki67.

Basal Cell Adenoma/Adenocarcinoma

Basal cell adenoma is an extremely rare benign salivary gland tumor that can only be distinguished from its malignant counterpart through the examination of histologic sections that allow for the detection of infiltrative growth or lymphangioinvasion.[53,54] These tumors exhibit a dual population of basaloid cells in small and intermediate sizes, often organized in clusters that show the smaller cells' peripheral nuclear palisading, hyaline extracellular matrix is also present.

The most common mutations associated with basal cell adenoma are

a. CTNNB1 mutations, which induce nuclear overexpression of beta-catenin and have a moderate sensitivity (around 80%) and a 96% specificity for this type of tumors when compared to PA and AdCC. Despite its high specificity, this marker has not proven to be completely useful in diagnostic practice due to the heterogeneous staining of the myoepithelial elements;
b. Rare (possible association with Brooke–Spiegler syndrome) mutation of the cylindromatosis gene determines the membranous variant of basal cell tumors and is characterized by greater clinical aggressiveness.

The genetic profile of basal cell adenocarcinoma shows

- PIK3CA-activating mutation a potential targeted gene.[54–59]
- The Wnt3a pathway, which is responsible for the development of numerous tissues (mammary glands, hair follicles, teeth, and airway

submucosal glands), regulates lymphoid enhancer binding factor 1 (LEF-1). Its detection is helpful in head and neck pathology. LEF-1 expression has been found to be common in basal cell neoplasms, both adenoma and its malignant counterpart; in fact, when compared to other salivary gland diseases, it is positive in 67%. However, not all research agrees that this signature is solely seen in basal cell tumors.[53]

The immunoprofile of basal adenoma and basal cell carcinoma is very similar, they express positivity for

- Pancytokeratin, CK7.
- CEAm and S100 (variable) in luminal cells.
- *P63*, *P40*, 34betaE12, CK14, CK5, calponin, SMA, vimentin, S100 in basal/myoepithelial cell.

Basal cell adenoma also more frequently, but not exclusively, expresses nuclear positivity for beta-catenin and BCL2.[59,60]

Adenoid Cystic Carcinoma

AdCC is distinguished by the presence of basaloid cells and a metachromatic extracellular matrix organized in the shape of globules, cylinders, or fingerlike projections. The basaloid cells are dispersed around the extracellular matrix, which has distinct borders.[54] The MYB gene rearrangement represents the most common genetic changes (>50%):

- t(6;9) fusion of MYB and NFIB
- t(8;9) fusion of MYBL1::NFIB

MYB can be recognized via IHC, and its positivity must be characterized by strong nuclear staining of abluminal myoepithelial cells and weaker and zonal staining of luminal ductal cells.[53] Strong and diffuse MYB nuclear staining is helpful in confirming an AdCC cytologic diagnosis. However, because it can appear in both benign and other malignant basaloid tumors, weak and focal staining of MYB should be viewed cautiously.[61]

FISH approaches can be employed in dubious or problematic circumstances.

Ductal cells predominantly express CD117 (c-KIT).[54] CD117 expression was seen in a broader spectrum of salivary and nonsalivary gland tumors, emphasizing the need for caution when utilizing CD117 expression as a diagnostic for AdCC.[53]

NOTCH1 mutation has recently been linked to a subtype of AdCC with more aggressive behavior and solid growth, which correlates with broad

Fig. 2. Acinic cell carcinoma as seen on a conventional smear (*A, B*) and liquid-based preparation

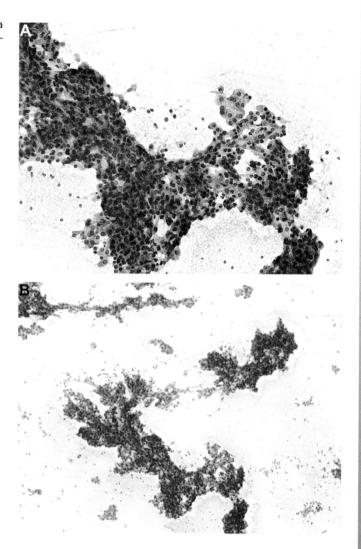

immunohistochemistry expression of activated NOTCH1 (N1CD1). Its diagnostic usefulness for adenoid cystic cancer, however, is limited.[54,62] Immunohistochemical markers for AdCC include sialoglycoprotein CD43, which may help to restrict the differential diagnosis, as well as nonspecific markers for myoepithelial cells (SMA, S100, calponin, p40, p63, and cytokeratins) and ductal cells (CK7 and CAM 5.2). A higher incidence of perineural invasion is linked to NCAM expression. Both a predictive and diagnostic test is Ki-67.[63]

ONCOCYTOID LESIONS

All cytologic forms that upon aspirate examination seem to be distinguished by a more expanded cytoplasm, even if not absolutely oncocytic, are included in the group of oncocytoid neoplasms. Both benign and cancerous kinds of tumors might be included in the diagnostic spectrum. As a result, ancillary approaches can be extremely

helpful in differential diagnosis or as proof of a certain diagnosis.[53]

Warthin Tumor

Warthin's tumor is a benign cystic salivary gland tumor with a stroma that resembles lymph nodes and abundant lymphocytes. It lacks *MAML2* fusion, which is positive in MEC.

The epithelial component is positive for pancytokeratin and EMA; the basal cells have a variable nuclear staining for *P*63 and *P*40.

The lymphoid population has a positive test for CD20 (B-cell marker) and CD3, CD4, CD8 (T-cell markers).[58]

Mucoepidermoid Carcinoma

According to the literature, MEC is among the most common type of salivary gland malignant tumor. The tumor is made up of many cell groups in

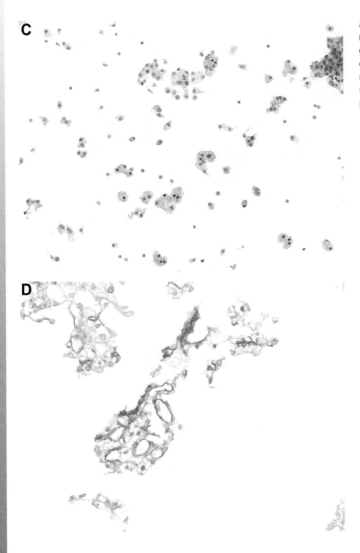

C

D

Fig. 2. (*continued*). (*C*) The cells are primarily seen in organized clusters, possess granular cytoplasm, and have a delicate, oncocytic appearance. (*D*) A DOG-1 immunostain performed on residual material from liquid-based preservative was positive (200x).

varying proportions: mucous, intermediate, and epidermoid cells.

The properties of aspirates are determined by their cytologic grade. MEC is categorized into 3 levels, each of which has a varied prognosis.

FN results are common in low grade, often cystic forms, because they are primarily composed of mucous cells and may appear merely as the contents of the cyst or with sparse tumor cells. Epidermoid-type cells with a squamoid appearance can be seen in high grade, mostly solid forms, which might cause differential diagnosis with other types of cancer.[53,54] The FISH approach can be definitive in the most challenging cases, especially when a preoperative diagnosis appears to be critical.[53] In fact, 60% to 90% of MECs have a t(11;19) (q21;p13) rearrangement of the MAML2 gene, which specifies the MAML2::CRTC1 fusion. A less common mutation

is the t(11;15) (q21;q26) translocation, which results in the MAML2::CRTC3 fusion.[53,54,64] MAML2 fusion with other genes such as KMT2A, YAP1, or SAMSN1 is uncommon. It has been found that the mutation rate in low-grade MECs is much higher than in high-grade MECs. It has recently been discovered that cases of MEC with negative MAML2 correspond with a poor prognosis. Identifying the MAML2 rearrangement in a primary salivary gland tumor is thus a critically crucial diagnostic signal for MEC, but its absence does not rule out the diagnosis. There is currently no IHC technique for identifying the MAML2 rearrangement.[64] Mucicarmine can be utilized to mark intracytoplasmic mucin in mucous cells if molecular investigations are not accessible. Furthermore, significant positivity for p63/p40 is typical of, but not unique to, the MEC. Typically, SOX10 is negative.[53,54]

Fig. 3. Secretory carcinoma on a liquid-based preparation, defined by isolated cells or small clusters of neoplastic cells with cytoplasmic vacuoles with different size and shape (Pap stain 200x).

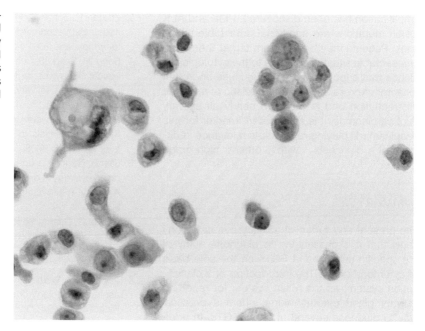

Acinic Cell Carcinoma

Acinic cell carcinoma is a relatively uncommon type of salivary gland cancer. The cells resemble those of normal non-neoplastic glandular tissue, but their architecture (solid, microcystic, papillary, cystic, or follicular) distinguishes them. This trait is detected in aspirated smears with the presence of grapelike clusters, discohesion, and delicate cytoplasm.[53] A gene rearrangement specific to acinic cell carcinoma was recently discovered, but it is not found in all cases:

- t(4;9) (q13;q31) determines NR4A3 overexpression.
- In 4% to 15% of cases, the MSANTD::HTN3 fusion was discovered, as well as nuclear overexpression of NR4A3.

FISH can identify these gene changes, although IHC has been found to be more sensitive.[64] SOX10 and DOG1 can be used as markers for serous acinar distinction in IHC. S100 and p63 are typically negative[53,54] (**Fig. 2A–D**).

Secretory Carcinoma

Secretory carcinoma, first described by Skalova and colleagues, is primarily seen in the parotid, submandibular, and oral cavities. Aspirate smear cells have a spherical histiocyticlike shape, ovoid nuclei, inconspicuous nucleoli, and a vast, vacuolated cytoplasm. The cells might form flaps, papillary clusters, or they can be scattered as single cells.[53,54] Approximately 80% of secretory carcinomas have the t(12;15) (p13;q25) gene rearrangement, which results in the ETV6::NTRK3 fusion. Rarely, rearrangements involving other partner genes (eg, RET, MET, or MAML3) have been reported.

The evidence of the ETV6 rearrangement by FISH can be employed in cytology to validate the diagnosis of secretory carcinoma.[53,54,64] The utility of pan-TRK IHC evaluation in the diagnosis of secretory carcinoma has been proven in the literature (nuclear staining separates secretory carcinoma with the NTRK3 fusion from its mimics).[53,54] Furthermore, RNA sequencing that validates the molecular rearrangement of NTRK3 helps to identify the target for systemic therapy in instances with more aggressive behavior, the formation of metastases, and high-grade characteristics.[64] S100 and mammaglobin coexpression is typical of secretory carcinoma[53,54] (**Fig. 3**).

Salivary Duct Carcinoma

Salivary duct carcinoma is an aggressive tumor that primarily affects men in their sixth decade.[54] It has an apocrine phenotype, similar to apocrine ductal carcinoma of the breast.[53] The cells exhibit significant atypia, with apocrine features, and are organized in big clusters, papillae, and flaps; necrosis is prevalent.[53] Salivary duct carcinoma frequently develops on a PA and may have the same PLAG1 and HMG2A gene rearrangements as this cancer. In one-third of cases, ERBB2 amplification has been discovered. PI3K and ALK fusion mutations are additional detectable mutations. Patients may benefit from target therapy in unresectable situations thanks to the cytologic evidence that supports it.[53,54,64] Because androgen receptor expression is a characteristic of apocrine differentiation and is found in nearly all salivary duct carcinomas, it is an excellent marker for this neoplasm, displaying remarkable relevance in differential diagnosis with other high-grade tumors.[53,54]

SUMMARY

The present and future of salivary cytopathology show that it is challenging to diagnose many of the specific subtypes of SGTs on the sole basis of cytomorphology. The introduction of a classification system, as the Milan system for reporting salivary gland cytopathology, offers a practical way to diagnose several of these SGTs. In addition, the present but especially the future of salivary research demonstrates that an accurate diagnosis is best achieved by a combination of cytomorphology with clinical findings and ancillary test results including molecular features.

CLINICS CARE POINTS

- Salivary cytology is a gold standard for the evaluation of salivary lesions.

- Morphology alone is able to diagnose the majority of salivary lesions.

- In some cases, as for the SUMP category and some others, the support of ancillary testing represents a valid additional diagnostic clue.

DISCLOSURE

The authors have nothing to disclose. This research did not receive any specific grant from any funding agency in the public, commercial, or not-profit sectors.

REFERENCES

1. Wang H, Fundakowski C, Khurana JS, et al. Fine-needle aspiration biopsy of salivary gland lesions. Arch Pathol Lab Med 2015;139(12):1491–7.

2. Griffith CC, Pai RK, Schneider F, et al. Salivary gland tumor fine-needle aspiration cytology: a proposal for a risk stratification classification. Am J Clin Pathol 2015;143(6):839–53.

3. Zbaren P, Schar C, Hotz MA, et al. Value of fine-needle aspiration cytology of parotid gland masses. Laryngoscope 2001;111(11 Pt 1):1989–92.

4. Song IH, Song JS, Sung CO, et al. Accuracy of core needle biopsy versus fine needle aspiration cytology for diagnosing salivary gland tumors. J Pathol Transl Med 2015;49(2):136–43.

5. Faquin WC, Powers CN. In: Salivary gland cytopathology. Essentials in cytopathology series5. New York: Springer; 2008.

6. Jain R, Gupta R, Kudesia M, et al. Fine needle aspiration cytology in diagnosis of salivary gland lesions: A study with histologic comparison. CytoJournal 2013;10:5.

7. Colella G, Cannavale R, Flamminio F, et al. Fine-needle aspiration cytology of salivary gland lesions: a systematic review. J Oral Maxillofac Surg 2010;68: 2146–53.

8. Jayaram G, Verma AK, Sood N, et al. Fine needle aspiration cytology of salivary gland lesions. J Oral Pathol Med 1994;23:256–61.

9. Zurrida S, Alasio L, Tradati N, et al. Fine-needle aspiration of parotid masses. Cancer 1993;72:2306–11.

10. Qizilbash AH, Sianos J, Young JE, et al. Fine needle aspiration biopsy cytology of major salivary glands. Acta Cytol 1985;29:503–12.

11. Mihashi H, Kawahara A, Kage M, et al. Comparison of preoperative fine-needle aspiration cytology diagnosis and histopathological diagnosis of salivary gland tumors. Kurume Med J 2006;53:23–7.

12. Fundakowski C, Castaño J, Abouyared M, et al. The role of indeterminate fine-needle biopsy in the diagnosis of parotid malignancy. Laryngoscope 2014; 124:678–81.

13. Layfield LJ, Tan P, Glasgow BJ. Fine-needle aspiration of salivary gland lesions. Comparison with frozen sections and histologic findings. Arch Pathol Lab Med 1987;111:346–53.

14. Kocjan G, Nayagam M, Harris M. Fine needle aspiration cytology of salivary gland lesions: Advantages and pitfalls. Cytopathology 1990;1:269–75.

15. Schindler S, Nayar R, Dutra J, et al. Diagnostic challenges in aspiration cytology of the salivary glands. Semin Diagn Pathol 2001;18:124–46.

16. Rajwanshi A, Gupta K, Gupta N, et al. Fine-needle aspiration cytology of salivary glands: diagnostic pitfalls–revisited. Diagn Cytopathol 2006;34:580–4.

17. Mukunyadzi P. Review of fine-needle aspiration cytology of salivary gland neoplasms, with emphasis on differential diagnosis. Am J Clin Pathol 2002;S100–15.

18. Daneshbod Y, Daneshbod K, Khademi B. Diagnostic difficulties in the interpretation of fine needle aspirate samples in salivary lesions: diagnostic pitfalls revisited. Acta Cytol 2009;53:53–70.

19. Mairembam P, Jay A, Beale T, et al. Salivary gland FNA cytology: role as a triage tool and an approach

to pitfalls in cytomorphology. Cytopathology 2016; 27:91–6.

20. Schmidt RL, Hunt JP, Hall BJ, et al. A systematic review and meta-analysis of the diagnostic accuracy of frozen section for parotid gland lesions. Am J Clin Pathol 2011;136:729–38.

21. Hughes JH, Volk EE, Wilbur DC, Cytopathology Resource Committee, College of American Pathologists. Pitfalls in salivary gland fine-needle aspiration cytology: lessons from the College of American Pathologists Interlaboratory Comparison Program in Nongynecologic Cytology. Arch Pathol Lab Med 2005;129:26–31.

22. Kim BY, Hyeon J, Ryu G, et al. Diagnostic accuracy of fine needle aspiration cytology for high-grade salivary gland tumors. Ann Surg Oncol 2013;20:2380–7.

23. Tyagi R, Dey P. Diagnostic problems of salivary gland tumors. Diagn Cytopathol 2015;43:495–509.

24. Layfield LJ, Gopez EV. Cystic lesions of the salivary glands: cytologic features in fine-needle aspiration biopsies. Diagn Cytopathol 2002;27:197–204.

25. Chai C, Dodd LG, Glasgow BJ, et al. Salivary gland lesions with a prominent lymphoid component: cytologic findings and differential diagnosis by fine-needle aspiration biopsy. Diagn Cytopathol 1997; 17:183–90.

26. Mooney EE, Dodd LG, Layfield LJ. Squamous cells in fine-needle aspiration biopsies of salivary gland lesions: potential pitfalls in cytologic diagnosis. Diagn Cytopathol 1996;15:447–52.

27. El-Naggar AK, Chan J, Takata T, et al. WHO classification of tumours. Pathology and genetics of head and neck tumours. 4th edition. Lyon: IARC Press; 2017.

28. Pusztaszeri MP, García JJ, Faquin WC. Salivary gland FNA: New markers and new opportunities for improved diagnosis. Cancer Cytopathol 2016; 124:307–16.

29. Pusztaszeri MP, Faquin WC. Update in salivary gland cytopathology: Recent molecular advances and diagnostic applications. Semin Diagn Pathol 2015;32:264–74.

30. Pusztaszeri M, Shadow P, Ushiku A, et al. MYB immunostaining is a useful ancillary test for distinguishing adenoid cystic carcinoma from pleomorphic adenoma in fine-needle aspiration biopsy specimens. Cancer Cytopathol 2014;122:257–65.

31. Foo WC, Jo VY, Krane JF. Usefulness of translocation-associated immunohistochemical stains in the fine-needle aspiration diagnosis of salivary gland neoplasms. Cancer Cytopathol 2016;124:397–405.

32. Griffith CC, Siddiqui MT, Schmitt AC. Ancillary testing strategies in salivary gland aspiration cytology: a practical pattern-based approach. Diagn Cytopathol 2017;45:808–19.

33. Rossi ED, Wong LQ, Bizzarro T, et al. The impact of FNAC in the management of salivary gland lesions: Institutional experiences leading to a risk-based

classification scheme. Cancer Cytopathol 2016; 124:388–96.

34. Baloch ZW, Faquin WC, Layfield LJ. Is it time to develop a tiered classification scheme for salivary gland fine-needle aspiration specimens? Diagn Cytopathol 2017;45:285–6.

35. Bajwa MS, Rose SJ, Mairembam P, et al. Feasibility of a novel classification for parotid gland cytology: A retrospective review of 512 cytology reports taken from 4 United Kingdom general hospitals. Head Neck 2016;38:1596–603.

36. Wei S, Layfield LJ, LiVolsi VA, et al. Reporting of fine needle aspiration specimens of salivary gland lesions: A comprehensive review. Diagn Cytopathol 2017;45:820–7.

37. Rossi ED Faquin WC, Baloch Z, Baloch Z, et al. The milan system for reporting salivary gland cytopathology: analysis and suggestions of initial survey. Cancer 2017;125:757–66.

38. Murai N, Taniguchi Z, Takahashi Y, et al. A study of salivary gland aspiration cytology reporting: guideline validity. Nihon Jibiinkoka Gakkai Kaiho 2011; 114:615–9.

39. Nayar R, Wilbur DC. The Pap test and Bethesda 2014. Cancer Cytopathol 2015;123:271e281.

40. Bajwa MS, Mitchell DA, Brennan PA. Is it time we adopted a classification for parotid gland cytology? Br J Oral Maxillofac Surg 2014;52:99–101.

41. Baloch ZW, LiVolsi VA, Asa SL, et al. Diagnostic terminology and morphologic criteria for cytologic diagnosis of thyroid lesions: a synopsis of the National Cancer Institute Thyroid Fine-Needle Aspiration State of the Science Conference. Diagn Cytopathol 2008;36:425–37.

42. Pitman MB, Centeno BA, Ali SZ, Papanicolaou Society of Cytopathology, Stelow E, Mino-Kenudson M, Castillo CFD, Schmidt CM, Brugge WR, Layfield LJ. Standardized terminology and nomenclature for pancreatobiliary cytology: the Papanicolaou Society of Cytopathology guidelines. Diagn Cytopathol 2014;42:338–50.

43. Layfield LJ, Baloch Z, Elsheikh T, et al. Standardized terminology and nomenclature for respiratory cytology: the Papanicolaou Society of Cytopathology guidelines. Diagn Cytopathol 2016;44:399–409.

44. Rosenthal DL, Wojcik EM, Kurtycz. The paris system for reporting urinary cytology. Cham: Springer; 2016.

45. Maleki Z, Miller JA, Arab SE, et al. "Suspicious" salivary gland FNA: risk of malignancy and interinstitutional variability. Cancer 2018;126:94–100.

46. Viswanathan K, Sung S, Scognamiglio T, et al. The role of the milan system for reporting salivary gland cytopathology: a 5-year institutional experience. Cancer Cytopathol 2018 May 24. https://doi.org/10.1002/cncy.22016, [Epub ahead of print].

47. Layfield LJ, Baloch ZW, Hirschowitz SL, et al. Impact on clinical follow-up of the Milan System for salivary

gland cytology: A comparison with a traditional diagnostic classification. Cytopathology 2018 May 3. https://doi.org/10.1111/cyt.12562, [Epub ahead of print].

48. Wang H, Malik A, Maleki Z, et al. "Atypical" salivary gland fine needle aspiration: Risk of malignancy and interinstitutional variability. Diagn Cytopathol 2017;45:1088–94.

49. Rohilla M, Singh P, Rajwanshi A, et al. Three-year cytohistological correlation of salivary gland FNA cytology at a tertiary center with the application of the Milan system for risk stratification. Cancer Cytopathol 2017;125:767e775.

50. Thiryayi SA, Low YX, Shelton D, et al. A retrospective 3-year study of salivary gland FNAC with categorisation using the Milan reporting system. Cytopathology 2018 Apr 23. https://doi.org/10.1111/cyt.12557, [Epub ahead of print].

51. Liu H, Ljungren C, Lin F, et al. Analysis of histologic follow-up and risk of malignancy for salivary gland neoplasm of uncertain malignant potential proposed by the milan system for reporting salivary gland cytopathology. Cancer Cytopathol 2018 Apr;18. https://doi.org/10.1002/cncy.22002, [Epub ahead of print].

52. Faquin WC, Rossi ED, editors. The Milan system for reporting salivary gland cytopathology. Cham: Springer; 2018.

53. Kimberly P, Griffith C. The role of ancillary techniques in salivary gland cytopathology specimens. Acta Cytol 2020;64(1–2):92–102.

54. Jo V, Krane JF. Ancillary testing in salivary gland cytology: a practical guide cancer. Cytopathol 2018 Aug;126(Suppl 8):627–42.

55. Xu B, Katabi N. Myoepithelial carcinoma. Surg Pathol Clin 2021 Mar;14(1):67–73.

56. Hashimoto K, Yamamoto H, Shiratsuchi H, et al. HER-2/neu gene amplification in carcinoma ex pleomorphic adenoma in relation to progression and prognosis: a chromogenic in-situ hybridization study. Histopathology (Oxf) 2012 May;60(6B): E131–42.

57. Ihrler S, Weiler C, Hirschmann A, et al. Intraductal carcinoma is the precursor of carcinoma ex pleomorphic adenoma and is often associated with dysfunctional p53. Histopathology (Oxf) 2007 Sep; 51(3):362–71.

58. Kuzenko YV, Romanuk AM, Dyachenko OO, et al. Pathogenesis of warthin's tumors. Interv Med Appl Sci 2016 Jun 1;8(2):41–8.

59. Robinson RA. Basal cell adenoma and basal cell adenocarcinoma. Surg Pathol Clin 2021 Mar;14(1): 25–42. Epub 2021 Jan 5.

60. Jo VY, Sholl LM, Krane JF. Distinctive patterns of CTNNB1 (β-Catenin) alterations in salivary gland basal cell adenoma and basal cell adenocarcinoma. Am J Surg Pathol 2016 Aug;40(8):1143–50.

61. Sun T, Akalin A, Dresser K, et al. The utility of MYB immunohistochemistry (IHC) in fine needle aspiration (FNA) diagnosis of adenoid cystic carcinoma (AdCC). Head Neck Pathol 2021 Jun;15(2):389–94.

62. Sajed DP, Faquin WC, Carey C, et al. Diffuse staining for activated NOTCH1 correlates with NOTCH1 mutation status and is associated with worse outcome in adenoid cystic carcinoma. Am J Surg Pathol 2017 Nov;41(11):1473–82.

63. Lewis AG, Tong T, Maghami E. Diagnosis and management of malignant salivary gland tumors of the parotid gland. Otolaryngol Clin North Am 2016 Apr;49(2):343–80.

64. Vnaderlaan P, Roy-Chowdhuri S, Griffith CC, et al. Molecular testing of cytology specimens: overview of assay selection with focus on lung, salivary gland, and thyroid testing. Journal of the American Society of Cytopathol 2022;11:403–14.

Head and Neck Fine Needle Aspiration
Current and Future Impact on Patient Care

Varsha Manucha, MD

KEYWORDS

- Precision cytopathology • Head and neck squamous cell carcinoma • Biomarkers • HPV • PDL-1

Key points

- Fine needle aspiration of the neck often provides the only material available to test for biomarkers in recurrent and metastatic head and neck carcinoma.
- The 2 most important biomarkers in head and neck squamous cell carcinoma are human papillomavirus and programmed death ligand 1, both successfully performed on cytology specimens.
- Combined approach of morphologic evaluation and machine learning algorithms has the potential to allow point-of-care testing on cytology specimens in head and neck carcinomas.
- Cytology specimens are superior to tissue biopsies for molecular testing, assessment of tumoral heterogeneity, and tumor mutational burden.

ABSTRACT

The discovery of multiple novel biomarkers in head and neck tumors has led to an increasing interest in utilizing head and neck cytology material as the primary specimens for testing diagnostic and prognostic biomarkers. Although human papillomavirus and programmed death ligand 1 are the most well-established biomarkers tested in cytology specimens, their utilization in cytology is limited by the absence of standardized protocols for specimen collection and fixation. This has led to a quest for innovative techniques to explore the genomic landscape in head and neck tumors and its application in cytology.

OVERVIEW

Recent advances in molecular genetics have resulted in the identification of numerous predictive and prognostic molecular biomarkers, thereby increasing the understanding of patient outcomes and treatment options for advanced-stage cancers.[1] Given the success of cytology specimens for biomarker analysis in the lung and thyroid, there is an increased interest in exploring the role of cytology in determining prognostic and predictive markers in tumors arising in other sites. The presence of metastasis in the neck indicates an advanced stage of the tumor, suggesting a role for targeted therapy options. Since the neck is an easily accessible site, fine needle aspiration (FNA) is a simple and inexpensive diagnostic test, often yielding the only material available for morphologic diagnosis and biomarker analysis.[2] The specificity and positive predictive value of FNA in the diagnosis of a lateral neck mass (nonthyroid and nonsalivary gland) have been shown to be up to 100% with 3.4% false-negative and 0.9% false-positive rates.[3,4] Metastatic squamous cell carcinoma is the predominant diagnosis in head and neck cytology, aside from the thyroid and salivary glands.

Department of Pathology, Univeristy of Mississippi Medical Center, 2500 North State Street, Jackson, MS 39216, USA

E-mail address: vmanucha@umc.edu

Surgical Pathology 17 (2024) 359–369

https://doi.org/10.1016/j.path.2024.04.004

This review will focus on the potential use of cytopathology specimens for the evaluation of biomarkers assays including immunohistochemistry, in situ hybridization, and molecular genetic tests in the diagnosis and management of metastatic squamous cell carcinoma of head and neck origin.

DISCUSSION

HUMAN PAPILLOMAVIRUS

The diagnosis of metastatic squamous cell carcinoma on FNA of a neck mass, an otherwise straightforward diagnosis, is complicated by the presence of often cystic necrosis, the presence of poorly differentiated (basaloid) morphology, and the absence of a known primary site, all 3 features commonly seen in tumors originating from the oropharynx. At least 64% of oropharyngeal primary squamous cell carcinomas are reported to be human papillomavirus (HPV)-associated, of which 90% are HPV16 DNA variants.[5] Given the strikingly better prognosis with improved responsiveness to chemotherapy as well as chemoradiotherapy and favorable survival rates, HPV is the most researched and well-established diagnostic and prognostic marker in head and neck squamous cell carcinoma (HNSCC). The detection of HPV using immunohistochemistry (IHC) and in situ hybridization (ISH) in cytologic samples obtained from FNA of metastatic lymph nodes has proven to be an accurate and cost-effective method for diagnosing HPV-related HNSCC, as compared to a biopsy of the oropharynx.[5] p16 IHC, a surrogate marker for HPV in oropharyngeal squamous cell carcinoma, has been shown to yield reliable results when performed on formalin-fixed paraffin-embedded sections of cell blocks (CBs) and demonstrates a strong correlation with tissue p16 staining (**Fig. 1**). However, unpredictable cellularity and variable fixation and processing steps limit the utility of CB as a testing specimen, which has led to the exploration of other testing options. Staining for p16 IHC on alcohol-fixed smears and ThinPrep are potential alternatives; however, despite the concordance rate of 90% or more with tissue p16 positivity, there is a risk of false-positive and false-negative results.[6] HPV DNA and RNA ISH have been successfully used in cytology CBs (see **Fig. 1**); however, similar to p16 IHC, the sensitivity, and specificity can vary depending on the use of different probes, types of amplification, and detection systems.[6] Molecular tests on cytology rinse material hold promise as a means to potentially eliminate the need for HPV testing in a CB. Tests such as polymerase chain reaction (PCR) amplification, Digene hybrid capture assay, Cobas HPV

tests, Cervista HPV test, and Aptima HPV assay in cytology specimens have shown high concordance with HPV status (p16 IHC/HPV DNA or RNA ISH) in corresponding tissue specimens. Furthermore, HPV genotyping using a combination of PCR amplification and line probe assay for concurrent detection and genotyping of HPV (Roche linear array and Innogenetics, Ghent, Belgium [INNO-LiPA] HPV) on FNA material have shown very high sensitivity (96%) and specificity (100%) and a high agreement ($\kappa = 0.796$) compared to HPV status of the paraffin-embedded histologic material.[7] Regardless of the specific test a laboratory chooses for HPV status testing, it is recommended by the College of American Pathologists that the laboratory validate the chosen test method before routine use.

Recent research has shown that HPV circulating tumor DNA (ctDNA) can be detected in most patients with HPV-mediated HNSCC, with a sensitivity of 89% to 95% and specificity of 95% to 100%.[8] This superior diagnostic performance in comparison to standard tissue sampling offers potential in prognostics, treatment prediction, minimal residual disease detection, and recurrence identification. While HPV ctDNA analysis is poised to revolutionize clinical practices for patients with HPV-mediated HNSCC, the role of p16 IHC/RNA ISH remains important as it represents a good compromise, between acceptable diagnostic accuracy and easy applicability for everyday clinical practice.[9]

IMMUNOHISTOCHEMISTRY IN DIAGNOSIS OF POORLY DIFFERENTIATED HEAD AND NECK CARCINOMA

In recent years, several molecular and immunohistochemical advancements have facilitated the accurate identification of a poorly differentiated carcinoma of head and neck origin. The diagnosis of HPV-associated squamous cell carcinoma and EBV-associated nasopharyngeal carcinomas can be accomplished through the HPV RNA ISH and Epstein-Barr virus–encoded small RNA on the Cell block (**Fig. 2**).[10] Utilization of IHC, including the use of insulinoma-associated protein 1 as a single stain or in combination with synaptophysin and chromogranin A, significantly aids in confirming the diagnosis of neuroendocrine carcinoma.[11,12] An additional IHC stain for KRT20 is significant when it reveals a dot-like perinuclear pattern in a neuroendocrine carcinoma, as this establishes a diagnosis of Merkel cell carcinoma. Merkel cell carcinoma is a highly aggressive primary cutaneous neuroendocrine carcinoma that may be encountered in FNA specimens from the

Fig. 1. Non-keratinizing squamous cell carcinoma in an FNA of a 3.5 cm neck mass without a known primary. (*A*) Diff-Quik, 200×. (*B*) P16 IHC, CB (plasma thrombin method), 200×.

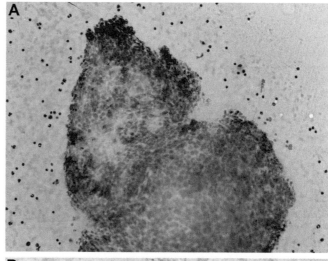

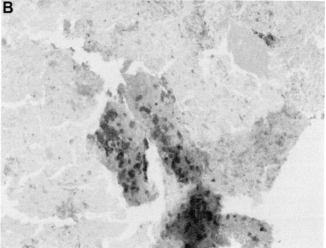

head and neck of elderly patients.[13] Notably, checkpoint inhibitor therapy has been shown to be highly effective and is rapidly emerging as first-line therapy in Merkel cell carcinoma.[14]

Other high-grade non keratinizing squamous cell carcinoma (NKSCC) with primitive tumor cells and conspicuous nucleoli should raise suspicion of nuclear protein in testis (NUT) carcinoma, while the presence of rhabdoid cells should raise a possibility of switch/sucrose nonfermenting complex (SWI/SNF)-related matrix-associated actin-dependent regulator of chromatin subfamily B member 1 (SMARCB1)–deficient sinonasal carcinoma. Both tumors can be diagnosed with ease in CB using NUT-1 (NUT family member 1 protein) and SMARCB1 immunostains.[15,16] Early and accurate diagnosis of these tumors is essential for prognostication, the initiation of appropriate management protocols, and the possible inclusion of patients in clinical trials evaluating novel treatment modalities. Enhancer of zeste homolog 2 (EZH2) inhibitors, for instance, have emerged as potential targeted therapy against SWI/SNF-deficient tumors.[15,16]

PROGRAMMED DEATH LIGAND 1

Cancer immunotherapy using programmed death ligand 1 (PD-1/PD-L1) immune checkpoint blockade represents the standard of care in metastatic and locally advanced non-small cell lung cancer and melanoma. The rate of tumor response to anti-PD-1 and/or anti-PD-L1 antibodies is predicted by evaluating the expression of PDL-1 on neoplastic cells and is now the most commonly used predictive biomarker.[17]

Recently, pembrolizumab plus platinum and 5-fluorouracil was approved as an appropriate first-line treatment of recurrent or metastatic HNSCC,

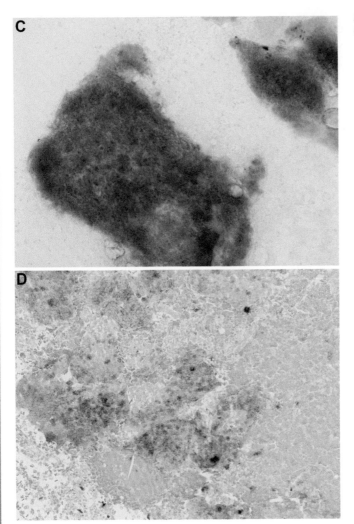

Fig. 1. (*C*) P16 IHC, direct smear, 200×. (*D*) ISH mRNA for high-risk HPV, CB.

and pembrolizumab monotherapy is an appropriate first-line treatment of PD-L1-positive recurrent or metastatic HNSCC.[18] The identification of HNSCC patients eligible for anti-PD-1 immunotherapy is performed through the evaluation of PD-L1 expression and assessment of combined positive score (CPS ≥1) by IHC, which has been validated on formalin-fixed paraffin-embedded tissue sections. A multicenter study demonstrated good interobserver reliability and a strong and significant correlation between the 2 most commonly used assays, 22C3 pharmDx assay (Agilent Technologies/Dako, Carpinteria, CA, USA) and the Ventana SP263 Assay (Ventana Medical Systems Inc, Tucson, Arizona), for evaluating PDL-1 expression in HNSCC.[19] In routine clinical practice, most advanced-stage and metastatic patients have only cytology samples from neck FNA available, for diagnosis, staging, and biomarker analysis. The recent discovery of intrinsic heterogeneity in

PD-L1 expression in tumors procured at different times of natural history and a higher degree of positivity for PDL-1 in metastatic lymph nodes makes the neck FNA even more relevant (**Table 1**).[20] The International Association for the Study of Lung Cancer pathology Committee states that all "cytologic preparations including cell blocks, ethanol fixed, and air-dried slides" can be used for immunocytochemistry.[21] Lozano and colleagues[22] demonstrated excellent concordance (97.3%) between paired Papanicolaou-stained cytology smears and formalin-fixed paraffin-embedded samples in non-small cell lung cancer using 22C3 pharmDx assay and the Ventana SP263 assay. However, assessing PDL-1 IHC represents a diagnostic challenge due to variations in the use of antibodies, platforms, scoring systems, cutoffs by tumor type, and interobserver variability in the interpretation of the results.[23,24] The challenge is further complicated in cytology specimens due to the diverse collection

Fig. 2. Nonkeratinizing squamous cell carcinoma in an FNA of a 4.8 cm neck mass with a nasal/nasopharyngeal mass. (*A*) Papanicolaou 200×. (*B*) p40 IHC, CB (plasma thrombin method), 200×.

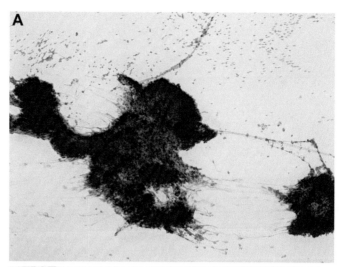

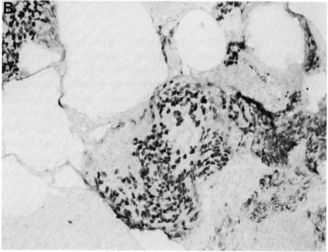

methods, CB preparation methods, and unpredictable sample cellularity. Furthermore, the interpretation of the CPS (includes both tumor cells and tumor-associated immune cells) is challenging in cytology specimens because of the inherent difficulty of differentiating tumor-associated lymphocytes from the lymphoid cells native to the aspirated lymph node in FNA specimens and or inflammatory cells that may be present because of peripheral blood contamination. Liu and colleagues[25] evaluated PDL1 (22C3 clone) expression with the CPS and TPS scores (percentage positive tumor cells relative to all viable tumor cells) in FNA CBs of metastatic HNSCC and found a substantial concordance (76.2%; κ = 0.607) and a 100% positive predictive value with paired histologic specimens but a lower negative predictive value (57.1% for CPS and 50% for TPS assessment). The increased false-negative results are most likely because of limited cellularity and intratumoral heterogeneity secondary to sampling error in a limited volume FNA specimen.[25] Therefore, a negative PDL-1 expression in a cytology specimen should be followed by a re-evaluation in a larger tissue specimen when feasible. Additionally, in FNA specimens where CPS scoring is difficult due to difficulty in differentiating between tumor-associated immune cells and inflammatory cells, concurrent evaluation of TPS score may prove beneficial.[25]

COMPUTATIONAL TECHNOLOGY WITH ARTIFICIAL INTELLIGENCE AND MACHINE LEARNING

The application of computational cytology and artificial intelligence beyond cervical Pap cytology has been limited in nongynecologic cytology practice because of the variation in the sample preparation

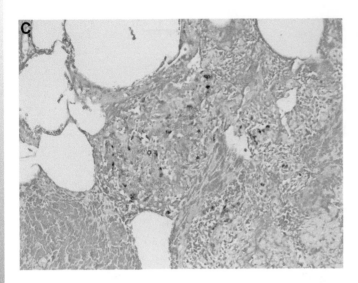

Fig. 2. (*C*) ISH Epstein–Barr encoding region (EBER), CB.

techniques, use of multiple stains, complex visual data in cytology preparations requiring z-stacking leading to increased image acquisition time and large file sizes, and labor-intensive task of annotating/labeling cytology images.[26] In head and neck cytopathology, a combined approach of morphologic evaluation with the application of a machine learning algorithm has yielded the greatest overall performance when applied to indeterminate cases in thyroid cytology, but its effectiveness in indeterminate cases in salivary gland cytology remains to be established.[27,28] Beyond the thyroid and salivary gland, the most exciting potential applications of computational cytology are in the diagnosis and management of cystic metastasis in HNSCC as a tool for point-of-care testing.[29] Demonstration of aneuploid DNA content using image cytometry DNA analysis in indeterminate cytology specimens correlates strongly with lymph node metastasis, however routine use is limited by

Table 1
Advantages, opportunities, and challenges of using neck fine needle aspiration for biomarker testing

Advantages	Opportunities	Challenges
• FNA is often the sole sample of surgically unresectable, high-grade, locally advanced, recurrent, or metastatic head and neck cancer • FNA has the ability to widely sample a tumor compared with a core needle biopsy allowing better assessment of intratumoral heterogeneity • Potential to use almost the whole spectrum of cytology specimens—smears, CBs, liquid-based preparation, supernatant, and fresh viable tumor cells • High-quality DNA and RNA	• To determine eligibility for specific targeted therapy, monitor tumor response, and assess tumor microenvironment using a safe and fast technique, even for otherwise sites inaccessible and unsafe for tissue sampling	• Inconsistent distribution of cellular material in cytology preparations (may require more than specimen type to be used to ensure tumor cell adequacy) • Unless formalin-fixed paraffin-embedded sections of CB are used, requires additional validation • Significant capital and time investment • Complex and variable preanalytical methods (variations in specimen collection, fixation, and processing) • Requirement of quality control protocols/audits for send-outs of commercial assay/other molecular test results

the demonstrated 45% intratumoral ploidy heterogeneity. [30–32] More recently, machine learning algorithms using morphologic (cellular/nuclear features), intensity-based cell metrics, and expression of molecular biomarkers have been developed to determine the probability of malignancy in the assessment of potentially malignant oral lesions. The cytology-on-a-chip approach uses minimally invasive oral brush cytology specimens and holds promise as a point-of-care diagnostics. [33,34] Other potential areas where artificial intelligence and neural network models can be utilized in cytology include quantitative assessment of cellularity in digitized CB, which has been shown to be more reliable using software than visual estimation by cytopathologists. Further clinical studies are warranted to assess its performance on FNA cytology specimens and validate its integration with existing technologies for clinical adaption and regulatory approval. [35]

TUMOR MUTATIONAL BURDEN

Tumor mutational burden (TMB)—the number of somatic mutations per DNA megabase—has emerged as an independent predictor of immune checkpoint inhibitor treatment outcomes across multiple tumor types including HNSCC. [36,37] In addition, the significantly higher TMB and the presence of distinct ultraviolet damage-associated catalogue of somatic mutations in cancer single base substitutions (COSMIC SBS) mutation signature in head and neck cutaneous squamous cell carcinoma at the metastatic site can assist in identifying the primary site and guide treatment decisions, despite the histologic and immunohistochemical similarities between head and neck cutaneous squamous cell carcinoma and oral squamous cell carcinoma, at the metastatic site. [38] With regards to TMB analysis in cytologic specimens, studies have shown that CBs provide similar results to histologic-matched specimens, while smears have been shown to be potentially superior to formalin-fixed paraffin-embedded samples due to their high-quality DNA and lack of formalin-fixation-induced artifacts, making them a promising alternative for TMB analysis. [39,40]

MULTIPLEX IMMUNOHISTOCHEMISTRY/ IMMUNOFLUORESCENCE

One of the challenges in utilizing cytology specimens for biomarker assay is the limited quantity of material available, which limits the number of tests that can be performed. However, the growing value of cytology specimens for the evaluation of biomarkers has led to a focus on doing more with

less. Multiplex IHC is a low-cost adjunct to diagnosis in cytology, which coupled with image analysis can aid in a definitive diagnosis and save tissue for biomarker analysis. [41]

Multiplex immunohistochemistry/immunofluorescence (M-IHC/IF) allows in situ visualization of multiple markers and has shown great promise in assessing biomarkers in situ, in single cells. When used as an adjunct to conventional cytomorphology, it can increase the specificity and sensitivity of tumor detection. [42] Quantitative fluorescence image analysis has been used for the detection of tumors as well as for monitoring recurrence, and therapeutic response and assessment of individual risk in exfoliated bladder tumor cells and more recently in pleural effusion specimens. [43,44]

Fast analytical screening technique FNA represents an example of single cell-based multiplex analysis technology that has been applied to HNSCC. In this technique, FNA samples undergo a cyclic process of fixation and staining with fluorescent-labeled antibodies. Deep learning algorithms or semi-manual image analysis routines are then used to quantify marker expression in each cell and generate unique FNA-specific biomarker scores. FAST PD-L1 score of FNA specimens is quicker (<2 hours from cell harvesting to report), serially deployable, and ultimately proves to be more cost-effective by eliminating the need for sedation or surgical intervention. [45]

NEXT-GENERATION SEQUENCING

In head and neck cancer, the mutation profile between HPV-negative and HPV-positive HNSCC is significantly different. The majority of HPV-negative HNSCC harbor tumor protein 53 gene (TP53), cyclin - dependent kinase inhibitor 2A (CDKN2A), phosphatase and tensin homolog (PTEN), phosphatidylinositol-4,5-biphosphate 3-kinase catalytic subunit alpha (PIK3CA), and the telomerase reverse transcriptase (TERT) promoter mutations in addition to mutations related to squamous differentiation (eg, neurogenic locus notch homolog protein 1 [NOTCH1], interferon regulatory factor 6 [IRF6], and tumor protein 63 [TP63]). On the other hand, in HPV-positive HNSCC, unique mutations in genes like DEAD-Box helicase 3 X - linked (DDX3X), fibroblast growth factor recptor 2/3 (FGFR2/3), and aberrations in phophatidylnositol-4,5-bisphosphate 3-kinase catalytic subunit alpha (PIK3CA), kristen rat sarcoma virus (KRAS), mixed lineage leukemis 2/3 protein (MLL2/3), and NOTCH1 have been observed. Additionally, mutations in genes such as NOTCH1, CDKN2A, and TP53 were identified as prognostic indicators for poor survival. [46]

Table 2
Biomarkers in head and neck squamous cell carcinoma

Bio Markers	Site	Cytology Specimen	Testing
Established			
HPV (diagnostic and prognostic marker)	Oropharynx	• FNA of neck mass • Smears, cell-block	P16 IHC ISH—HR HPV PCR HPV DNA
EBV genomic DNA and EBV RNA from the EBER (diagnostic marker)	Nasopharynx	• FNA of neck mass • Cell-block	EBV RNA ISH
PDL-1 (prognostic and predictive marker)	Recurrent advanced stage HNSCC (mucosal)	FNA of neck mass • CB, smears	PDL1 22C3 IHC
In development			

NOTCH1 (prognostic markers	HPV-positive squamous cell carcinoma	• FNA of neck mass
		• Monolayer liquid-based smears, direct smears, and residual CytoLyt
		  CBs
		    (recommended and more commonly validated)
			Next-generation sequencing

CDKN2A, TP53 (prognostic markers	HPV-negative squamous cell carcinoma	• FNA of neck mass
		• Monolayer liquid-based smears, direct smears, and residual CytoLyt
		  CBs
		    (recommended and more commonly validated)
			Next-generation sequencing

Tumor mutational burden (predictive marker)	Head and neck cutaneous squamous cell carcinoma	• FNA of neck mass • CBs, smears	Next-generation sequencing
Tumor microenvironment (predictive and prognostic marker	HNSCC	• Formalin-fixed paraffin-embedded sections of the CB	M-IHC/IF

Ideally, all advanced and metastatic carcinoma should undergo routine genomic testing. FNA typically contains a higher tumor fraction, ensures a wider sampling of the targeted lesion, and offers better-quality DNA and RNA. The inclusion of rapid onsite evaluation ensures effective triage and procurement of adequate tissue for subsequent analysis. CBs, smears, liquid-based cytology, cell-free supernatant, and fresh cells can all be utilized for next-generation sequencing.[47] Although newer generation throughput PCR assay allows for exponential amplification of even very small quantities of template DNA, the success of molecular analysis still depends upon the presence of an adequate number of viable tumor cells in the specimen.[48] FNA specimens carry a risk of hemodilution that may result in a lower amount of input material, thereby resulting in diminished sensitivity of the analytical assay. Other potential issues in using small input quantities are the inadvertent introduction of "mutation" through PCR artifact and formalin-induced artifact that can lead to sequence alterations.[48] The tumor cells can, however, be enriched in the cytology specimen by performing microdissection of tumor cells on smears, CB sections, and monolayer slides including cytospins.[49]

The most important limitation (after the cost) of the widespread implementation of cytology specimens for broad ancillary molecular genetic testing is the lack of standardized preanalytical protocols in the collection, fixation, and processing of cytology specimens (**Table 2**).

SUMMARY

Intratumoral heterogeneity between primary and metastatic and/or recurrent tumors and between different metastatic sites is the main cause of targeted and nontargeted therapy resistance. It is, therefore, imperative that biomarker testing is performed on recurrent tumors and even at different metastatic sites. In comparison to tissue biopsies, cytology specimen is preferred to assess tumor microenvironment for 3 main reasons. (1) Cytology is the first-line diagnostic test for neck FNA because of its minimally invasive nature and high diagnostic accuracy; (2) The wider area of lesion sampling; and (3) Easier laser capture microdissection and a higher likelihood of capturing entire rather than partial nuclei.[1,50]

The cytologists and cytopathologists will continue to play an important role in conducting the initial morphology-based examination, determining the indicated/necessary biomarkers or ancillary studies, and finally integrating all the diagnostic information to guide appropriate patient management.

DISCLOSURE

The author has no commercial or financial conflicts of interest and any funding sources.

REFERENCES

1. Sanchez A, Bocklage T. Precision cytopathology: expanding opportunities for biomarker testing in cytopathology. J Am Soc Cytopathol 2019;8(2):95–115.
2. Göret CC, Göret NE, Özdemir ZT, et al. Diagnostic value of fine needle aspiration biopsy in nonthyroidal head and neck lesions: a retrospective study of 866 aspiration materials. Int J Clin Exp Pathol 2015;8(8):8709–16.
3. Ashraf MJ, Raad H, Azarpira N, et al. Fine-needle aspiration cytological diagnosis of neck masses. Acta Cytol 2015;59(1):68–76.
4. Steel BL, Schwartz MR, Ramzy I. Fine needle aspiration biopsy in the diagnosis of lymphadenopathy in 1,103 patients. Role, limitations and analysis of diagnostic pitfalls. Acta Cytol 1995;39(1):76–81.
5. Larsen MHH, Channir HI, von Buchwald C. Human papillomavirus and squamous cell carcinoma of unknown primary in the head and neck region: a comprehensive review on clinical implications. Viruses 2021;13(7):1297.
6. Manucha V, Adeniran AJ, Asiry S, et al. American society of cytopathology clinical practice committee. High-risk human papillomavirus testing in cytology aspiration samples from the head and neck part 1: a review of the literature on available testing options. J Am Soc Cytopathol 2022;11(5):295–305.
7. Jalaly JB, Hosseini SM, Shafique K, et al. Current Status of p16 Immunohistochemistry and HPV Testing in Fine Needle Aspiration Specimens of the Head and Neck. Acta Cytol 2020;64(1–2):30–9.
8. Haring CT, Rocco JW. Emerging role of blood-based biomarker testing in HPV-mediated head and neck squamous cell carcinoma. Cancer Cytopathol 2023;132(1):7–9.
9. Kühn JP, Schmid W, Körner S, et al. HPV Status as prognostic biomarker in head and neck cancer-which method fits the best for outcome prediction? Cancers (Basel) 2021 Sep 21;13(18):4730.
10. Garady C, Saieg MA, Ko HM, et al. Epstein-Barr virus encoded RNA detected by in situ hybridization using cytological preparations. Cytopathology 2014;25(2):101–7.
11. Xu B, Chetty R, Perez-Ordoñez B. Neuroendocrine neoplasms of the head and neck: some suggestions for the new WHO classification of head and neck tumors. Head Neck Pathol 2014;8(1):24–32.
12. Maleki Z, Nadella A, Nadella M, et al. INSM1, a Novel biomarker for detection of neuroendocrine neoplasms: Cytopathologists' View. Diagnostics (Basel) 2021;11(12):2172.
13. Shield PW, Crous H. Fine-needle aspiration cytology of Merkel cell carcinoma-a review of 69 cases. Diagn Cytopathol 2014;42(11):924–8.
14. Bellizzi AM. Immunohistochemistry in the diagnosis and classification of neuroendocrine neoplasms: what can brown do for you? Hum Pathol 2020;96:8–833.
15. Dutta R, Nambirajan A, Mittal S, et al. Cytomorphology of primary pulmonary NUT carcinoma in different cytology preparations. Cancer Cytopathol 2021;129(1):53–61.
16. Kezlarian BE, Lin O, Dogan S. SMARCB1-deficient carcinomas of the head and neck region: a cytopathologic characterization. J Am Soc Cytopathol 2020;9(6):494–501.
17. Lecis D, Sangaletti S, Colombo MP, et al. Immune checkpoint ligand reverse signaling: looking back to go forward in cancer therapy. Cancers (Basel) 2019 May 4;11(5):624.
18. Burtness B, Harrington KJ, Greil R, et al. Pembrolizumab alone or with chemotherapy versus cetuximab with chemotherapy for recurrent or metastatic squamous cell carcinoma of the head and neck

(KEYNOTE-048): a randomised, open-label, phase 3 study. Lancet 2019;394(10212):1915–28.

19. Cerbelli B, Girolami I, Eccher A, et al. Evaluating programmed death-ligand 1 (PD-L1) in head and neck squamous cell carcinoma: concordance between the 22C3 PharmDx assay and the SP263 assay on whole sections from a multicentre study. Histopathology 2022;80(2):397–406.

20. Paolino G, Pantanowitz L, Barresi V, et al. PD-L1 evaluation in head and neck squamous cell carcinoma: Insights regarding specimens, heterogeneity and therapy. Pathol Res Pract 2021;226:153605.

21. Tejerina E, Garca Tobar L, Echeveste JI, et al. PD-L1 in Cytological samples: a review and a practical approach. Front Med (Lausanne) 2021;7(8):668612.

22. Lozano MD, Abengozar-Muela M, Echeveste JI, et al. Programmed death-ligand 1 expression on direct Pap-stained cytology smears from non-small cell lung cancer: comparison with cell blocks and surgical resection specimens. Cancer Cytopathol 2019;127(7):470–80.

23. Crosta S, Boldorini R, Bono F, et al. PD-L1 Testing and squamous cell carcinoma of the head and neck: a multicenter study on the diagnostic reproducibility of different protocols. Cancers (Basel) 2021;13(2):292.

24. Girolami I, Pantanowitz L, Barberis M, et al. Challenges facing pathologists evaluating PD-L1 in head & neck squamous cell carcinoma. J Oral Pathol Med 2021;50(9):864–73.

25. Liu Z, Williams M, Stewart J, et al. Evaluation of programmed death ligand 1 expression in cytology to determine eligibility for immune checkpoint inhibitor therapy in patients with head and neck squamous cell carcinoma. Cancer Cytopathol 2022;130(2):110–9.

26. McAlpine ED, Pantanowitz L, Michelow PM. Challenges developing deep learning algorithms in cytology. Acta Cytol 2021;65(4):301–9.

27. Elliott Range DD, Dov D, Kovalsky SZ, et al. Application of a machine learning algorithm to predict malignancy in thyroid cytopathology. Cancer Cytopathol 2020;128(4):287–95.

28. Obad-Kovačević D, Kardum-Skelin I, Jelić-Puškarić B, et al. Parotid gland tumors: correlation between routine cytology and cytomorphometry by digital image analysis using conventional and newly introduced cytomorphometric parameters. Diagn Cytopathol 2013;41(9):776–84.

29. Lollie TK, Krane JF. Applications of computational pathology in head and neck cytopathology. Acta Cytol 2021;65(4):330–4.

30. Nordemar S, Tani E, Högmo A, et al. Image cytometry DNA-analysis of fine needle aspiration cytology to aid cytomorphology in the distinction of branchial cleft cyst from cystic metastasis of squamous cell carcinoma: a prospective study. Laryngoscope 2004;114(11):1997–2000.

31. Oya R, Ikemura K. Can flow cytometrically determined DNA ploidy and S-phase fraction predict regional metastasis in squamous cell carcinoma of the oral cavity? Head Neck 2002;24(2):136–42.

32. Hass HG, Schmidt A, Nehls O, et al. DNA ploidy, proliferative capacity and intratumoral heterogeneity in primary and recurrent head and neck squamous cell carcinomas (HNSCC)–potential implications for clinical management and treatment decisions. Oral Oncol 2008;44(1):78–85.

33. McRae MP, Modak SS, Simmons GW, et al. Point-of-care oral cytology tool for the screening and assessment of potentially malignant oral lesions. Cancer Cytopathol 2020;128(3):207–20.

34. Abram TJ, Floriano PN, Christodoulides N, et al. Cytology-on-a-chip' based sensors for monitoring of potentially malignant oral lesions. Oral Oncol 2016;60:103–11.

35. McRae MP, Simmons G, McDevitt JT. Challenges and opportunities for translating medical microdevices: insights from the programmable bio-nano-chip. Bioanalysis 2016;8(9):905–19.

36. Aggarwal C, Ben-Shachar R, Gao Y, et al. Assessment of tumor mutational burden and outcomes in patients with diverse advanced cancers treated with immunotherapy. JAMA Netw Open 2023;6(5):e2311181.

37. Klempner SJ, Fabrizio D, Bane S, et al. Tumor mutational burden as a predictive biomarker for response to immune checkpoint inhibitors: a review of current evidence. Oncologist 2020 Jan;25(1):e147–59.

38. Gupta R, Strbenac D, Satgunaseelan L, et al. Comparing genomic landscapes of oral and cutaneous squamous cell carcinoma of the head and neck: quest for novel diagnostic markers. Mod Pathol 2023;36(8):100190.

39. Pepe F, Pisapia P, Gristina V, et al. Tumor mutational burden on cytological samples: A pilot study. Cancer Cytopathol 2021 Jun;129(6):460–7.

40. Alborelli I, Bratic Hench I, Chijioke O, et al. Robust assessment of tumor mutational burden in cytological specimens from lung cancer patients. Lung Cancer 2020;149:84–9.

41. Chan RCK, Li JJX, Yeung W, et al. Virtual multiplex immunohistochemistry: application on cell block of effusion and aspiration cytology. Diagn Cytopathol 2020;48(5):417–23.

42. Lau RP, Kim TH, Rao J. Advances in Imaging Modalities, Artificial intelligence, and single cell biomarker analysis, and their applications in cytopathology. Front Med (Lausanne) 2021;8:689954.

43. Bonner RB, Hemstreet GP, Fradet Y, et al. Bladder cancer risk assessment with quantitative fluorescence image analysis of tumor markers in exfoliated bladder cells. Cancer 1993;72(8):2461–9.

44. Zhu Y, Wang A, Allard GM, et al. Immunofluorescent and molecular characterization of effusion

tumor cells reveal cancer site-of-origin and disease-driving mutations. Cancer Cytopathol 2022; 130(10):771–82.

45. Pai SI, Faquin WC, Sadow PM, et al. New technology on the horizon: Fast analytical screening technique FNA (FAST-FNA) enables rapid, multiplex biomarker analysis in head and neck cancers. Cancer Cytopathol 2020;128(11):782–91.

46. Stransky N, Egloff AM, Tward AD, et al. The mutational landscape of head and neck squamous cell carcinoma. Science 2011;333(6046):1157–60.

47. da Cunha Santos G, Saieg MA, Troncone G, et al. Cytological preparations for molecular analysis: A review of technical procedures, advantages and limitations for referring samples for testing. Cytopathology 2018;29(2):125–32.

48. Aisner DL, Sams SB. The role of cytology specimens in molecular testing of solid tumors: techniques, limitations, and opportunities. Diagn Cytopathol 2012; 40(6):511–24.

49. Bellevicine C, Malapelle U, Vigliar E, et al. How to prepare cytological samples for molecular testing. J Clin Pathol 2017;70(10):819–26.

50. Beca F, Schmitt F. Growing indication for FNA to study and analyze tumor heterogeneity at metastatic sites. Cancer Cytopathol 2014;122(7):504–11.

Thyroid Fine-Needle Aspiration
The Current and Future Landscape of Cytopathology

Jaylou M. Velez Torres, MD[a], Louis J. Vaickus, MD, PhD[b,c],
Darcy A. Kerr, MD[b,c],*

KEYWORDS

- Thyroid nodule • Thyroid cancer • Fine-needle aspiration cytology
- Bethesda system for reporting thyroid cytopathology • Molecular testing • Indeterminate
- Artificial intelligence

Key points

- Fine-needle aspiration cytology is the most widely used technique for sampling thyroid nodules.

- Molecular testing has emerged as a reliable ancillary tool to improve preoperative risk stratification of thyroid nodules, and results can help guide patient treatment.

- Thyroid cytology has limitations, including indeterminate thyroid nodules and false-positive and false-negative results.

- Advances in thyroid cytology have led to a decrease in the number of unnecessary surgeries and a reduction in health care costs while improving patient outcomes.

- Artificial intelligence and other emerging technologies are being explored as a means of further improving the efficiency and diagnostic accuracy of thyroid cytology.

ABSTRACT

Thyroid cytology is a rapidly evolving field that has seen significant advances in recent years. Its main goal is to accurately diagnose thyroid nodules, differentiate between benign and malignant lesions, and risk stratify nodules when a definitive diagnosis is not possible. The current landscape of thyroid cytology includes the use of fine-needle aspiration for the diagnosis of thyroid nodules with the use of uniform, tiered reporting systems such as the Bethesda System for Reporting Thyroid Cytopathology. In recent years, molecular testing has emerged as a reliable preoperative diagnostic tool that stratifies patients into different risk categories (low, intermediate, or high) with varying probabilities of malignancy and helps guide patient treatment.

OVERVIEW

THYROID FINE-NEEDLE ASPIRATION CYTOLOGY REPORTING SYSTEMS

Fine-needle aspiration cytology (FNAC) is a fast, minimally invasive, cost-efficient, and well-established technique that plays a critical role in

---

[a] University of Miami Hospital, Miller School of Medicine, 1400 NW 12th Avenue, Room 4078, Miami, FL 33136, USA; [b] Department of Pathology and Laboratory Medicine, Dartmouth-Hitchcock Medical Center, One Medical Center Drive, Lebanon, NH 03756, USA; [c] Geisel School of Medicine at Dartmouth, Hanover, NH 03755, USA
* Corresponding author. Geisel School of Medicine at Dartmouth, Hanover, NH 03755.
E-mail address: Darcy.A.Kerr@hitchcock.org
Twitter: @JaylouVelez (J.M.V.T.); @darcykerrMD (D.A.K.)

Surgical Pathology 17 (2024) 371–381
https://doi.org/10.1016/j.path.2024.04.005
1875-9181/24/© 2024 Elsevier Inc. All rights reserved.

the preoperative evaluation of patients with thyroid nodules. It can reliably distinguish benign versus malignant thyroid nodules and guide treatment.[1,2] In recent years, various thyroid cytology reporting systems have been proposed to improve communication between cytopathologists and treating physicians and facilitate data sharing among institutions. In 2007, the Bethesda System (TBS) for Reporting Thyroid Cytopathology was established, with updates in 2018 (second edition) and 2023 (third edition). TBS is endorsed by the American Thyroid Association (ATA)[3] and has been widely adopted in the United States and throughout North America, as well as by a range of other countries globally. However, several alternative thyroid cytology reporting systems currently exist, such as the 2014 Italian SIAPEC-AIT classification, the 2016 UK Royal College of Pathologists (RCPath) thyroid reporting system, and the 2019 Japanese reporting system for thyroid aspiration cytology (JRSTAC2019). Each current classification system provides different, tiered diagnostic categories, each with an implied risk of malignancy (ROM) and recommended management (**Table 1**).[4–9]

TBS is comparable with other internationally recognized systems, particularly the Italian and UK RCPath classifications. Despite some differences in diagnostic terminology, they use similar morphologic criteria, such as architectural atypia and cytologic atypia, but differ in their classification of indeterminate aspirates and therapeutic recommendations.[4,10] The subdivision of indeterminate categories into 2 groups is common to all the above-mentioned reporting systems. Both the UK and TBS terminologies include cases with mild nuclear atypia in both indeterminate categories, Thy3a and Thy3f, or atypia of undetermined significance (AUS) and follicular neoplasm (FN), respectively, leading to similar ROMs.[7] On the other hand, in the Italian system, cases with nuclear atypia are placed in the indeterminate high-risk category (TIR 3B), which explains the greater separation in the ROM between the lower (TIR 3A) and higher-risk categories (TIR 3B).[6] For management recommendations, molecular testing plays a more prominent role in TBS than other classifications. In the Japanese JRSTAC system, active surveillance is more commonly recommended compared to the diagnostic surgeries favored in the other systems.[11]

Given the wide adoption of TBS, the numerous publications available regarding its performance, and the fact that this reporting system is currently utilized in the authors' institutions, the subsequent sections largely use this reporting framework. However, the discussion is also conceptually applicable to the other classification systems.

CURRENT PRACTICE

THYROID FINE-NEEDLE ASPIRATION CYTOLOGY AND THE BETHESDA SYSTEM

Ultrasound with FNAC of nodules meeting sampling criteria is the standard of care for evaluating thyroid nodules. The American College of Radiology's Thyroid Imaging Reporting and Data System (ACR TI-RADS) risk stratifies thyroid nodules according to ultrasonographic features such as composition, echogenicity, shape, margin, and echogenic foci.[12] ACR TI-RADS thyroid nodules with scores of 1 and 2 are not recommended for FNAC as they are likely benign. However, ACR TI-RADS nodules with scores of 3, 4, and 5 are recommended for either FNAC or ultrasonography surveillance, depending on their size.[13] FNAC risk stratifies nodules and is reported to have a high diagnostic accuracy (94.5%) with a sensitivity, specificity, positive predictive value, and negative predictive value of 84.2%, 97.2%, 88.3%, and 96%, respectively, according to TBS.[14] However, cytomorphology has its limitations, and potential diagnostic pitfalls exist.[15] While most thyroid aspirates are accurately classified as benign or malignant, up to 30% fall into indeterminate categories.[16] Moreover, false-positive results may occur due to morphologic overlap between benign and malignant neoplastic and/or non-neoplastic lesions. In contrast, false-negative results may occur in larger-size nodules (>4 cm), limited cellularity, or macrofollicular-patterned thyroid carcinomas.[17–20] Further challenges arise when subclassifying lesions based on nuclear atypia. The third edition of TBS recommends further subdividing the AUS category according to the presence or absence of nuclear atypia, as studies have demonstrated that the presence of nuclear atypia is associated with different molecular alterations and higher ROMs.[21,22] However, the assessment of nuclear atypia in cytology aspirates is subjective, and there are limited data regarding appropriate diagnostic criteria for determining whether nuclear atypia is present.[23]

To avoid overuse, TBS recommends limiting AUS interpretation to 10% or less of all thyroid FNAC.[22] While this recommendation aims to assure quality, it lacks robust supportive data. Further, it does not account for differences in cancer prevalence between different patient populations and has proven to be an unrealistic target for a number of laboratories.[24] In addition, due to the inherent heterogeneity of the AUS category and variable diagnostic thresholds, differences in its utilization are inevitable, which result in significant variability in AUS rates (range 3%–22%).[24,25]

Table 1
Comparison between Bethesda, Italian, British, and Japanese thyroid cytology classification systems

2023 Bethesda System		2014 Italian SIAPEC-AIT		2016 RCPath Classification		2019 JRSTAC	
Diagnostic Category (ROM%)	Management	Diagnostic Category (ROM%)	Management	Diagnostic Category (ROM%)	Management	Diagnostic Category (ROM%)	Management
I. Non-diagnostic-including cyst fluid only (2%–20%)	Repeat FNA with US	TIR1. Non-diagnostic (29.8%) TIR 1C. Non-diagnostic-cystic	Repeat FNA with US Repeat FNA with US	Thy1. Non-diagnostic (5%–22%) Thy1c. Non-diagnostic—cystic[a]	US assessment ± repeat FNA.	1. Unsatisfactory (5.6%)	Repeat FNA
II. Benign (0%–6%)	Clinical follow-up	TIR 2 Benign (<3%)	Clinical follow-up	Thy2. Non-neoplastic (3%–9%) Thy2c. Non-neoplastic-cystic[a]	Correlate with clinical and US findings	2. Cyst fluid only (0.2%)	Sonographic follow-up is recommended
III. Atypia of undetermined significance (20%–32%)	Repeat FNA, molecular testing, lobectomy, or surveillance	TIR 3A. Low-risk indeterminate (12%–22%)	Clinical follow-up with repeat FNA	Thy3a. Neoplastic possible, atypia/non-diagnostic (20%–31%)	US assessment ± repeat FNA[b]	3. Benign (1.2%)	Clinical follow-up
IV. Follicular neoplasm (25%–50%)	Molecular testing, lobectomy	TIR 3B. High-risk indeterminate (40%–55%)	Surgery	Thy3f. Neoplasm possible, suggesting follicular neoplasm (24%–39%)	Diagnostic hemithyroidectomy	4. Undetermined significance (13%)	Repeat FNA[e]
V. Suspicious for malignancy (50%–80%)	Molecular testing, lobectomy or total thyroidectomy	TIR 4. Suspicious for malignancy (60%–80%)	Surgery	Thy4. Suspicious for malignancy (70%–87%)	Diagnostic hemithyroidectomy[c,d]	5. Follicular neoplasm (22.3%–26.2%)	Active surveillance

(continued on next page)

Table 1
(continued)

2023 Bethesda System		2014 Italian SIAPEC-AIT		2016 RCPath Classification		2019 JRSTAC	
Diagnostic Category (ROM%)	Management	Diagnostic Category (ROM%)	Management	Diagnostic Category (ROM%)	Management	Diagnostic Category (ROM%)	Management
VI. Malignant (85%–100%)	Total thyroidectomy or lobectomy	TIR 5. Malignant (>95%)	Surgery	Thy5. Malignant (97%–99%)	Therapeutic surgery[c]	6. Suspicious for malignancy (95.8%–98.8%)	Active surveillance or surgical resection[f]
						7. Malignant (99.2%–99.3%)	Active surveillance or surgical resection

Abbreviations: FNA, fine needle aspiration; ROM, risk of malignancy; US, ultrasound.
[a] Not enough number of cases to calculate ROM.
[b] If Thy3a on repeat FNAC needs multidisciplinary assessment.
[c] Must be discussed at multidisciplinary meeting.
[d] If the ultrasound examination reveals a solid area in the cystic lesions, repeated fine needle aspiration cytology of the solid area is recommended.
[e] Surgery if suspicious ultrasound or cytologic features of atypia, nodules extending to the mediastinum.
[f] Active surveillance for nodules with suggested low-risk DTC is acceptable.

Furthermore, for laboratories or cytopathologists that exceed this target, there are no clear recommendations on how to reduce their AUS rate. Importantly, lowering AUS rates without adjusting individual diagnostic thresholds may compromise the diagnostic sensitivity of thyroid FNAC.[26] Consequently, it is necessary to investigate potential tools to assess and manage the overutilization of AUS. Krane and colleagues proposed the AUS:-malignant (AUS:M) ratio as a laboratory quality control measure to help assess AUS utilization (which should fall within the range of 1.0–3.0).[24] By monitoring the AUS:M ratio over time, institutions can evaluate the performance of their cytopathologists and provide feedback to adjust their diagnostic criteria. A benefit of this tool is that it accounts for the cancer prevalence among different patient populations. There are, however, some limitations; cytopathologists may interpret AUS differently, even within the same institution. Furthermore, it does not consider the possibility of false positive or false negative cases as the calculation does not rely on histologic follow-up. Another approach is to compare molecular test (MT) results with AUS rates. This correlation can reveal both over-calling and under-calling of different diagnostic categories across TBS. Therefore, it can be used to help adjust the individual diagnostic threshold as well as facilitate the standardization of cytology practices across laboratories.[25,27]

ROLE OF MOLECULAR TESTING IN INDETERMINATE THYROID NODULES

Indeterminate thyroid aspirates pose a diagnostic challenge due to their heterogeneous nature. TBS defines the AUS category as aspirates that contain follicular cells with architectural and/or cytologic atypia without sufficient evidence to be classified as FN, suspicious for malignancy (SFM), or malignant (M). Its estimated ROM ranges from 10% to 30%.[22] In contrast, cellular aspirates composed of follicular cells with an altered architectural pattern (significant crowding and/or predominance of microfollicles) are classified as FN and have an estimated ROM of 25% to 40%.[22]

Managing patients with indeterminate cytology can be challenging. MT has arisen as a reliable pre-operative diagnostic tool that stratifies patients into different risk categories (low, intermediate, or high) with varying probabilities of malignancy.[28] Studies have shown that MT-positive nodules have a higher surgical resection rate than MT-negative nodules in both AUS (MT+ 72% vs MT- 12%) and FN categories (MT+ 91% vs MT- 27%).[21,29] Furthermore, MT

has reduced the number of diagnostic thyroidectomies (lobectomy or total thyroidectomy) performed in patients with AUS and FN indeterminate thyroid nodules by up to 61%.[29] Molecular-based risk stratification (Table 2) has the ability to predict aggressive cancer behavior, including the likelihood of distant metastases, and this information can be utilized in the pre-operative setting to enable a more customized treatment.[30,31] Those nodules with an intermediate to high-risk molecular profile may require more aggressive treatment, such as a total thyroidectomy. Conversely, patients with low-risk molecular profiles may benefit from de-escalation active surveillance protocols.[31]

ROLE OF MOLECULAR TESTING IN MALIGNANT THYROID NODULES

The current 2015 ATA guidelines recommend that thyroid lobectomy alone may be sufficient as initial management for patients with low-risk differentiated thyroid carcinoma (DTC; ie, papillary thyroid carcinoma [PTC] and follicular thyroid carcinoma [FTC]).[3] In contrast, total thyroidectomy is recommended for patients with high-risk DTC who are more likely to develop distant metastases.[3] However, thyroid FNAC and other preoperative clinical parameters only manage to identify a minority of patients (18%) with indications for total thyroidectomy, and up to half of the remaining patients ultimately require a completion thyroidectomy, indicating a failure to provide an optimal surgical treatment at the outset.[32] Unfortunately, the factors determining whether a tumor will recur are often unknown before surgery. In this regard, preoperative risk stratification using MT may be one of the few available clinical parameters that could help identify patients who are at a higher risk for recurrence and may require total thyroidectomy.[33] Molecular testing is not only capable of detecting

---

Table 2
Molecular-based risk stratification

Molecular Risk Group	Molecular Alterations
Low	*RAS* and *RAS*-like[a]
Intermediate	*BRAF* V600E, *BRAF*-like alterations,[b] and CNA
High	Early mutation and late hit mutation (eg, *TERT, TP53, AKT1,* and *PIK3CA*)

Abbreviation: CNA, copy number alterations.
[a] *BRAF* K601E and *PAX8::PPARG.*
[b] *ALK* fusions, *NTRK*1/3 fusions, and *RET::PTC.*

genetic alterations associated with a high probability of malignancy (eg, *BRAF* V600E) but can also identify genetic profiles associated with more aggressive thyroid carcinoma (eg, *TERT* promoter mutations or alterations in *TP53* or *PIK3CA*).[33] In contrast, a preoperatively detected low-risk molecular profile is associated with an exceedingly low (~0.12%) risk of distant metastasis and should only require thyroid lobectomy.[30] Molecular testing is not routinely performed in FNA diagnosis of malignancy, and only a very small percentage of cases submitted for ThyroSeq represent SFM (0.7%) aspirates.[31] Nevertheless, recent advances in our understanding of the association between genetic alterations and cancer phenotypes have prompted the consideration for molecular testing in M and SFM aspirates. The availability of pre-operative MT may help to inform optimal surgical management, offering the prospect of tailoring treatment strategies to match the patient's specific risk.[3,30]

Molecular Testing for Identification of Therapeutically Targetable Alterations in Thyroid Carcinoma

Most Bethesda SFM or M nodules contain *BRAF*-like alterations and are enriched in intermediate- and high-risk genetic profiles, including therapeutically relevant mutations and gene fusions.[31] In this context, MT can help determine which tumors have actionable alterations and are suitable for targeted therapy. Although most DTCs are cured by surgery alone, tumors with high-risk histology, residual disease, and distant or loco-regional metastases may require further treatment. The most commonly used adjuvant treatment for DTC is radioactive iodine (RAI). However, de novo or acquired RAI resistance may develop, necessitating alternative treatments. According to one study, up to 12% of RAI-refractory thyroid carcinomas harbor actionable kinase fusions.[34] Kinase fusion-related thyroid carcinomas (KFTC) represent a spectrum of molecularly diverse tumors with overlapping clinicopathologic features and a tendency for aggressive behavior.[35] Among KFTC, *RET* rearrangement accounts for approximately 50% of cases, followed by *NTRK* 1/2/3 (~30%), *ALK* (~5%), *MET*, *ROS1*, and *FGFR* 1/2 rearrangements.[36] Selective kinase inhibitors (eg, larotrectinib, entrectinib, selpercatinib, and pralsetinib) have shown significant efficacy with favorable side effects in treating KFTCs, making it increasingly important to identify these tumors.[35] Furthermore, as a result of findings from a clinical trial examining dabrafenib plus trametinib in patients with *BRAF* V600E-

mutated anaplastic thyroid carcinoma (ATC), the FDA approved the first targeted treatment for patients with ATC in 2018.[37] Due to the positive response of this combination against *BRAF* V600E-mutated ATCs, a highly aggressive and nearly uniformly fatal disease, *BRAF* V600E mutation testing is indicated for all ATCs.[38] FDA-approved therapeutic options also exist for treating *RET*-mutated medullary thyroid carcinoma (MTC) and *RET*-fusion positive PTC and for metastatic and unresectable thyroid carcinomas carrying *NTRK* fusions.[39,40] Additionally, FDA-approved on- and off-label targeted therapies are available for patients with thyroid carcinomas carrying *ALK* or *ROS* fusions.[41–43]

Role of Molecular Testing in Medullary Thyroid Carcinoma

Approximately 75% of cases of MTC are sporadic and have a peak incidence between the fourth and sixth decades of life. In contrast, hereditary forms comprise 25% of cases and have an autosomal dominant inheritance pattern.[44] Up to 67% of sporadic MTCs have somatic *RET* mutations followed by *RAS* mutations (43%), whereas almost 98% of hereditary MTCs have a *RET* germline mutation.[45,46] A recent study reported that 82% of MTC-positive FNAs (aspirates with high calcitonin and neuroendocrine gene expression) tested with ThyroSeq v3 GC showed gene mutations including *RET* (54%), *HRAS* (21%), *KRAS* (4.8%), and *BRAF* non-V600E alterations (2.4%) such as *BRAF* K601E, and G469A.[31] For patients that harbor a *RET* mutation, germline genetic testing should be considered. In contrast, the 28% of patients with MTC harboring *RAS* or *BRAF* mutation can be reassured of the sporadic nature of their disease with no need for additional germline testing.[47]

ROLE OF MOLECULAR TESTING IN PEDIATRIC THYROID NODULES

The incidence of pediatric thyroid cancer is increasing, and it represents the second-most common malignancy in adolescents.[14,48] Thyroid nodules are less prevalent in children than adults (~2% vs 30%); however, they carry a greater ROM (~25% vs 5%).[49] Malignant pediatric thyroid nodules have a unique molecular landscape when compared with adults, dominated by gene fusions, most commonly *RET* and *NTRK1/3*, and gene mutations involving *DICER1*, *PTEN*, and *TSHR*.[50,51] On the other hand, *BRAF/RAS* and high-risk (*TP53/TERT*) alterations are uncommon in this age group.[50,51] Although thyroid carcinomas with underlying *DICER1* mutations are usually indolent, recent studies have shown that pediatric poorly differentiated thyroid carcinoma (PDTC) and thyroblastoma, both aggressive tumors, also harbor *DICER1* mutations.[52,53] Further, pediatric patients with FTC or PDTC are recommended to undergo genetic testing for *DICER1* germline mutations since these tumors may be the first manifestation of *DICER1* syndrome.[54] As in adults, knowing the genetic profile of a pediatric thyroid tumor in the preoperative setting can help guide treatment and reduce diagnostic or completion thyroidectomies, resulting in fewer complications.[55]

THYROID FINE NEEDLE ASPIRATION IMPLICATIONS RELATED TO THE RECENT FIFTH EDITION WHO CLASSIFICATION OF ENDOCRINE TUMORS

Medullary Thyroid Carcinoma

The most important update for MTC was the endorsement of a grading scheme. Recently, an international study validated the significant relationship between grade and survival and recommended a two-tiered grading of MTC.[56] This was based on the strong association between worse patient outcomes and high-grade pathologic features defined as having at least one of the following features: tumor necrosis, elevated mitotic count ($\geq$5 per 2 mm^2), or Ki67 proliferation index ($\geq$5%).[38,56] Nevertheless, these criteria have not been widely assessed in MTC cytology aspirates, and further studies are needed to determine how applicable the grading scheme is to cytology specimens.

High-Grade Differentiated Thyroid Carcinomas

The fifth edition of the WHO Classification introduced a new high-grade carcinoma analogous to PDTC termed "differentiated high-grade thyroid carcinoma" (DHGTC) for PTCs and FTCs/oncocytic carcinomas with $\geq$5 mitoses per 2 mm^2 and/or tumor necrosis. These tumors retain morphologic features of specific DTCs but also exhibit high-grade features and are associated with an aggressive clinical course similar to that of conventional PDTC. The tumors classified as DHGTC have retained PTC-like nuclear features or a follicular growth pattern and exhibit features that do not fulfill the Turin criteria for a diagnosis of PDTC.[38] Establishing a cytologic diagnosis of PDTC poses a challenge due to morphologic overlap with FNs. Nevertheless, important clues for the FNA diagnosis of PDTC include increased cellularity, an insular/trabecular growth pattern, and presence of mitotic activity or necrosis.[57] Similarly,

some authors have suggested that FNAs might offer insights into the diagnosis of aggressive PTC subtypes such as tall cell, columnar cell, and hobnail.[58] Additional research is needed to determine how likely DHGTC is to be recognized on cytology aspirates.

Low-Risk Follicular Neoplasms

The diagnostic category of low-risk FNs refers to borderline tumors that are morphologically and clinically intermediate between benign and well-differentiated malignant tumors, with an extremely low risk of loco-regional and/or distant recurrence. There are several low-risk follicular-derived neoplasms listed in the WHO classification, including noninvasive follicular thyroid neoplasm with papillary-like nuclear features (NIFTP), thyroid tumors of uncertain malignant potential (UMP), and hyalinizing trabecular tumors (HTT).[38] A majority of FNA specimens from either UMP or NIFTP will be classified as AUS or FN.[59] However, in a minority of cases, NIFTP might be classified as suspicious for PTC or as PTC due to the presence of nuclear atypia.[60,61] Additionally, the majority of HTTs will fall under indeterminate diagnostic categories of TBS, including AUS (22%), FN (33%), and SFM (28%).[62] However, a minority of cases could be misdiagnosed as PTC due to the presence of overlapping nuclear features, including frequent nuclear pseudo-inclusions and grooves.[62] Nevertheless, the presence of significant stromal hyaline material, particularly intra-trabecular hyalinization, may serve as a helpful clue suggestive of HTT, given that this finding is relatively uncommon in PTC.[63]

FUTURE DIRECTIONS

While thyroid FNAC is a highly effective technique, there is still an opportunity to improve upon its limitations. Uniform reporting systems such as TBS have enhanced communication and data sharing. However, it is important to acknowledge the inherent subjectivity in cytopathologic diagnoses and, in particular, to highlight the need for a consistent definition of nuclear atypia within this framework. The establishment of more precise, standardized criteria for determining whether nuclear atypia is present could have a significant impact on reducing the frequency of indeterminate diagnoses, ultimately leading to a decrease in repeat FNAs and unnecessary surgeries. Despite the lack of formal criteria or defined thresholds for assessing nuclear atypia in cytology aspirates, nuclear scoring systems developed for histologic applications have been applied to thyroid cytology aspirates.[64,65] The nuclear scoring of various features have been shown to help distinguish between benign adenomas, NIFTP, and PTC.[65,66] Moreover, studies looking for phenotypic patterns that might be predictive of specific molecular alterations have underscored the capacity of nuclear scoring to differentiate neoplasms driven by *BRAF*-like alterations from those with *RAS*-like alterations.[66] Nonetheless, further research is still needed in this area.

A significant challenge in thyroid pathology is the reliance on histopathologic diagnoses as the gold standard for determining whether a tumor is benign or malignant, using parameters such as capsular/vascular invasion and assessing PTC-like nuclear features. However, as many pathologists in this field can attest, these distinctions can be highly subjective.[67] This issue has been acknowledged and incorporated into the WHO classification within the category of thyroid tumors of UMP, tumors with persistent uncertainty regarding capsular or vascular invasion even after meticulous sampling and comprehensive examination. Based on their nuclear characteristics, thyroid tumors that fall under the UMP category are further divided into 2 subtypes: follicular tumor of UMP, which lacks PTC-like nuclear features, and well-differentiated tumor of UMP, which exhibit varying degrees of nuclear features resembling PTC.[38] Considering these challenges, there is a critical need for long-term follow-up studies that can provide greater insight into the biologic behavior of these tumors over time. Such studies could help clarify the factors that contribute to the development and progression of these tumors while also identifying potential markers that can help improve our diagnostic accuracy.

As noted above, MT has shown great promise in the preoperative evaluation of thyroid nodules, enabling genetic profile-informed personalized treatment strategies. While the cost of the test may be a barrier in some settings, studies have demonstrated that MT can be a cost-effective strategy for managing thyroid nodules. As the technology advances and becomes more affordable, MT will likely become an integral part of the evaluation and management of thyroid nodules.[68] Furthermore, just as Afirma and ThyroSeq demonstrating improved benign call rates and enhanced assessment of oncocytic cell lesions in subsequent test iterations, existing molecular platforms are expected to continue to improve over time.[69,70]

Artificial intelligence (AI) will likely play an increasing role in thyroid FNA in the future. From a radiographic perspective, the development of radiomics algorithms has the potential to increase diagnostic accuracy of preoperative imaging techniques and may influence the composition of thyroid nodules selected for FNA.[71] From a cytology interpretation standpoint, the technical obstacles and lack of optimized scanners for cytology samples have hindered the advancement of AI-assisted algorithms for analyzing digital images of cytology specimens. Nonetheless, a number of studies have investigated the use of AI-based approaches in evaluating thyroid FNAC specimens.[72,73] AI-based algorithms have demonstrated improved diagnostic accuracy and could be a valuable ancillary tool in the diagnosis of thyroid cytopathology to reduce cytopathologist workload by automating some aspects of the analysis.[74] With proper training of the model, AI has the potential to offer an affordable, sustainable ancillary tool. While there are challenges in developing and optimizing AI algorithms for pathology, the potential benefits make it a promising area of research and development. With ongoing advancements in technology and increasing availability of digital pathology platforms, the integration of AI into pathology practice is becoming more feasible and practical.

CLINICS CARE POINTS

- Structured reporting systems in thyroid fine-needle aspiration cytology guide the clinical management of patients with thyroid nodules.

- Molecular testing of cytologically indeterminant nodules reduces the number of unnecessary surgeries for low-risk and benign nodules.

- In high-risk nodules, molecular testing can inform surgical approaches and identify targetable alterations such as tyrosine kinase fusions.

- Artificial intelligence is likely to play an increasing role in selecting thyroid nodules for biopsy and interpretation of their cytologic features.

DISCLOSURE

The authors have nothing to disclose.

REFERENCES

1. Rosario PW, de Castro Nicolau T. The value of ultrasonography for the indication of fine-needle aspiration in autonomous thyroid nodules. Diagn Cytopathol 2021;49:363–6.

2. Maxwell C, Sipos JA. Clinical diagnostic evaluation of thyroid nodules. Endocrinol Metab Clin North Am 2019;48:61–84.

3. Haugen BR, Alexander EK, Bible KC, et al. 2015 American Thyroid Association Management Guidelines for Adult Patients with Thyroid Nodules and Differentiated Thyroid Cancer: The American Thyroid Association Guidelines Task Force on Thyroid Nodules and Differentiated Thyroid Cancer. Thyroid 2016;26:1–133.

4. Nardi F, Basolo F, Crescenzi A, et al. Italian consensus for the classification and reporting of thyroid cytology. J Endocrinol Invest 2014;37:593–9.

5. Torregrossa L, Poma AM, Macerola E, et al. The Italian Consensus for the Classification and Reporting of Thyroid Cytology: Cytohistologic and molecular correlations on 37,371 nodules from a single institution. Cancer Cytopathol 2022;130:899–912.

6. Trimboli P, Crescenzi A, Castellana M, et al. Italian consensus for the classification and reporting of thyroid cytology: the risk of malignancy between indeterminate lesions at low or high risk. A systematic review and meta-analysis. Endocrine 2019;63: 430–8.

7. Poller DN, Bongiovanni M, Trimboli P. Risk of malignancy in the various categories of the UK Royal College of Pathologists Thy terminology for thyroid FNA cytology: A systematic review and meta-analysis. Cancer Cytopathol 2020;128:36–42.

8. Kamma H, Kameyama K, Kondo T, et al. Pathological diagnosis of general rules for the description of thyroid cancer by Japanese Society of Thyroid Pathology and Japan Association of Endocrine Surgery. Endocr J 2022;69:139–54.

9. Sakamoto A, Hirokawa M, Ito M, et al. Introduction of histological classification and cytology reporting format of the Japanese General Rules for the Description of Thyroid Cancer with a special focus on the differences of the WHO Histological Classification and The Bethesda System of Thyroid Cytology. Endocr J 2021;68:621–30.

10. Pizzimenti C, Mazzeo F, Militi GB, et al. Reporting thyroid cytology in a globalized. World 2021;2: 311–9.

11. Hirokawa M, Suzuki A, Higuchi M, et al. The Japanese reporting system for thyroid aspiration cytology 2019 (JRSTAC2019). Gland Surg 2020;9:1653–62.

12. Grant EG, Tessler FN, Hoang JK, et al. Thyroid ultrasound reporting lexicon: white paper of the acr thyroid imaging, reporting and data system (TIRADS) committee. J Am Coll Radiol 2015;12:1272–9.

13. Floridi C, Cellina M, Buccimazza G, et al. Ultrasound imaging classifications of thyroid nodules for malignancy risk stratification and clinical management: state of the art. Gland Surg 2019;8:S233–44.

14. Alshahrani AS, Algazlan AG, Junaid M, et al. Association of fine-needle aspiration of thyroid nodules with final histopathology in diagnosing thyroid malignancy: a single institute retrospective study. Cureus 2022;14:e31733.

15. Castro MR, Gharib H. Thyroid fine-needle aspiration biopsy: progress, practice, and pitfalls. Endocr Pract 2003;9:128–36.

16. Rossi ED, Pantanowitz L, Faquin WC. The Role of Molecular Testing for the Indeterminate Thyroid FNA. Genes (Basel) 2019;10.

17. Pinchot SN, Al-Wagih H, Schaefer S, et al. Accuracy of fine-needle aspiration biopsy for predicting neoplasm or carcinoma in thyroid nodules 4 cm or larger. Arch Surg 2009;144:649–55.

18. McCoy KL, Jabbour N, Ogilvie JB, et al. The incidence of cancer and rate of false-negative cytology in thyroid nodules greater than or equal to 4 cm in size. Surgery 2007;142:837–44, discussion 844 e831-833.

19. Mezei T, Kolcsar M, Pascanu I, et al. False positive cases in thyroid cytopathology - the experience of a single laboratory and a systematic review. Cytopathology 2021;32:493–504.

20. Chung D, Ghossein RA, Lin O. Macrofollicular variant of papillary carcinoma: a potential thyroid FNA pitfall. Diagn Cytopathol 2007;35:560–4.

21. Gajzer DC, Tjendra Y, Kerr DA, et al. Probability of malignancy as determined by ThyroSeq v3 genomic classifier varies according to the subtype of atypia. Cancer Cytopathol 2022;130:881–90.

22. Cibas ES, Ali SZ. The 2017 bethesda system for reporting thyroid cytopathology. J Am Soc Cytopathol 2017;6:217–22.

23. Borges FA, Camilo-Junior DJ, de Almeida EHC, et al. Score system for cytological evaluation of fine-needle aspiration specimens to predict the diagnosis of papillary thyroid carcinomas. Ann Diagn Pathol 2023;64:152129.

24. Krane JF, Vanderlaan PA, Faquin WC, et al. The atypia of undetermined significance/follicular lesion of undetermined significance:malignant ratio: a proposed performance measure for reporting in The Bethesda System for thyroid cytopathology. Cancer Cytopathol 2012;120:111–6.

25. VanderLaan PA, Nishino M. Molecular testing results as a quality metric for evaluating cytopathologists' utilization of the atypia of undetermined significance category for thyroid nodule fine-needle aspirations. J Am Soc Cytopathol 2022;11:67–73.

26. Renshaw AA. Subclassification of atypical cells of undetermined significance in direct smears of fine-needle aspirations of the thyroid: distinct patterns and associated risk of malignancy. Cancer Cytopathol 2011;119:322–7.

27. Martinez Coconubo D, Levy JJ, Kerr DA, et al. Use of molecular testing results to analyze the overuse of atypia of undetermined significance in thyroid cytology. J Am Soc Cytopathol 2023;12(6):451–60.

28. Vuong HG, Nguyen TPX, Hassell LA, et al. Diagnostic performances of the Afirma Gene Sequencing Classifier in comparison with the Gene Expression Classifier: A meta-analysis. Cancer Cytopathol 2021;129:182–9.

29. Carty SE, Ohori NP, Hilko DA, et al. The clinical utility of molecular testing in the management of thyroid follicular neoplasms (Bethesda IV Nodules). Ann Surg 2020;272:621–7.

30. Yip L, Gooding WE, Nikitski A, et al. Risk assessment for distant metastasis in differentiated thyroid cancer using molecular profiling: A matched case-control study. Cancer 2021;127:1779–87.

31. Chiosea S, Hodak SP, Yip L, et al. Molecular profiling of 50,734 bethesda III-VI Thyroid nodules by thyroSeq v3: Implications for personalized management. J Clin Endocrinol Metab 2023;12(6):451–60.

32. Wang TSJCT. Current ATA thyroid Cancer guidelines are poor predictors of the extent of thyroidectomy 2018;30:56–8.

33. Hier J, Avior G, Pusztaszeri M, et al. Molecular testing for cytologically suspicious and malignant (Bethesda V and VI) thyroid nodules to optimize the extent of surgical intervention: a retrospective chart review. J Otolaryngol Head Neck Surg 2021; 50:29.

34. van der Tuin K, Ventayol Garcia M, Corver WE, et al. Targetable gene fusions identified in radioactive iodine refractory advanced thyroid carcinoma. Eur J Endocrinol 2019;180:235–41.

35. Chu YH, Wirth LJ, Farahani AA, et al. Clinicopathologic features of kinase fusion-related thyroid carcinomas: an integrative analysis with molecular characterization. Mod Pathol 2020;33:2458–72.

36. Chu YH, Sadow PM. Kinase fusion-related thyroid carcinomas: distinct pathologic entities with evolving diagnostic implications. Diagn Histopathol (Oxf) 2021;27:252–62.

37. Subbiah V, Kreitman RJ, Wainberg ZA, et al. Dabrafenib and trametinib treatment in patients with locally advanced or metastatic BRAF V600-mutant anaplastic thyroid cancer. J Clin Oncol 2018;36:7–13.

38. Baloch ZW, Asa SL, Barletta JA, et al. Overview of the 2022 WHO classification of thyroid neoplasms. Endocr Pathol 2022;33:27–63.

39. Doebele RC, Drilon A, Paz-Ares L, et al. Entrectinib in patients with advanced or metastatic NTRK fusion-positive solid tumours: integrated analysis of three phase 1-2 trials. Lancet Oncol 2020;21: 271–82.

40. Oliveira LCB, Mulligan LM. Selpercatinib: First approved selective RET inhibitor. Cell 2023;186: 1517.

41. Fullmer T, Cabanillas ME, Zafereo M. Novel therapeutics in radioactive iodine-resistant thyroid cancer. Front Endocrinol (Lausanne) 2021;12:720723.

42. Leroy L, Bonhomme B, Le Moulec S, et al. Remarkable response to ceritinib and brigatinib in an anaplastic lymphoma kinase-rearranged anaplastic thyroid carcinoma previously treated with crizotinib. Thyroid 2020;30:343–4.

43. Liu SV, Macke LA, Colton BS, et al. Response to entrectinib in differentiated thyroid cancer with a ROS1 fusion. JCO Precis Oncol 2017;1.

44. Ponder BA, Ponder MA, Coffey R, et al. Risk estimation and screening in families of patients with medullary thyroid carcinoma. Lancet 1988;1:397–401.

45. Moura MM, Cavaco BM, Leite V. RAS protooncogene in medullary thyroid carcinoma. Endocr Relat Cancer 2015;22:R235–52.

46. Romei C, Mariotti S, Fugazzola L, et al. Multiple endocrine neoplasia type 2 syndromes (MEN 2): results from the ItaMEN network analysis on the prevalence of different genotypes and phenotypes. Eur J Endocrinol 2010;163:301–8.

47. Ciampi R, Mian C, Fugazzola L, et al. Evidence of a low prevalence of RAS mutations in a large medullary thyroid cancer series. Thyroid 2013;23:50–7.

48. Vaccarella S, Lortet-Tieulent J, Colombet M, et al. Global patterns and trends in incidence and mortality of thyroid cancer in children and adolescents: a population-based study. Lancet Diabetes Endocrinol 2021;9:144–52.

49. Wang H, Mehrad M, Ely KA, et al. Incidence and malignancy rates of indeterminate pediatric thyroid nodules. Cancer Cytopathol 2019;127:231–9.

50. Baran JA, Halada S, Bauer AJ, et al. Indeterminate thyroid fine-needle aspirations in pediatrics: exploring clinicopathologic features and utility of molecular profiling. Horm Res Paediatr 2022;95: 430–41.

51. Gallant JN, Chen SC, Ortega CA, et al. Evaluation of the molecular landscape of pediatric thyroid nodules and use of a multigene genomic classifier in children. JAMA Oncol 2022;8:1323–7.

52. Sauer M, Barletta JA. Proceedings of the North American society of head and neck pathology, Los Angeles, CA, March 20, 2022: DICER1-related thyroid tumors. Head Neck Pathol 2022;16:190–9.

53. Chernock RD, Rivera B, Borrelli N, et al. Poorly differentiated thyroid carcinoma of childhood and adolescence: a distinct entity characterized by DICER1 mutations. Mod Pathol 2020;33:1264–74.

54. Lee YA, Im SW, Jung KC, et al. Predominant DICER1 pathogenic variants in pediatric follicular thyroid carcinomas. Thyroid 2020;30:1120–31.

55. Buryk MA, Monaco SE, Witchel SF, et al. Pre-operative cytology with molecular analysis to help guide surgery for pediatric thyroid nodules. Int J Pediatr Otorhinolaryngol 2013;77:1697–700.

56. Xu B, Fuchs TL, Ahmadi S, et al. International medullary thyroid carcinoma grading system: a validated

grading system for medullary thyroid carcinoma. J Clin Oncol 2022;40:96–104.

57. Pietribiasi F, Sapino A, Papotti M, et al. Cytologic features of poorly differentiated 'insular' carcinoma of the thyroid, as revealed by fine-needle aspiration biopsy. Am J Clin Pathol 1990;94:687–92.

58. Gupta S, Sodhani P, Jain S, et al. Morphologic spectrum of papillary carcinoma of the thyroid: role of cytology in identifying the variants. Acta Cytol 2004;48:795–800.

59. Rossi ED, Baloch Z. The Impact of the 2022 WHO classification of thyroid neoplasms on everyday practice of cytopathology. Endocr Pathol 2023;34:23–33.

60. LiVolsi VA, Baloch Z. Non-invasive follicular tumor with papillary-like nuclear features: a practice changer in thyroid pathology. Arch Pathol Lab Med 2021; 145:659–63.

61. Rossi ED, Faquin WC, Baloch Z, et al. Non-invasive follicular thyroid neoplasm with papillary-like nuclear features (NIFTP): update and diagnostic considerations-a review. Endocr Pathol 2019;30:155–62.

62. Dell'Aquila M, Gravina C, Cocomazzi A, et al. A large series of hyalinizing trabecular tumors: cytomorphology and ancillary techniques on fine needle aspiration. Cancer Cytopathol 2019;127:390–8.

63. Rossi ED, Papotti M, Faquin W, et al. The diagnosis of hyalinizing trabecular tumor: a difficult and controversial thyroid entity. Head Neck Pathol 2020;14: 778–84.

64. Nikiforov YE, Seethala RR, Tallini G, et al. Nomenclature revision for encapsulated follicular variant of papillary thyroid carcinoma: a paradigm shift to reduce overtreatment of indolent tumors. JAMA Oncol 2016;2:1023–9.

65. Strickland KC, Howitt BE, Barletta JA, et al. Suggesting the cytologic diagnosis of non-invasive follicular thyroid neoplasm with papillary-like nuclear features (NIFTP): A retrospective analysis of atypical and suspicious nodules. Cancer Cytopathol 2018;126: 86–93.

66. Shahi M, Bloechl SJ, Vogel RI, et al. Semiquantitative assessment of cytomorphologic features can predict mutation status of thyroid nodules with indeterminate cytologic diagnosis. Hum Pathol 2019;93: 81–9.

67. Kakudo K. Different threshold of malignancy for RAS-like thyroid tumors causes significant differences in thyroid nodule practice. Cancers (Basel) 2022;14.

68. Tessler I, Leshno M, Feinmesser G, et al. Is there a role for molecular testing for low-risk differentiated thyroid cancer? a cost-effectiveness analysis. Cancers (Basel) 2023;15.

69. Nikiforova MN, Mercurio S, Wald AI, et al. Analytical performance of the ThyroSeq v3 genomic classifier for cancer diagnosis in thyroid nodules. Cancer 2018;124:1682–90.

70. Yang Z, Zhang T, Layfield L, et al. Performance of afirma gene sequencing classifier versus gene expression classifier in thyroid nodules with indeterminate cytology. J Am Soc Cytopathol 2022;11:74–8.

71. Kong D, Zhang J, Shan W, et al. Evaluation of radiomics models based on computed tomography for distinguishing between benign and malignant thyroid nodules. J Comput Assist Tomogr 2022;46: 978–85.

72. Wong CM, Kezlarian BE, Lin O. Current status of machine learning in thyroid cytopathology. J Pathol Inform 2023;14:100309.

73. Alabrak MMA, Megahed M, Alkhouly AA, et al. Artificial intelligence role in subclassifying cytology of thyroid follicular neoplasm. Asian Pac J Cancer Prev 2023;24:1379–87.

74. Hirokawa M, Niioka H, Suzuki A, et al. Application of deep learning as an ancillary diagnostic tool for thyroid FNA cytology. Cancer Cytopathol 2023;131:217–25.

Urinary Tract Cytopathology
Current and Future Impact on Patient Care

Merce Jorda, MD, PhD, MBA[a],*, Oleksandr N. Kryvenko, MD[b],
Fiona Hanly, MS[c], Yiqin Zuo, MD, PhD[d]

KEYWORDS

- The paris system • TPS • Urine cytology • Diagnostic synergy • Ancillary studies
- Artificial intelligence

Key points

- Urine cytology is a simple, non-invasive, cost-efficient, and sensitive test to detect high-grade urothelial carcinoma.

- The Paris System for Reporting Urinary Cytology is a standardized, evidence-based system focused on detecting high-grade urothelial carcinoma.

- The integration of urine cytology and tissue sample findings is important to avoid false negative and false positive results.

- Recent advances in artificial intelligence-assisted solutions may provide a more objective evaluation of criteria by developing automated computational models to assist using The Paris System.

ABSTRACT

Urine cytology is a non-invasive, cost-efficient, and sensitive test to detect high-grade urothelial carcinoma. The Paris System (TPS) for Reporting Urinary Cytology is an evidence-based system that uses the risk of malignancy to guide patient management. Since its inception, TPS has standardized urine cytology reports, facilitating communication among pathologists and between pathologists and clinicians. It is imperative to correlate the urine cytology findings with the concurrent tissue sample to avoid false-negative and false-positive results when possible. Several ancillary tests and artificial intelligence algorithms are being developed to increase the accuracy of urine cytology interpretation.

INTRODUCTION

Urine cytology is a non-invasive, cost-efficient, and sensitive test used to detect high-grade urothelial carcinoma (HGUC).[1] There are several clinical settings where urine cytology is indicated,

---

[a] Department of Pathology & Laboratory Medicine, Desai Sethi Urology Institute, Sylvester Comprehensive Cancer Center, University of Miami Miller School of Medicine, 1400 Northwest 12th Avenue, Miami, FL 33136, USA; [b] Department of Radiation Oncology, Sylvester Comprehensive Cancer Center, University of Miami Miller School of Medicine, 1400 Northwest 12th Avenue, Miami, FL 33136, USA; [c] University of Miami Miller School of Medicine, 1400 Northwest 12th Avenue, Miami, FL 33136, USA; [d] Department of Pathology & Laboratory Medicine, Sylvester Comprehensive Cancer Center, University of Miami Miller School of Medicine, 1400 Northwest 12th Avenue, Miami, FL 33136, USA
* Corresponding author. Department of Pathology & Laboratory Medicine, University of Miami Miller School of Medicine, Miami, Florida. 1400 Northwest 12th Avenue, Room 4061, Miami, FL 33136.
E-mail address: mjorda@med.miami.edu

Surgical Pathology 17 (2024) 383–394
https://doi.org/10.1016/j.path.2024.06.001
1875-9181/24/© 2024 Elsevier Inc. All rights reserved, including those for text and data mining, AI training, and similar technologies.

the most relevant being at the initial evaluation of unexplained hematuria and the follow-up of patients with a previous diagnosis of urothelial cancer.[2] Bladder cancer is the most prevalent urothelial malignancy, whereas upper urinary tract cancers are less frequent.[3] Bladder urothelial carcinoma most often presents as a non-muscle invasive disease, either of low-grade or high-grade. The recurrence rate of non-muscle invasive urothelial carcinoma after initial therapy is high and the cancer may progress to muscle-invasive disease.[4] Urine cytology has low sensitivity in detecting low-grade urothelial carcinoma (LGUC), however, it performs well in detecting HGUC[5,6]; hence, positive urine cytology should be further investigated regardless of biopsy results.[1] Despite urine cytology's proven value in the diagnosis of HGUC, the lack of standardized diagnostic and reporting criteria has been the cause of its low credibility among urologists. This perception changed after the implementation of The Paris System for Reporting Urinary Cytology in 2015.[7]

THE PARIS SYSTEM OF REPORTING RINARY CYTOLOGY

During the 2013 International Congress of Cytology in Paris, and with the support from both the International Academy of Cytology and the American Society of Cytopathology, several committees were formed with the goal of forming an international consensus on reporting urinary tract cytology samples. In late 2015, the consensus group published its guidelines, known as The Paris System (TPS) for Reporting Urinary Cytology.[7] TPS is a standardized, evidence-based system applicable to either voided or instrumented specimens and for specimens sampled from both the lower and upper urinary tract. As with any other standardized reporting system, the main purpose was to collect, examine, and utilize evidence-based data regarding the risk of malignancy (ROM) to guide patient management. TPS was developed to standardize reporting, facilitating communication among pathologists and between pathologists and clinicians.[7–9]

Genomic studies have identified 2 separate urothelial carcinoma pathways associated with 2 distinct molecular signatures: LGUC, associated with good prognosis and low chance of progression, and HGUC, associated with high incidence of recurrence, high rate of progression, and elevated mortality rate.[10,11] In this context, TPS has been a significant step forward in better

reporting urine cytology because its main focus is the most clinically important diagnosis—HGUC. From its implementation, TPS has proven to enhance correlation with histology, especially in the lower urinary tract, while decreasing the "atypical" or "indeterminate" diagnoses.[12–16] The first edition of TPS (TPS-1.0) comprised 7 diagnostic categories: non-diagnostic/unsatisfactory, negative for high-grade urothelial carcinoma (NHGUC), atypical urothelial cells (AUC), suspicious for high-grade urothelial carcinoma (SHGUC), HGUC, low-grade urothelial neoplasm (LGUN), and other primary or secondary malignancies.[7] The diagnostic criteria of TPS 1.0 are displayed in **Table 1**.[7] The frequency of each diagnostic category is extremely variable and depends primarily on the patient population. The initial estimates of ROM for TPS-1.0 were based on pre-TPS-1.0 published data. The Paris Group understood that once TPS came into use, the ROM for each category would change with new data. An international panel of experts in the field of urine cytopathology conducted a survey supported by the American Society of Cytopathology to seek opinions, gather evidence, and identify practice patterns regarding urine cytology before and after the introduction of TPS-1.0.[17] Results from this survey were utilized in the development of the second edition of TPS (TPS-2.0). TPS 2.0 included modifications of the diagnostic criteria to enhance sensitivity.[18] The diagnostic criteria of the TPS-2.0 are displayed in **Table 1**.[18] Like TPS-1.0, TPS-2.0 focuses on the detection of HGUC. The main changes from TPS-1.0 were in the diagnoses of AUC and HGUC. In the TPS-2.0, the major criterion for the diagnosis of AUC was defined as the presence of non-superficial and non-degenerated urothelial cells with an increased nuclear-to-cytoplasmic (N/C) ratio (=> 0.5) secondary to nuclear enlargement. The "nuclear enlargement" was added after observing that the enlarged nuclear size, and not only the increased N/C ratio (=> 0.5), could increase the positive predictive value for the diagnosis of AUC.[19] About the changes in the diagnostic criteria for HGUC, they were intended to tackle the existence of HGUC with hypochromatic nuclei,[20] low N/C ratio,[21] and different subtypes of HGUC, such as plasmacytoid and micropapillary.[22] Additionally, the diagnosis of LGUN was included in the category of NHGUC. Unlike TPS-1.0, TPS-2.0 addresses squamous dysplasia/atypia, but it does not include it in the AUC category; TPS-2.0 designates those changes as atypical squamous cells. Finally, TPS-2.0 includes a diagnostic flow algorithm with an emphasis on the N/C ratio as a triage point.

Table 1
Diagnostic criteria of The Paris System 1.0 and 2.0 for all diagnostic categories

Diagnostic Category	Risk of High-Grade Malignancy (ROHM) for TPS 1.0 Categories		Risk of High-Grade Malignancy (ROHM) for TPS 2.0 Categories	
	Diagnostic Criteria	ROM	Diagnostic Criteria	ROHM
Non-diagnostic/ Unsatisfactory	Voided urine <25 mL with ThinPrep <30 mL with SurePath preparations. Acellular (voided urine), <2 well-visualized urothelial cells per high-power field in 10 consecutive high-power fields (instrumented urine) if not atypical, and samples with completley obscured cellularity (voided and instrumented urine)	<5%–10%	Voided urine <25 mL with ThinPrep <30 mL with SurePath preparations. Acellular (voided urine), <2 well-visualized urothelial cells per high-power field in 10 consecutive high-power fields (instrumented urine) if not atypical, and samples with completley obscured cellularity (voided and instrumented urine)	<5%–10%
NHGUC	Benign urothelial, glandular, squamous cells, benign tissue fragments, changes due to instrumentation, lithiasis, polyoma virus, therapy.	0%–10%	Benign urothelial, glandular, squamous cells, benign tissue fragments, changes due to instrumentation, lithiasis, polyoma virus, therapy.	8%–24%
AUC	*Required:* Major Criteria and 1 Minor Criteria *Major criteria:* presence of non-superficial and non-degenerated urothelial cells with N/C ratio (=> 0.5) *Minor criteria:* hyperchromasia, irregular clumpy chromatin, irregular nuclear contours	8%–35%	*Required:* Major Criteria and 1 Minor Criteria *Major criteria:* presence of non-superficial and non-degenerated urothelial cells with increased N/C ratio due to nucleomegaly (=> 0.5) *Minor criteria:* hyperchromasia, irregular clumpy sschromatin, irregular nuclear contours	24%–53%
SHGUC	*Required:* Major Criteria and 1 Minor Criteria *Major criteria:* Few cells (<5–10) non-superficial and non-degenerated urothelial cells with N/C ratio (>0.7) and hyperchromasia *Minor criteria:* irregular clumpy chromatin, irregular nuclear contours	50%–90%	*Required:* Major Criteria and 2 Minor Criteria *Major criteria:* Few cells (<5–10) non-superficial and non-degenerated urothelial cells with high N/C ratio (>0.7) *Minor criteria:* hyperchromasia, irregular clumpy chromatin, irregular nuclear contours	59%–94%
Positive for HGUC	*Required:* Major Criteria and 1 Minor Criteria *Major Criteria:* Many cells (<10) non-superficial and non-degenerated urothelial cells with N/C ratio (>0.7) and hyperchromasia *Minor Criteria:* irregular clumpy chromatin, irregular nuclear contours	>90%	*Required:* Major Criteria and 2 Minor Criteria *Major Criteria:* Many cells (<10) non-superficial and non-degenerated urothelial cells with high N/C ratio (>0.7) *Minor criteria:* hyperchromasia, irregular clumpy chromatin, irregular nuclear contours	76%–100%

(continued on next page)

Table 1
(continued)

Diagnostic Category	Risk of High-Grade Malignancy (ROHM) for TPS 1.0 Categories		Risk of High-Grade Malignancy (ROHM) for TPS 2.0 Categories	
	Diagnostic Criteria	ROM	Diagnostic Criteria	ROHM
Low-Grade Urothelial Neoplasm (LGUN)	Presence of fibrovascular cores in instrumented urine samples	appr. 10%	N/A	N/A
Other Malignancies	N/A	>90%	N/A	>90%

Abbreviations: ROHM, risk of high-grade malignancy; ROM, risk of malignancy.

THE DIAGNOSTIC SYNERGY OF BLADDER TISSUE SAMPLES AND URINARY CYTOLOGY

The use of TPS criteria for HGUC has been used globally. In large cohort studies with histology follow-ups, the risk of high-grade malignancy is above 90%, demonstrating its high positive predictive value.[18] Cellblock material can be helpful in a subset of cases, however, TPS-2.0 does not comment on criteria that should be applied to cell blocks. The risk of high-grade malignancy (ROHM) using TPS-2.0 ranges from 76% to 100%. On the other hand, transurethral resection of bladder tumor (TURBT) is the essential first step in the current algorithm for the management of bladder cancer. However, despite its importance, TURBT has several limitations, including cost, hospitalization, anesthesia, and potential complications.

According to the 2022 WHO Classification of Urinary and Male Genital Tumors (5th edition), urothelial carcinoma exhibits more than 13 subtypes, each with well-defined features, and approximately one-third of consecutive urothelial carcinomas show subtype morphologies and/or divergent differentiation on the resection sample.[23] The current recommendation is to provide an estimated percentage of non-conventional histology for its potential change in patient management. Identifying subtypes can be difficult in small tissue samples and especially in urine cytology since subtypes possess characteristic features that often do not align with the criteria for diagnosing HGUC, as defined by TPS. Therefore, there may be instances of false-negative urine cytology reports in cases with subtype or divergent morphologies.[24]

According to the National Comprehensive Cancer Network Guidelines, version 1.2024, non-muscle invasive bladder cancer can be stratified as low-risk, intermediate-risk, and high-risk, driving patient management.[25] HGUC, despite falling in the intermediate or high-risk category requires intervention, either intravesical therapy or chemotherapy/cystectomy. Thus, increasing the accuracy of urine cytology is of the utmost importance given it is one of the main diagnostic and follow-up methods for this entity.

The impact of TPS on the rate of discrepant cases in the NHGUC category (false negative urine cytology) that had a subsequent diagnosis of HGUC on concurrent tissue samples is not well studied.[26] Likewise, the rate of discrepant cases with a tissue diagnosis of NHGUC (false negative tissue sample) that had concurrent urine cytology showing HGUC is not well known.

False negative urine cytology results are more often preventable (60%) than non-preventable (40%).

Preventable false negative urine cytology results are due to malignant cells obscured by blood, debris, and/or inflammation; paucity of malignant urothelial cells; poor cellular preservation; and interpretative error. TPS aids in decreasing the false negative rate in urine cytology and it does not alter the negative predictive value for detecting HGUC compared to our pre-TPS era.[27] Interpretative errors can occur due to failure to recognize conventional HGUC or non-conventional HGUC subtypes. TPS-1.0 required the presence of hyperchromasia along with N/C ratio >0.7 for the diagnosis of HGUC. However, it is known that a subset of HGUC cases consists of cells with extremely hypochromatic nuclei, with finely rather than coarsely clumped chromatin, and they did not meet TPS-1.0 diagnostic criteria (hyperchromatic, coarsely clumped chromatin).[28] (**Fig. 1**) In TPS-2.0, hyperchromasia is no longer considered a mandatory criterion for diagnosing HGUC. Other interpretative errors can be due to unrecognized non-conventional HGUC subtypes, including plasmacytoid and micropapillary HGUC. Both are aggressive subtypes of HGUC, which are often associated with advanced-stage disease and poor patient outcomes. Both subtypes are chemotherapy-sensitive and much less responsive to intravesical Bacillus-Calmette-Guerin therapy when compared to conventional HGUC.[29] Therefore, its identification has critical diagnostic and therapeutic significance. Plasmacytoid HGUC is characterized by infiltrative, large plasmacytoid cells with hyperchromatic nuclei and irregular nuclear membranes, and most cases do not fit the elevated N/C ratio required as a diagnostic criterion in TPS due to the presence of abundant cytoplasm (**Fig. 2**). Most cases do not fit the AUC, SHGUC, or HGUC categories. Micropapillary HGUC may show both micro papillae and single malignant cells with abundant cytoplasm in urinary cytology, which, again, may not fit the AUC, SHGUC, or HGUC categories.[22] (**Fig. 3**) On the other hand, careful attention is needed to not miss non-urothelial carcinomas in urinary samples (**Fig. 4**).

Non-preventable false negative urine cytology results are caused by urothelial carcinomas that do not shed cells and/or do not significantly involve the mucosal service. The nested subtype of urothelial carcinoma usually does not have a surface component and often presents with small irregularly distributed nests that simulate Von Brunn nests with bland cytology. Therefore, nested subtypes of urothelial carcinoma may be overlooked in urinary cytology.

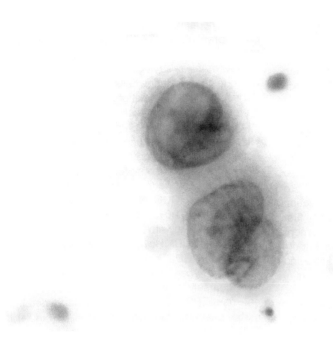

Fig. 1. High-Grade Urothelial Carcinoma: Instrumented urine. The cells display hyperchromasia. [Papanicolaou Stain, Original magnification 60 ×].

False negative bladder tissue results may occur in several clinical settings. Frequently, tissue samples obtained after intravesical therapy may demonstrate abundant denudation, and the HGUC cells may only be present in the urine specimen. In those occasions, urine cytology is the diagnostic gold standard (**Fig. 5**). Additionally, a situation where urine cytology can be the diagnostic method for HGUC is in the setting of in situ urothelial carcinoma (CIS). CIS usually produces positive cytology but is often missed on tissue samples. Given the considerable risk of progression to invasive urothelial carcinoma, its visualization and complete resection during diagnostic tissue sampling and surveillance cystoscopies are crucial to improving outcomes.[30] Of importance is to mention that CIS and papillary HGUC findings are similar in urine cytology (**Fig. 6**). Cystoscopy and tissue sampling are typically performed using traditional white-light cystoscopy, which has limited sensitivity in detecting suspicious lesions. Consequently, enhanced imaging techniques such as Blue-light cystoscopy have been developed showing improvement in detecting non-muscle invasive bladder cancer and increasing detection rates of carcinoma in-situ and papillary lesions.[31]

False positive urine cytology results can be caused by polyoma virus infection; the presence

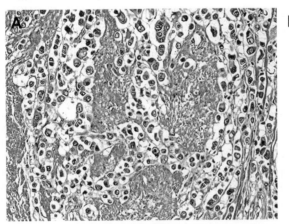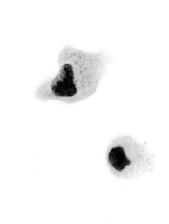

Fig. 2. Urothelial Carcinoma, Plasmacytoid Subtype. (*A*) Single cell infiltrative pattern with large plasmacytoid cells [H&E. Original magnification 40 ×]. (*B*) Instrumented urine with cells with large cytoplasm and not increased nuclear-to-cytoplasmic (N/C) ratio [Papanicolaou Stain, Original magnification 60 ×].

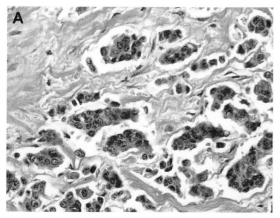
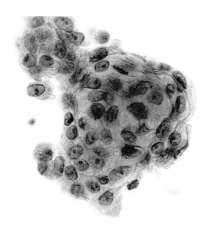

Fig. 3. Urothelial Carcinoma, Micropapillary Subtype. (*A*) Small clusters of tumor cells without fibrovascular surrounded by lacunae [H&E. Original magnification 40 ×]. (*B*) Instrumented urine with Papillary-like groups of urothelial cells with a slightly increased N/C ratio. [Papanicolaou Stain, Original magnification 60 ×].

of basal/intermediate cells; pseudocarcinomatous urothelial hyperplasia; and nephrogenic adenoma. In cases *of polyomavirus (Simian virus)* infection, the infected cells have a high N/C ratio, but the nuclei are round, and the nuclear membrane is smooth. Ground glass inclusions diagnostic of *polyomavirus* are present. Cells with those characteristics, despite having a high N/C ratio, are categorized as NHGUC in TPS-2.0.[18] In case of doubt, immunohistochemistry for SV40 can be utilized to avoid a false positive diagnosis of HGUC. *The presence of basal/intermediate cells*, which may appear to have an increased N/C ratio, may also be a reason for a false positive urine cytology result. In those cases, however, the cells have

fine chromatin, smooth nuclear contours, and monotony of cellular population, and therefore, would not fulfill TPS criteria for AUC, SHGUC, or HGUC.[18] The cells would also lack a nucleomegaly. *Pseudocarcinomatous urothelial hyperplasia* architecturally and cytologically mimics cancer and consists of a reactive urothelial proliferation with a pseudo-infiltrative growth pattern that can mimic invasive urothelial carcinoma.[32] In a sizable proportion of cases, the cells exhibited mild nuclear hyperchromasia, irregular nuclear membrane, and increased N: C ratio (>0.5) or variable combinations thereof, triggering an AUCs and HGUC diagnosis (**Fig. 7**).[33] Finally, *nephrogenic adenoma* is another potential pitfall that may

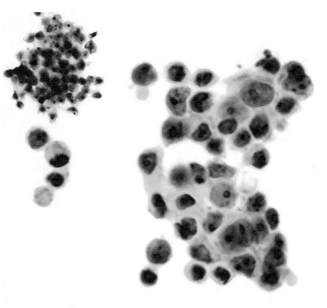

Fig. 4. Prostatic adenocarcinoma. Instrumented urine with cells exhibiting nucleoli, and they are positive for NKX3.1. [Papanicolaou-Stained smear. Original magnification 60 × and NKX3.1 immunocytochemistry].

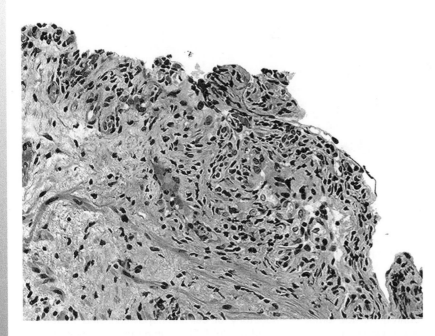

Fig. 5. High-grade urothelial carcinoma. Transurethral resection with complete denudation. [H&E. Original magnification 40 ×].

provide a false positive diagnosis in urine cytology. The cytologic findings may overlap with those of reactive and neoplastic conditions of the urothelium. Immunocytochemistry for PAX8 and Napsin A has been described as having high sensitivity and specificity for the diagnosis of this entity and can be used in urine cytology preparations (**Fig. 8**). However, some studies may suggest that previously described cytologic characteristics of this entity are not distinctive and may not represent lesional cells in urine samples.[34]

ANCILLARY STUDIES IN URINARY CYTOLOGY

Today, urine cytology and cystoscopy with tissue sampling are the gold standard for the diagnosis of urothelial carcinoma. However, each diagnostic method individually, and when combined, may still fail to diagnose a substantial number of patients with urothelial cancer. It is highly desirable to develop tests with sufficient negative predictive value to reduce the frequency of surveillance procedures.[35] Several US Food and Drug Administration (FDA)-approved assays now exist to diagnose urothelial carcinoma. They can be based on cytologic preparations (cell-based tests), or in non-morphological analysis of urinary fluids (liquid-based tests). Cell-based tests allow for the result to be directly correlated with cytomorphologic findings, but only if the cells of interest are present. This may potentially place those tests at a similar disadvantage as urinary tract cytology, affecting their sensitivity value. On the other hand, liquid-based tests do not require an additional slide to be prepared, and they may even be implemented as point-of-care testing. Some tests detect the expression of altered or abnormally expressed subcellular material (proteins, DNA, RNA, etc.) often disassociated from the tumor cells, and that may have a positive result even if tumor cells are absent in the tested specimen. Additionally, liquid-based test results are mostly available to the urologist but not to the cytopathologist, prohibiting integration with the cytomorphology.[35] Of the cell-based tests, UroVysion fluorescence in situ hybridization (U-FISH; Abbott Laboratories, Abbot Park, II, USA) is the one more frequently used. U-FISH is a multitarget fluorescence in situ hybridization assay that combines centromeric probes to chromosomes 3, 7, and 17 with a locus-specific probe to band 9p21. In a meta-analysis study, the sensitivity and specificity of FISH were 72% and 83%, respectively, as compared with 42% and 96%, respectively, for urinary cytology.[36] Overall performance varies between laboratories, and its utility is considered controversial due to the high cost and low positive predictive value when applied to unselected patients with hematuria. However, U-FISH could have a future role in patients with atypical cytology and equivocal or negative cystoscopy.

At the molecular level, muscle-invasive urothelial carcinoma is a heterogeneous disease characterized by genomic instability and a high mutation rate. The WHO 2022 Classification of Urinary and Male Genital Tumors (5th edition)[23] highlights the potential impact of the novel molecular taxonomy on the diagnosis and future management of urinary

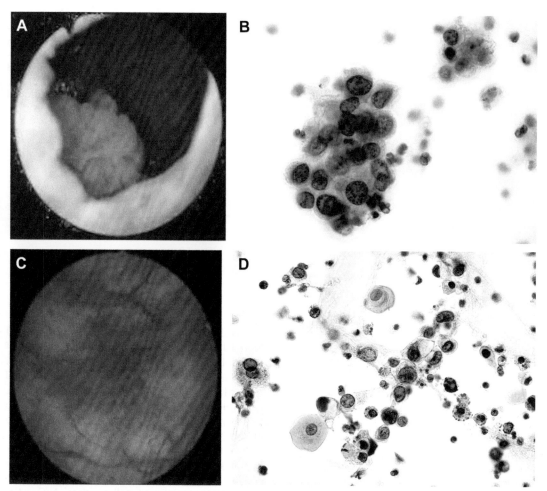

Fig. 6. High-grade urothelial carcinoma. (*A*) Cystoscopy with papillary tumor. (*B*) Instrumented urine with high-grade urothelial carcinoma [Papanicolaou-stained smear. Original magnification 60 ×]; (*C*) Cystoscopy with erythematous lesion suggestive of in situ urothelial carcinoma. (*D*) Instrumented urine with high-grade urothelial carcinoma [Papanicolaou-stained smear. Original magnification 60 ×].

tract cancers. In 2020, an international multidisciplinary team of experts reconciled the published classification schemes in a "Consensus Molecular Classification of Muscle-invasive Bladder Cancer" and concluded that data were insufficient to support the routine use of molecular subtyping to guide bladder cancer management at that time.[37] The molecular subtypes of bladder cancer include 3 subgroups within the luminal subtype, stroma-rich, basal-squamous, and a distinct neuronal cluster, for a total of 6 subtypes.[38] In a more simplistic approach, cluster analysis enables the grouping of non-neuronal- associated muscle-invasive urothelial carcinoma into 2 major subtypes, luminal, and basal, which also differ in their immunohistochemistry profiles. Markers of urothelial luminal differentiation are GATA3, keratin 20, Uroplakin, FGFR3, FOXA1, and PPARG, while keratin 5/6,

keratin 14, CD44, desmocollins, and desmogleins are markers of basal subtype.[23] Initial immunohistochemical subtyping studies using a limited antibody panel demonstrated that immunophenotyping is a feasible and cost-effective method for detecting subtypes of invasive bladder cancer.[38] Non-invasive urothelial carcinomas are predominantly luminal subtype. Incorporating immunohistochemical panels into daily urine cytology sign-out will be soon a cost-effective approach developed by the consensus classification.

Recent studies have shown that bladder-specific next-generation sequencing panels may increase the sensitivity and specificity of urine cytology for the diagnosis of low-grade and high-grade urothelial carcinomas and may serve as a noninvasive surveillance method in the follow-up of patients with urothelial carcinoma.[39]

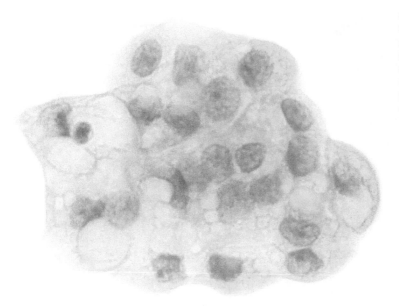

Fig. 7. Pseudocarcinomatous Urothelial Hyperplasia. Instrumented urine with cells with nuclear hyperchromasia, irregular nuclear membrane, and increased N:C ratio (>0.5) [Papanicolaou Stain, Original magnification 60 ×].

ARTIFICIAL INTELLIGENCE APPLIED TO URINE CYTOLOGY

Recent advances in artificial intelligence (AI)-assisted solutions may provide a more objective evaluation of criteria by developing automated computational models to assist cytotechnologists and cytopathologists using TPS. Machine learning has been used in cytopathology with the automation-assisted screening of the Papanicolaou test for cervical cancers, which was one of the first and most successful clinical applications of machine learning in pathology.[40] Recent AI works have focused on whole slide images of gynecologic and non-gynecologic cytopathology. Deep-learning algorithms that use artificial neural networks have produced superior results. Recently, some studies applied AI technology to urine cytology for computational and quantitative analysis of urine cytology with promising results. A recent study successfully developed a deep-learning-based algorithm to automatically classify AUCs into low-risk and high-risk categories, with quantitative analysis of cell number, N/C ratio,

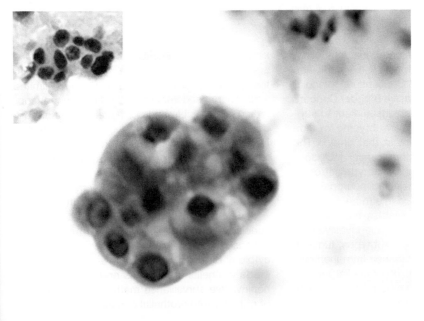

Fig. 8. Nephrogenic Adenoma. Instrumented urine with vacuolated polygonal cells arranged in small groups [Papanicolaou-stained smear. Original magnification 60 ×]; PAX-8 positive [PAX-8 immunostaining on smear. Original magnification 60 ×].

and nuclear size, using whole-slide images for urine cytology. This initial study demonstrated that using the AI algorithm effectively supported the clinical workflow of urine cytology reporting based on TPS criteria.[41]

CLINICS CARE POINTS

- The diagnosis of high-grade urothelial carcinoma requires intervention, either intravesical therapy or chemotherapy/cystectomy.
- Thus, increasing the accuracy of urine cytology is of the utmost importance given it is one of the main diagnostic and follow-up methods for this entity.

DISCLOSURE

The authors have nothing to disclose.

REFERENCES

1. Bastacky S, Ibrahim S, Wilczynski SP, et al. The accuracy of urinary cytology in daily practice. Cancer 1999;87:118e128.
2. Van den Bussche CJ. A Review of the Paris System for Reporting Urinary Cytology. Cytopathology 2016; 27:153–6.
3. Sung H, Ferlay J, Siegel RL, et al. Global Cancer Statistics 2020: GLOBOCAN Estimates of Incidence and Mortality Worldwide for 36 Cancers in 185 Countries. CA Cancer J. Clin 2021;71:209–49.
4. Gupta M, VandenBussche CJ, Bivalacqua TJ. Urinary Cytology and the Paris System for Reporting Urinary Cytology: Implications for Urological Management. Cytopathology 2018;29:368–70.
5. Barkan GA, Wojcik EM. Genitourinary cytopathology (kidney and urinary tract). Cancer Treat Res 2014; 160:149e183.
6. McIntire PJ, Khan R, Hussain H, et al. Negative predictive value and sensitivity of urine cytology prior to implementation of The Paris System for Reporting Urinary Cytology. Cancer Cytopathol 2019;127:125e131.
7. Rosenthal DL, Wojcik E, Kurtycz DF. The Paris System for reporting urinary cytology. 1st edition. New York: Springer; 2015.
8. Barkan GA, Wojcik EM, Nayar R, et al. The Paris System for Reporting Urinary Cytology: the quest to develop a standardized terminology. Acta Cytol 2016;60:185e197.
9. Cowan ML, VandenBussche CJ. The Paris System for Reporting Urinary Cytology: Early Review of the Literature Reveals Successes and Rare Shortcomings. J. Am. Soc. Cytopathol 2018;7:185–94.
10. Wu XR. Urothelial tumorigenesis: a tale of divergent pathways. Nat Rev Cancer 2005;5:713e725.
11. Knowles MA, Hurst CD. Molecular biology of bladder cancer: new insights into pathogenesis and clinical diversity. Nat Rev Cancer 2015;15:25e41.
12. Bertsch EC, Siddiqui MT, Ellis CL. The Paris System for Reporting Urinary Cytology Improves Correlation with Surgical Pathology Biopsy Diagnoses of the Lower Urinary Tract. Diagn Cytopathol 2018;46:221–7.
13. Torous VF, Brancely D, VanderLaan PA. Implementation of the Paris System for Reporting Urinary Cytology Results in Lower Atypical Diagnostic Rates. J. Am. Soc. Cytopathol 2017;6:205–10.
14. Hang J-F, Charu V, Zhang ML, et al. Digital Image Analysis Supports a Nuclear-to-Cytoplasmic Ratio Cutoff Value of 0.5 for Atypical Urothelial Cells. Cancer Cytopathol 2017;125:710–6.
15. Rohra P, Ocampo Gonzalez FA, Yan L, et al. Effect of the Paris System for Reporting Urinary Cytology with Histologic Follow-Up. Diagn Cytopathol 2021;49:691–9.
16. Tian W, Shore KT, Shah RB. Significant Reduction of Indeterminate (atypical) Diagnosis after Implementation of The Paris System for Reporting Urinary Cytology: A Single-Institution Study of More than 27,000 Cases. Cancer Cytopathol 2021;129:114–20.
17. Kurtycz DFI, Wojcik EM, Rosenthal DL. Perceptions of Paris: an international survey in preparation for The Paris System for Reporting Urinary Cytology 2.0 (TPS 2.0). J Am Soc Cytopathol 2024;12:66–74.
18. Wojcik EM, Kurtycz DFI, Rosenthal DL. The Paris System for reporting urinary cytology. 2nd edition. New York: Springer; 2022.
19. Vosoughi A, Ordobazari A, Lora-Gonzalez M, et al. The Paris System "atypical urothelial cells" category: can the current criteria be improved? J Am Soc Cytopathol 2021;10:3–8.
20. Pierconti F, Martini M, Straccia P, et al. Hypochromatic Large Urothelial Cells in Urine Cytology Are Indicative of High-Grade Urothelial Carcinoma. APMIS 2018;126:705–9.
21. Kurtycz DFI, Sundling KE, Barkan GA. The Paris System of Reporting Urinary Cytology: Strengths and Opportunities. Diagn. Cytopathol 2020;48:890–5.
22. Suo L, Vega I, Thrall M. Cyto-histo correlations of plasmacytoid and micropapillary variants of high-grade urothelial carcinoma: do they fit well in the paris system for reporting urinary cytology? J. Am. Soc. Cytopathol 2021;10:20–4.
23. Urinary and Male Genital Tumours. WHO classification of tumors. 5th edition. Lyon, France: International Agency for Research on Cancer; 2022.
24. Arshia A, Hassan FA, Hensley PJ, et al. Urinary tract cytology showing variant morphology and divergent differentiation. Cytopathology 2024;35:199–212.

25. NCCN Guidelines Version 1.2024. Non-Muscle Invasive Bladder Cancer bladder. Guidelines Detail (nccn.org) Accessed February 24, 2024.

26. Yuan L, Gero M, Zia S, et al. Cyto-histo correlation and false-negative urine: Before and after the Paris system for reporting urinary cytology. Diagn Cytopathol 2023;51:744–50.

27. McIntire P, Kilic I, Pambuccian S, et al. The Paris System for Reporting Urinary Cytology reduces atypia rates and does not alter the negative predictive value of urine cytology. J Am Soc Cytopathol 2021; 10:14–9.

28. Renshaw A, Gould E. High-grade urothelial carcinoma with hypochromatic chromatin in urine cytology. J Am Soc Cytopathol 2021;10:25–8.

29. Lobo N, Shariat SF, Guo CC, et al. What Is the significance of variant histology in urothelial carcinoma? Eur Urol Focus 2020;6:653e–63e.

30. Chang SS, Boorjian SA, Chou R, et al. Diagnosis and treatment of non-muscle invasive bladder cancer: AUA/SUO guideline. J Urol 2016;196(4):1021–9.

31. Cahilla EM, Chuab K, Doppalapudib SK, et al. The use of blue-light cystoscopy in the detection and surveillance of non-muscle invasive bladder cancer. Curr Urol 2022;16:121–6.

32. Pseudocarcinomatous urothelial hyperplasia of the bladder: clinical findings and follow-up of 70 patients. Kryvenko ON, Epstein JI. J Urol 2013 Jun; 189(6):2083–6.

33. Velez Torres JM, Lora Gonzalez M, Martinez Duarte E, et al. Urine Cytology Findings in Cases of Pseudocarcinomatous Urothelial Hyperplasia of the Bladder Often Represent a Diagnostic Challenge. Arch Pathol Lab Med 2023;147:716–21.

34. McCroskey Z, Pambuccian SE, Wojcik EM, et al. Can We Identify Nephrogenic Adenoma in Urine Cytology Specimens? Am J Clin Pathol 2016;145:373–8.

35. Allison DB, VandenBussche ChJ. A review of urine ancillary tests in the era of the paris system. Acata Cytol 2020;64:182–92.

36. Hajdinjak T. UroVysion FISH test for detecting urothelial cancers: Meta-analysis of diagnostic accuracy and comparison with urinary cytology testing. Seminars and Original Investigations 2008;26:646–51.

37. Kamoun A, de Reynies A, Allory Y, et al. Bladder Cancer Molecular Taxonomy Group. A consensus molecular classification of muscle-invasive bladder cancer. Eur Urol 2020;77:420–33.

38. Terlevic R, Ulamec M, Stimac G, et al. Molecular classification of muscle-invasive bladder cancer based on a simplified immunohistochemical panel using GATA3, CK5/6, and p16. Biomolecules and Biomedicine 2023;23:968–75.

39. Sun T, Hutchinson L, Tomaszewicz K, et al. A bladder-specific NGS panel increases the sensitivity and specificity of urine cytology's diagnostic utility in both low- and high-grade tumors and may serve as a noninvasive surveillance method in the follow-up of patients with UC harboring known mutations. Cancer Cytopathol 2021;129:537–47.

40. Landau MS, Pantanowitz L. Artificial intelligence in cytopathology: a review of the literature and overview of commercial landscape. J Am Soc Cytopathol 2019;8:230–324.

41. Ou Y, Tsao TY, Chang M, et al. Evaluation of an artificial intelligence algorithm for assisting the Paris System in reporting urinary cytology: A pilot study. Cancer Cytopathol 2022;130:872–80.

Pulmonary Cytopathology
Current and Future Impact on Patient Care

Jonas J. Heymann, MD[a],*, Danielle D'Ambrosio, MD[b],
Katya S. Dombrowski, MD[c], Niyati Desai, MD[d],
Peter B. Illei, MD[c]

KEYWORDS

- Lung cancer • Fine needle aspiration • Cytology • Cytopathology • Small biopsy
- Pulmonary cytopathology • Molecular testing • Predictive biomarkers

---

Key points

- Previously developed professional society guidelines for evaluation of cytopathology specimens derived from lung, as well as systems for nomenclature and reporting the results of such evaluations are rapidly being replaced and updated.

- Development of new modalities of procurement necessitate that cytopathologists recognize a broad range of morphologic features for lung malignancies.

- In order to optimize targeted and other therapy in patients for whom primary lung tumor resection is unavailable, it is necessary to detect a broad range of genetic alterations.

- Ancillary studies available to detect genetic alteration range from immunohistochemistry and immunocytochemistry through in situ hybridization and polymerase chain reaction to next-generation sequencing.

- Professional society guidelines for effective tissue utilization in small lung biopsy samples have recently become available.

ABSTRACT

Small biopsies of lung are routinely obtained by many methods, including several that result in cytologic specimens. Because lung cancer is often diagnosed at a stage for which primary resection is not an option, it is critical that all diagnostic, predictive, and prognostic information be derived from such small biopsy specimens. As the number of available diagnostic and predictive markers expands, cytopathologists must familiarize themselves with current requirements for specimen acquisition, handling, results reporting, and molecular and other ancillary testing, all of which are reviewed here.

OVERVIEW

Lung cancer is the most common cause of cancer-related death in both men and women. Most tumors are diagnosed at a stage for which surgical

---

[a] Department of Pathology and Laboratory Medicine, New York–Presbyterian Hospital–Weill Cornell Medicine, 1300 York Avenue, New York, NY 10065, USA; [b] Department of Pathology, New York University Grossman School of Medicine, 560 First Avenue, New York, NY 10016, USA; [c] Department of Pathology, The Johns Hopkins University School of Medicine, 600 North Wolfe Street, Baltimore, MD 21287, USA; [d] Department of Pathology and Cell Biology, New York–Presbyterian Hospital–Columbia University Irving Medical Center, 630 West 168th Street, New York, NY 10032, USA
* Corresponding author.
E-mail address: jjh7002@med.cornell.edu

Surgical Pathology 17 (2024) 395–410
https://doi.org/10.1016/j.path.2024.06.002
1875-9181/24/© 2024 Elsevier Inc. All rights are reserved, including those for text and data mining, AI training, and similar technologies.

resection provides maximal benefit only after neo-adjuvant therapy or at a stage too advanced for surgical resection to provide clinical benefit at all. For patients with such tumors, therapeutic options depend almost entirely on the diagnostic, predictive, and prognostic information derived from small biopsies, including cytopathology specimens.

It is useful for cytopathologists to be aware of previous ("old") guidelines, as they have informed the development of updated ("new") guidelines. This is particularly true in the case of molecular testing (MT), which has been used to identify biomarkers that predict response or resistance of adenocarcinoma (ADCA) and other forms of non–small cell carcinoma (NSCLCA) to specific therapeutic agents. Guidelines have been and remain clear that traditional cytomorphology and immunohistochemistry (IHC) should inform pathologists' choice of MT. New guidelines, in particular, highlight the importance of tissue triage and specimen preparation and selection for various MT modalities. Such guidelines have and continue to inform the current and future impact of pulmonary cytopathology on patient care.

Herein, the authors briefly review past and current guidelines for handling cytology and other small biopsy specimens while paying special attention to new techniques for specimen acquisition, result reporting, and MT. This includes the World Health Organization (WHO) Reporting System for Lung Cytopathology, which is the most recently published reporting system at the time of article publication. Quantification of programmed cell death ligand-1 (PD-L1) expression on primary lung carcinoma cells is beyond the scope of this review, and it will only be reviewed briefly.

PREVIOUS GUIDELINES

ANCILLARY STUDIES IN THE CYTOLOGIC DIAGNOSIS OF RESPIRATORY LESIONS

The Papanicolaou Society of Cytopathology (PSC) published a set of guidelines for the utilization of ancillary studies for respiratory cytology specimens in 2016.[1] Their guidelines included specimens that typically yield scant material, such as sputum, bronchial washings, and bronchial brushings, in addition to typically higher-yield transthoracic, computed tomography (CT) -guided, and transbronchial fine needle aspiration biopsies (FNA). The last of these at the time included only endobronchial ultrasound-guided (EBUS) FNA. The PSC also included recommendations for classification, microbiologic culture, immunocytochemistry (ICC) and IHC, molecular techniques,

and postdiagnosis management and follow-up. Recommendations were reached by consensus among members of a committee based on expertise, literature review, and external feedback.

Among the 9 recommendations were several anticipated recommendations from other organizations that form the current basis of pulmonary cytopathology practice. Notably, the PSC recommended that to preserve tissue in cases of NSCLCA for subsequent MT, preferably one marker of ADCA and one for squamous cell carcinoma (SCCA) should be selected. Furthermore, MT could be performed on cell blocks (CBs) or direct smear preparations following appropriate validation. The significance of such recommendations would grow as additional molecular targets were identified in subsequent years.

TARGETED TREATMENT OF LUNG CANCER

The College of American Pathologists (CAP), Association for Molecular Pathology (AMP), and International Association for the Study of Lung Cancer (IASLC) jointly published a set of MT guidelines for selection of patients with lung cancer for treatment with targeted tyrosine kinase inhibitors (TKIs) in 2018.[2–4] Their guidelines were endorsed shortly thereafter by the American Society of Clinical Oncology (ASCO), albeit with slight modifications.[5] After extensive literature review, an expert CAP/AMP/IASLC panel developed recommendations to address a discrete set of specific questions and provided the strength of each recommendation.

Among the 5 recommendations and 10 expert consensus opinions were several anticipated recommendations from other organizations that form the current basis of pulmonary cytopathology practice. Notably, per CAP/AMP/IASLC guidelines, pathologists may use either CBs *or other cytologic preparations* as suitable specimens for MT (ASCO also endorsed CBs *or smear preparations*, specifically). Furthermore, per CAP/AMP/IASLC guidelines, *EGFR*, *ALK*, and *ROS1* testing *must* be performed for all patients with lung ADCA, whereas *BRAF*, *MET*, *RET*, *ERBB2*, and *KRAS should* be included in any expanded testing panel, if adequate material is available. Importantly, ASCO instead included *BRAF* in its list of genes that *must* be tested, highlighting the rapid pace of discovery that would need to be addressed by professional society guidelines in subsequent years.

In addition, disease-specific guidelines published by the National Comprehensive Cancer Network (NCCN) include recommendations for biomarker testing that are reviewed and, if needed, revised on a regular basis (several times a year). The NCCN guidelines are considered most up-to-date and followed by most oncologists in the United States (see emerging techniques: molecular testing, in later discussion).

PROGRAMMED CELL DEATH PROTEIN-1 IMMUNOHISTOCHEMISTRY

Immune checkpoint blockade (ICB) has become a therapeutic option for patients with numerous tumors across organ systems, including small cell lung carcinoma (SCLCA) and NSCLCA lacking targetable driver alterations.[6] The most commonly used ICB agents for such tumors target programmed cell death protein-1 (PD-1) or its ligand, PD-L1.[7] Multiple biomarkers have been proposed to predict response to PD-1/PD-L1 inhibition with variable success, which presents pathologists and clinicians alike with predictive and therapeutic uncertainty. In addition, the most commonly used biomarker of response is the percent of tumor cells expressing any level of membranous PD-L1 by IHC also referred to as "tumor proportion score," which has been shown to be both temporally and spatially heterogenous,[8] and for which multiple different assays may be applied across different platforms. The full complexity of the preanalytical, analytical, and postanalytical aspects of PD-L1 testing is beyond the scope of this review, and it will be reviewed only briefly.

IHC assays designed to predict response to PD-1/PD-L1 inhibition were not developed in tandem. Rather, each was developed as a complementary/companion diagnostic IHC test for a specific ICB agent. The Blueprint Project was an industrial-academic collaborative partnership to compare commercially available PD-L1 IHC assays. In its first phase, the Blueprint collaborators found that the percentage of PD-L1–stained tumor cells was comparable for 3 assays (22C3, 28-8, and SP263), whereas a fourth assay (SP142) exhibited fewer stained tumor cells.[9] A pair of harmonization studies published at approximately the same time had only slightly different findings.[10,11] In its second phase, the Blueprint collaborators found that a fifth assay (73-10) stained a *greater* number of tumor cells. Importantly for patients whose tumors have been sampled by cytologic methods only, there was good agreement among pathologists assessing PD-L1 status on CBs,[12] a finding that has been reproduced in subsequent studies.[13–19] In the end, it would be prudent for pathologists to heed the results of a subsequent meta-analysis of head-to-head comparisons of PD-L1 IHC assays that demonstrated the importance of properly validated laboratory-developed tests

when Food and Drug Administration–approved companion diagnostics are not available.[20] There is also one anti-PD-1 ICB agent (pembrolizumab) that has received tumor agnostic approval for patients with tumors harboring high nonsynonymous tumor mutation burden (TMB),[21] a biomarker for which quantification may be feasible on cytology specimens.[22] However, as TMB determination requires broad and deep next-generation sequencing (NGS),[23] and the clinical actionability threshold remains controversial,[24] PD-L1 IHC retains primacy for determination of ICB for the time being. Similarly, pembrolizumab therapy was approved for microsatellite instability (MSI)-high solid tumors irrespective of site of origin, although MSI is vanishingly rare in primary lung carcinoma.

UPDATED GUIDELINES

CLASSIFICATION OF LUNG CARCINOMA IN SMALL BIOPSY AND CYTOLOGY SPECIMENS

To address diagnostic and therapeutic advances specifically in lung ADCA, the IASLC, American Thoracic Society (ATS), and European Respiratory Society (ERS) jointly sponsored development of a new multidisciplinary classification system, which they first published in 2011.[25] The new classification system provided terminology for nonresection (ie, cytologic and other small biopsy) specimens to facilitate a uniform approach to both treatment and clinical trial enrollment. Although detailed, the system particularly emphasized the need for pathologists to provide as specific a morphologic classification as possible with integration of IHC, histochemistry, and MT data. Their classification persisted through the publishing of the 2015 edition of the WHO Classification of Tumors of the Lung, Pleura, Thymus, and Heart[26] and up to the current (2021) edition with only minor modifications.[27] Recommended terminology for cytology specimens is summarized in an abridged form in **Table 1**.

There are idiosyncrasies to the IASLC/ATS/ERS system of which cytopathologists, in particular, should be aware. First and foremost, for primary lung ADCA the IASLC/ATS/ERS recommends listing the morphologic patterns present, a task that is especially difficult in cytologic specimens. Instead, the tumor may be diagnosed as ADCA, possibly with a comment that this may represent, at least in part, ADCA in situ. Similarly, because mucinous ADCA with or without (lepidic pattern) invasion may be especially difficult to specify in cytologic specimens, the tumor may be diagnosed as ADCA "with mucinous features" with a mention

Table 1
Morphologic classification of lung carcinoma in cytology specimens

Morphology/Stains	Terminology for Cytology Specimens	Terminology for Resection Specimens
Morphology only	Squamous cell carcinoma	Squamous cell carcinoma
Morphology only (stains may be used to demonstrate lung origin)	Adenocarcinoma • Adenocarcinoma with lepidic pattern • Adenocarcinoma with mucinous features/mucinous adenocarcinoma • Adenocarcinoma with colloid features • Adenocarcinoma with fetal features • Adenocarcinoma with enteric features	Adenocarcinoma (list at least predominant pattern) • Adenocarcinoma in situ or minimally invasive or invasive adenocarcinoma with a lepidic component • Adenocarcinoma in situ or minimally invasive or invasive adenocarcinoma, mucinous type • Colloid adenocarcinoma • Fetal adenocarcinoma • Enteric adenocarcinoma
Morphology supported by IHC	Non–small cell carcinoma, favor squamous cell carcinoma	Squamous cell carcinoma
Morphology supported by IHC	Non–small cell carcinoma, favor adenocarcinoma	Adenocarcinoma
Morphology with no clear IHC pattern	Non–small cell carcinoma, NOS	Large cell carcinoma
Morphology (may be supported by IHC)	Small cell carcinoma	Small cell carcinoma
Morphology supported by IHC	Non–small cell carcinoma with neuroendocrine morphology and positive neuroendocrine markers, possible large cell neuroendocrine carcinoma	Large cell neuroendocrine carcinoma
Morphology only	Non–small cell carcinoma, NOS • Comment that adenocarcinoma and squamous components are present, and that this could represent adenosquamous carcinoma	Adenosquamous carcinoma (if both components ≥10%)
Morphology supported by IHC	Non–small cell carcinoma, NOS • Specify the results of IHC, and comment that this could represent adenosquamous carcinoma	Adenocarcinoma, squamous cell carcinoma, or large cell carcinoma with unclear immunohistochemical features
Morphology only	Non–small cell carcinoma with spindle cell and/or giant cell carcinoma • Mention if adenocarcinoma or squamous carcinoma is present • Comment that this could represent a pleomorphic carcinoma	Pleomorphic, spindle cell, and/or giant cell carcinoma

Abbreviation: NOS, not otherwise specified.

of the differential diagnosis. Second, neuroendocrine IHC markers should be performed only in cases where there is suspected neuroendocrine morphology. Finally, the IASLC's Cytology Working Group has recently recognized that failure to specify morphologic subtypes is inevitable in some cases, highlighting the necessity of IHC.[28]

STANDARDIZED TERMINOLOGY AND NOMENCLATURE FOR RESPIRATORY CYTOLOGY

In 2016, the PSC proposed a standardized terminology scheme for respiratory cytology that correlates cytologic diagnosis with biologic behavior and patient management.[29] Its classification and terminology scheme recommended a 6-tiered system. Although the Society acknowledged that sensitivities and specificities for malignancy differ among procurement techniques,[30] its system endorsed and incorporated bronchial brushings, bronchial washings, percutaneous FNA, conventional transbronchial FNA, and EBUS FNA. In addition, although the system did not address the use of MT, the PSC suggested that it would be addressed in a subsequent guideline.

The 6-tiered reporting system incorporated "nondiagnostic," "negative (for malignancy)," "atypical," "neoplastic, benign neoplasm, low-grade carcinoma," "suspicious for malignancy," and "malignant" categories. Literature review at the time of publication, which has since been revised,[31] yielded the following respective categorical risks of malignancy (RoM): 40%; 24% to 43%; 54%; not applicable (never before used); 82%; 77% to 100%. The categories also included the following caveats: cytopathologists should provide a specific "benign (negative)" diagnosis whenever practical; assignment to the "benign neoplasm" category may be facilitated by clinical and imaging findings, as well as ancillary testing; reviewer experience is a criterion for assignment to the "suspicious" category; and tumors metastatic or secondary to the lung are included in the "malignant" category. As it was (and still is) the most contentious category, the "neoplastic" category was subdivided into "neoplastic (benign)," which included pulmonary hamartoma, sclerosing pneumocytoma, granular cell tumor, squamous papilloma, and hemangioma and "neoplasm—undetermined malignant potential," which included epithelioid hemangioendothelioma, primary pulmonary meningioma, Langerhans' cell histiocytosis, solitary fibrous tumor, inflammatory myofibroblastic tumor, and myoepithelial neoplasms. PEComa (clear cell sugar tumor) and sclerosing pneumocytoma could be included in either

subdivision. Good data on the extent to which the PSC system was adopted across laboratories are not available.

TOWARD AN INTERNATIONAL CLASSIFICATION FOR RESPIRATORY CYTOLOGY

In 2020, the Japan Lung Cancer Society and Japanese Society of Clinical Cytology proposed a reporting system designed to enhance communication among clinicians and pathologists at different institutions.[32] Their classification and terminology scheme recommended a 4-tiered system, although in their system, nondiagnostic/inadequate cases are not categorized because they are excluded in an initial step. Although the societies proposed that their system be applicable across procurement techniques and preparations, it was validated in a study that included solely alcohol-fixed, Papanicolaou-stained direct smear preparations of a narrow range of specimens, most of which were obtained from bronchial brushing. Interobserver agreement among 7 reviewers was only fair for their 4-tiered reporting system incorporating "negative for malignancy," "atypical cells," "suspicious for malignancy," and "malignancy." However, RoM was stratified evenly across categories.

FUTURE TRENDS: A GLOBALLY APPLICABLE REPORTING SYSTEM FOR LUNG CYTOPATHOLOGY

In 2022, the editorial board of the International Academy of Cytology (IAC) joined that of the International Agency for Research on Cancer (IARC) to develop an international standard for reporting lung cytopathology based on a 5-tiered system.[33,34] Their plans for the standard were ambitious in scope, aiming to facilitate communication with clinicians, provide options for diagnostic management, improve patient care, and facilitate research, beyond simply standardizing the reporting of cytopathology. In addition, the IAC and IARC purported to establish a system that could be used in all medical infrastructure settings, including those in low- and middle-income countries. Accordingly, the system they developed, The WHO Reporting System for Lung Cytopathology, provides recommendations for reporting using a range of cytologic preparations procured by different methods (except pleural effusion fluid procured by thoracentesis, which has its own reporting system) with and without rapid on-site evaluation (ROSE) and assessed with variable levels of access to IHC, ICC, and molecular techniques. In order to facilitate correlation with histology, the cytopathology reporting system is cross-referenced to the fifth edition (2021) of the WHO Classification of Thoracic Tumors[35] and indexed in a similar manner. Finally, the system correlated specific cytomorphologic criteria with both RoM and recommendations for clinical management. The reporting system synthesized expert opinion with literature review, as well as with results of an international survey developed by the IAC but promoted and disseminated by multiple professional societies.

The 5-tiered reporting system incorporates "insufficient/inadequate/nondiagnostic," "benign," "atypical," "suspicious for malignancy," and "malignant" categories that are intended to be used only as part of a structured report that includes demographic information, type of specimen, clinical and imaging information, specific diagnosis, macroscopic description, details of ROSE, microscopic description, and results of ancillary testing. (A working group consisting of members of the IAC and the International Collaboration on Cancer Reporting is currently working but has not yet established which of these represent "core" and which represent "noncore" components of the report.) The joint Editorial Board acknowledged the paucity of evidence for current RoM figures and recommended that it be refined based on future research. Nevertheless, literature review at the time of publication yielded the following respective categorical RoM for FNA specimens: 43% to 53%; 19% to 64%; 46% to 55%; 75% to 88%; 87% to 100%. Literature review yielded a separate set of figures for RoM of sputum, bronchial washing, and bronchial brushing specimens. Furthermore, the "benign" category is subdivided into "inflammatory processes" and "benign neoplastic lesions," whereas the "malignant" category is subdivided into "specific malignant lesions," "neuroendocrine neoplasms," "lymphoproliferative diseases," and "other malignancies." Such complexity renders diagnostic crosswalk between the PSC and WHO reporting systems difficult (Fig. 1).

EMERGING TECHNIQUES: SPECIMEN ACQUISITION

Recent advances in acquisition of cytologic and other small biopsy specimens provide interventional pulmonologists and pulmonary radiologists with a greater number of options for tissue procurement. In order to optimize tissue collection and triage for diagnostic and predictive evaluation, cytopathologists should familiarize themselves with the breadth of specimens they may be called on to assess. As in the past, specimens are generally acquired through one of 3 routes. Transthoracic FNA, often in combination with transthoracic core needle biopsy, has traditionally been used to sample peripheral lung lesions. Bronchoscopic techniques have traditionally been used to sample endobronchial and other centrally located lesions. Newer image-guided platforms enable bronchoscopists to navigate more accurately and farther into the pulmonary parenchyma and to access mediastinal and hilar lymph nodes at the same time. EBUS-guided aspiration biopsy has become standard of care for staging mediastinal lymph nodes. Pleural fluid aspiration is an extremely valuable tool that may provide concurrent therapeutic benefit to patients, but it is beyond the scope of this review. Recommendations for pleural fluid cytology evaluation and implementation have been thoroughly reviewed elsewhere.[36,37]

CT guidance allows for acquisition of FNA, core needle biopsy, or both. Transthoracic FNA allows for performance of ROSE, extraction of tumor cells from a broader area, extraction of higher-quality nucleic acid from liquid-based[38,39] or direct smear[40–42] preparations, and a better safety profile, all potentially without sacrificing diagnostic specificity or ability to conduct MT.[43] Core needle biopsy allows for evaluation and quantification of architectural patterns, particularly in ADCA specimens, and can often provide sufficient tumor samples for enrollment in clinical trials and samples for biomarker testing requiring tissue sections (ie, PD-L1 quantification). If both modalities are used, it is advisable to correlate the findings between them, especially when they are assigned to different pathologists, in order to optimize biomarker testing and harmonize diagnoses in order to prevent confusing clinicians and patients.[44]

Flexible fiber-optic bronchoscopy allows for acquisition of exfoliative or FNA cytology specimens and/or histologic specimens. Exfoliative specimens include bronchial washing and bronchial brushing specimens, which may be obtained with or without fluoroscopic guidance. Biopsy needles are now available in a variety of shapes and sizes that may alternately produce cytologic or histologic specimens. Regardless of the choice of needle, fluoroscopy or ultrasound may be used to guide the bronchoscope to the lesion.[45] More recently, multiple systems collectively marketed under the term "electromagnetic navigation"[46,47] have been developed to aid bronchoscopic navigation to small, peripheral lesions. Such systems use 3-dimensional reconstruction of CT data in combination with low-frequency electromagnetic waves, which are emitted from a device placed under the bronchoscopy table and detected in real

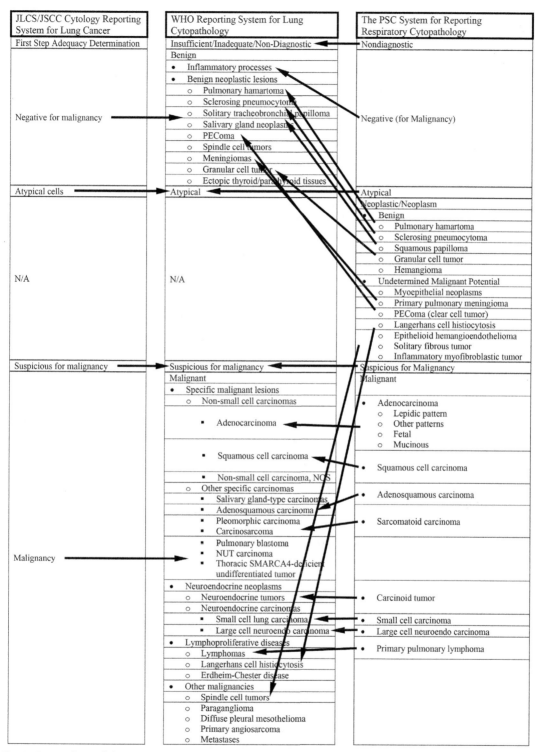

Fig. 1. Comparison of diagnostic categories and subcategories in the joint Japan Lung Cancer Society/Japanese Society of Clinical Cytology (JLCS/JSCC) Cytology System for Reporting Lung Cancer, the WHO Reporting System for Lung Cytopathology, and the PSC System for Reporting Respiratory Cytology. Mapping of entities in the JLCS/JSCC and PSC systems onto those in the WHO system are represented by black arrows, which demonstrate relative complexity of diagnostic crosswalk from the PSC system compared with that from the JLCS/JSCC system.

time. Ultrathin bronchoscopy[48] and radial probe EBUS[49] have also emerged as tools to optimize bronchoscopic tumor sample yield, with variable results.[50]

In order to improve sampling accuracy and diagnostic yield, bronchoscopists have also taken advantage of advances in robotic bronchoscopy.[51] The primary diagnostic advantage of a robotic bronchoscope is increased stability of the bronchoscope.[52] Similar to conventional bronchoscopes, early versions of robotic bronchoscopy lacked real-time guidance. Newer robotic bronchoscopy systems take advantage of additional technologies,[53] including computational correction to preprocedural planning CT ("CT-to-body divergence")[54,55] through intraprocedural tomosynthesis[56,57] with[58] or without[59] artificial intelligence, cone-beam CT,[60–62] or O-arm CT.[63]

EMERGING TECHNIQUES: MOLECULAR TESTING

Cytogenetic and molecular genetic analyses have proved to be among the most powerful of the tools in the pathologists' proverbial toolbox, able to provide diagnostic, predictive, prognostic, and increasingly, quality assurance information and educational feedback.[64–69] Depending on the test used, their results may be difficult to interpret. Therefore, it is important that pathologists deploy them wisely. Because of the often-limited nature of cytologic specimens, choosing wisely is especially important for cytopathologists. There are 3 specific questions cytopathologists may address:

1. What information can I provide to clinicians to help guide therapy (ie, what are the key genetic and/or genomic targets)?
2. What methodology is best suited to interrogating the selected targets?
3. How can I optimize my specimen for the selected methodology?
   Evidence-based answers to these questions in the context of pulmonary cytopathology is most well-developed for NSCLCA in general and ADCA in particular.

Key Molecular Therapeutic Targets

Although diagnostic and prognostic genetic and genomic information may be derived from lung FNA specimens, the primary goal of MT on NSCLCA is to identify alterations that predict response (or resistance) to specific, targeted therapy. Clinical and translational research has and continues to identify novel targets.[70–72] Because approximately two-thirds of patients with NSCLCA

present with advanced stage or otherwise unresectable disease,[73] it is critically important to identify such targets using the cytologic and other small biopsy specimens that often comprise the entirety of diagnostic material. Specific alterations and their clinical relevance have been extensively reviewed previously.[74,75] As of the time of preparation for this review, category 1 and 2A recommended targets identified by the NCCN in advanced stage or unresectable NSCLCA are listed in **Table 2** along with the methodologies by which they may be interrogated. Numerous other investigational targets have been identified, selected examples of which are listed in **Table 3**. With the advent of additional therapies, identification of such alterations will benefit patients with NSCLCA in laboratories equipped to do so.

Methodologies for Interrogation of Molecular Therapeutic Targets

Given the breadth of alterations that may and must be identified to effect optimal care of patients with NSCLCA, it is essential to select methods of MT that can identify a broad range of molecular alterations. NGS is particularly well-suited to this task, as it can identify single-nucleotide variants (SNVs), insertion-deletion mutations (indels), copy number variants (CNVs), and fusions, although it is important to remember that the sensitivity of detection for the last is higher for NGS of RNA than of DNA. NGS may also detect alterations in messenger RNA, microRNA, and methylation patterns, the clinical significance of which are active areas of investigation.[76–79] Fortunately, NGS has been extensively validated on cytologic and other small biopsy specimens.[41,43,80,81]

Alternatives to NGS include ICC, IHC, in situ hybridization (ISH), anchored, multiplex polymerase chain reaction (PCR), and quantitative real-time PCR (qPCR). The various advantages and disadvantages of each method are presented in **Table 4**. At present, ICC and IHC can be used for detection at various levels of sensitivity of a limited set of diagnostic and predictive alterations, including *BRAF* V600E, loss of several members of the SWI/SNF complex (*SMARCA2* [BRM], *SMARCA4* [BRG1], *SMARCB1* [INI1]), and fusions of *NUTM1*, *NTRK1-3*, *ALK*, and *ROS1*, and detection of the last must be confirmed by an orthogonal method. ISH can be used to detect both fusions and CNVs. Unlike NGS, in which multiple genes can be interrogated at once, use of each ISH probe requires an additional cytopreparation or CB section. Anchored, multiplex PCR does not suffer from this limitation, and it has the added benefit above and beyond

Table 2
Primary molecular targets to be interrogated in cytologic and other small biopsies of advanced or unresectable non–small cell lung carcinoma

Gene	Alteration Type	Specific Alterations	Appropriate Methods of Detection	Predictive Capability
EGFR	SNV, Indel	Activating mutation in TK domain (exons 18–21)	NGS, qPCR	TKIs
EGFR	Indel	Activating mutation in exon 20	NGS, qPCR	Bispecific Abs
EGFR	SNV	T790M	NGS, qPCR	*Resistance* to first-generation TKIs
ALK	Fusion	Multiple partners	NGS, FISH, IHC	TKIs
KRAS	SNV	Activating mutations in exons 2, 3, 4	NGS, qPCR	Lack of targetable molecular driver
KRAS	SNV	G12C (exon 2)	NGS, qPCR	Small molecule inhibitor (2nd line)
ROS1	Fusion	Multiple partners	NGS, FISH, IHC[a]	TKIs
BRAF	SNV	V600E	NGS, IHC	Small molecule inhibitors
NTRK1/2/3	Fusion	Multiple partners	NGS, IHC	TKIs
MET	Fusion	Fusion of exons 13 and 15 ("exon 14 skipping")	NGS	TKIs; RNAseq is more sensitive than DNAseq
RET	Fusion	Multiple partners	NGS, FISH	TKIs
ERBB2	Indel	Activating mutation in TK domain	NGS	Ab-drug conjugate
PD-L1[b]	Overexpression	N/A	IHC	ICB
TMB[b]	Nonsynonymous mutation	N/A	NGS	ICB

Abbreviations: Ab, antibody; DNAseq, NGS of DNA; FISH, fluorescence in situ hybridization; N/A, not applicable; NGS, next-generation (massively parallel) sequencing; RNAseq, NGS of ribonucleic acid; TK, tyrosine kinase.
[a] Immunohistochemical detection of ROS1 fusion must be confirmed by an orthogonal method.
[b] Non-gene molecular target.

traditional next-generation RNA sequencing of being able to interrogate fusion genes in a partner-agnostic fashion.[82] Depending on assay design, qPCR can detect a broad range of SNVs, indels, and fusions with great analytical sensitivity and rapid turnaround time. However, it can detect only a limited number of alterations in a single-assay run. Currently, it is predominantly used to detect the most common alterations in those genes most commonly altered in NSCLCA (*EGFR* and *KRAS*) to allow for both rapid initiation of therapy and exclusion of the presence of other, less-common driver alterations.[83] It is worth noting that an unusually high proportion of nonmucinous pulmonary ADCAs harbor a G12C alteration in exon 2 of *KRAS*, an alteration for which targeted second-line therapy is available.

The molecular landscape of mucinous lung ADCA, however, resembles that of its extrapulmonary counterparts, more commonly harboring *KRAS* G12D, G12V, or other non-G12C alterations at codons 12, 13, and 61.

CAP/IASLC/AMP guidelines make the following recommendations regarding choice of using IHC versus molecular methods to detect alterations in the genes below[3]:

1. *EGFR*: IHC should not be used.
2. *ROS1*: IHC may be used as a screening test but should be confirmed with molecular or cytogenetic testing.
3. *ALK*: IHC (D5F3 or 5A4 clone may be used) as an alternative to ISH. The ALK1 clone should not be used for this purpose.

Table 3
Investigational molecular targets that may be interrogated with sufficient material and resources in cytologic and other small biopsies of advanced or unresectable non–small cell lung carcinoma

Genes (alterations) for which alteration may confer resistance to TKIs	Genes for which LoF alteration may confer resistance to ICB	Genes (alteration) for which alteration may become targetable in the future
• *ALK* (SNV)	• *STK11*	• *BRAF* (fusion)
• *PIK3CA* (SNV)	• *KEAP1*	• *BRAF* (non-V600 SNV)
• *AXL* (overexpression, amplification)	• *PBRM1*	• *NRG1* (fusion)
• *EGFR* (amplification)		• *LTK* (fusion)
• *ERBB2* (amplification)		• *ERBB4* (fusion)
• *MET* (amplification)		• *FGFR1/3* (fusion)
		• *MAP2K1* (SNV)
		• *NF1* (LoF alteration)
		• *RIT1* (SNV)

Abbreviation: LoF, loss-of-function.

4. *BRAF, RET, ERBB2, KRAS, MET*: IHC is not recommended. These genes may be interrogated as part of a molecular panel.

Optimization of Cytologic Specimens for Molecular and Other Additional Testing: Guidelines for Effective Tissue Utilization in Small Samples

Advanced techniques yielding small tissue samples are developing concurrently with an expansion of options for diagnostic, predictive, and prognostic testing. Although small samples are excellent for patient safety, recovery, and comfort, they present a challenge to pathologists to provide ample information from very small amounts of tissue. Pathologists must be as definitive as possible, and they must triage and preserve tissue for further testing. CAP and several other organizations have provided guidelines on best practices to acquire sufficient diagnostic tissue and tissue for additional testing, specifically for these small samples. The guidelines are briefly summarized below[84]:

1. EBUS–transbronchial needle aspiration (TBNA) may be used in the evaluation of central lesions to include parenchymal lesions and mediastinal/hilar lymph nodes. Image-guided techniques may be used for more peripheral lesions.
2. ROSE should be performed during needle procedures, particularly for the purpose of adequacy and triage of tissue for ancillary studies, and particularly in transthoracic procedures and for peripheral lesions. Touch preparation may be used to assess adequacy and to triage core needle or forceps biopsies.
3. Three to 5 passes of needle procedures, and/or 3 core biopsies should be obtained, unless adequacy is achieved sooner. Additional passes for CB and ancillary studies should be performed as needed. Needles as small as 25 gauge (transthoracic), 22 gauge (TBNA), and 20 gauge (core needle biopsy) may be used.
4. As much pleural fluid should be obtained as is feasible and submitted fresh for cytologic evaluation.
5. If suspicion of tuberculosis is present, ultrasound-guided techniques may increase the yield of bronchoalveolar lavage (BAL) and transbronchial biopsy. Tissue should be collected for cytology, culture (including liquid media where available), mycobacterial smear, and PCR.
6. Ancillary studies such as IHC, fluorescence in situ hybridization, and/or mutational analysis should be performed on cytology preparations if the assays are appropriately validated for the specimen type.

The range of possibilities in both collection and processing of cytologic specimens derived from the lung presents both opportunities for and challenges to cytopathologists in optimizing such specimens for appropriate MT. The primary opportunity lies with cytopathologists' ability to select among preparations for the ones most likely to generate tumor-derived nucleic acid of high quality and quantity. The primary challenge is that differences in preanalytical variables among different clinical specimens impact downstream biomarker analysis. As of the time of preparation for this review, the vast majority of published research concerning MT on cytologic specimens derived from lung is focused on FNA specimens. The American Society for Cytopathology has convened an "Optimizing Cytology and Small Biopsy Specimen

Table 4
Comparison of molecular testing methodologies

	NGS (DNA)	NGS (RNA)	ICC	IHC	ISH	Anchored, Multiplex PCR	qPCR
Detectable alterations	SNV Indel CNV Fusion	Fusion	Fusion PD-L1	SNV (*BRAF* V600E) Protein loss Fusion PD-L1	CNV Fusion	Fusion	SNV Indel
Acceptable specimens	DS CS LBC CB cfNA	DS CS LBC CB cfNA	DS CS LBC	CB	DS CS LBC CB	DS CS LBC CB cfNA	DS CS LBC CB cfNA
Turnaround time	Slow	Slow	Rapid	Rapid	Moderate	Slow	Rapid
Analytical sensitivity	High	High	High	Depends on target	Depends on target	High	Very high
Clinical sensitivity	Depends on assay	High	N/A	N/A	N/A	Very high	Low
Additional considerations	Low sensitivity for many fusions May quantify TMB	Known fusion partners only	Must sacrifice one slide for each Ab Very limited number of fusions	No additional validation needed Limited number of fusions	Nuclear truncation artifact on CB sections	Partner-agnostic fusion detection	May be used for sequential testing

Abbreviations: Ab, antibody; cfNA, cell-free nucleic acid; CS, cytospin; DS, direct smear preparation; ISH, in situ hybridization; LBC, liquid-based cytologic preparation.

Processing for Ancillary Studies Task Force" tasked with creating evidence-based recommendations for optimizing cytologic specimens, including both exfoliative and FNA specimens across organ systems for a broad array of ancillary studies. Until the Task Force's findings are available, it is advisable to perform MT on FNA-derived material, where possible.

Formalin-fixed, paraffin-embedded (FFPE) CBs, direct smear preparations, and needle rinses comprise most cytologic specimens from which tumor-derived nucleic acid may be extracted. FFPE CBs are particularly convenient, because they may generate multiple sections, which in turn may be used for a variety of applications, including IHC. In addition, utilization of CB sections does not require additional validation beyond that required for histologic FFPE sections. In contrast, although direct smear preparations do require additional validation, they yield nucleic acid of particularly high quality upon extraction.[42,85,86] It may also be easier to identify and select tumor cells in direct smear preparations than in CBs.[41] The great disadvantage of MT on direct smear preparations is that their use requires sacrifice of the slides, preferentially preceded by digital archiving, which may be burdensome.[87,88] Nucleic acid may also be extracted directly from cell-free needle rinse supernatant after preparation of a liquid-based cytology slide or cell pellet.[89–93] Finally, in order to maximize its yield, nucleic acid extracted from CBs, direct smears, and needle rinse supernatants may be combined.[81] Regardless of the preparation from which nucleic acid is extracted for MT, the goal remains the same: provide clinicians with as much high-quality information as possible to inform their choice of targeted or other therapy for their patients with advanced lung cancer.

DISCLOSURE

The authors have nothing to disclose.

REFERENCES

1. Layfield LJ, Roy-Chowdhuri S, Baloch Z, et al. Utilization of ancillary studies in the cytologic diagnosis of respiratory lesions: The Papanicolaou Society of Cytopathology consensus recommendations for respiratory cytology. Diagn Cytopathol 2016;44(12):1000–9.
2. Lindeman NI, Cagle PT, Aisner DL, et al. Updated molecular testing guideline for the selection of lung cancer patients for treatment with targeted tyrosine kinase inhibitors: Guideline from the College of American Pathologists, the International Association for the Study of Lung Cancer, and the Association for Molecular Pathology. J Thorac Oncol 2018;13(3):323–58.
3. Lindeman NI, Cagle PT, Aisner DL, et al. Updated molecular testing guideline for the selection of lung cancer patients for treatment with targeted tyrosine kinase inhibitors: guideline From the College of American Pathologists, the International Association for the Study of Lung Cancer, and the Association for Molecular Pathology. Arch Pathol Lab Med 2018;142(3):321–46.
4. Lindeman NI, Cagle PT, Aisner DL, et al. Updated Molecular Testing Guideline for the Selection of Lung Cancer Patients for Treatment With Targeted Tyrosine Kinase Inhibitors: Guideline From the College of American Pathologists, the International Association for the Study of Lung Cancer, and the Association for Molecular Pathology. J Mol Diagn : J Mod Dynam 2018;20(2):129–59.
5. Kalemkerian GP, Narula N, Kennedy EB, et al. Molecular Testing Guideline for the Selection of Patients With Lung Cancer for Treatment With Targeted Tyrosine Kinase Inhibitors: American Society of Clinical Oncology Endorsement of the College of American Pathologists/International Association for the Study of Lung Cancer/Association for Molecular Pathology Clinical Practice Guideline Update. J Clin Oncol 2018;36(9):911–9.
6. Hanna NH, Schneider BJ, Temin S, et al. Therapy for Stage IV Non-Small-Cell Lung Cancer Without Driver Alterations: ASCO and OH (CCO) Joint Guideline Update. J Clin Oncol 2020;38(14):1608–32.
7. Yu H, Boyle TA, Zhou C, et al. PD-L1 expression in lung cancer. J Thorac Oncol 2016;11(7):964–75.
8. McLaughlin J, Han G, Schalper KA, et al. Quantitative assessment of the heterogeneity of PD-L1 Expression in Non-Small-Cell Lung Cancer. JAMA Oncol 2016;2(1):46–54.
9. Hirsch FR, McElhinny A, Stanforth D, et al. PD-L1 immunohistochemistry assays for lung cancer: results from phase 1 of the Blueprint PD-L1 IHC Assay Comparison Project. J Thorac Oncol 2017;12(2):208–22.
10. Scheel AH, Dietel M, Heukamp LC, et al. Harmonized PD-L1 immunohistochemistry for pulmonary squamous-cell and adenocarcinomas. Mod Pathol 2016;29(10):1165–72.
11. Gaule P, Smithy JW, Toki M, et al. A quantitative comparison of antibodies to programmed cell death 1 ligand 1. JAMA Oncol 2017;3(2):256–9.
12. Tsao MS, Kerr KM, Kockx M, et al. PD-L1 immunohistochemistry comparability study in real-life clinical samples: results of blueprint phase 2 Project. J Thorac Oncol 2018;13(9):1302–11.
13. Heymann JJ, Bulman WA, Swinarski D, et al. PD-L1 expression in non-small cell lung carcinoma: Comparison among cytology, small biopsy, and surgical

resection specimens. Cancer Cytopathol 2017; 125(12):896–907.

14. Torous VF, Rangachari D, Gallant BP, et al. PD-L1 testing using the clone 22C3 pharmDx kit for selection of patients with non-small cell lung cancer to receive immune checkpoint inhibitor therapy: are cytology cell blocks a viable option? J Am Soc Cytopathol 2018;7(3):133–41.

15. Arriola AGP, Bashover E, Joseph C, et al. The usefulness of various cytologic specimen preparations for PD-L1 immunostaining in non-small cell lung carcinoma. J Am Soc Cytopathol 2018;7(6):324–32.

16. Russell-Goldman E, Kravets S, Dahlberg SE, et al. Cytologic-histologic correlation of programmed death-ligand 1 immunohistochemistry in lung carcinomas. Cancer Cytopathol 2018;126(4):253–63.

17. Stoy SP, Rosen L, Mueller J, et al. Programmed death-ligand 1 testing of lung cancer cytology specimens obtained with bronchoscopy. Cancer Cytopathol 2018;126(2):122–8.

18. Hernandez A, Brandler TC, Zhou F, et al. Assessment of programmed death-ligand 1 (PD-L1) immunohistochemical expression on cytology specimens in non-small cell lung carcinoma. Am J Clin Pathol 2019;151(4):403–15.

19. Gagné A, Wang E, Bastien N, et al. Impact of specimen characteristics on PD-L1 testing in non-small cell lung cancer: validation of the IASLC PD-L1 Testing Recommendations. J Thorac Oncol 2019; 14(12):2062–70.

20. Torlakovic E, Lim HJ, Adam J, et al. "Interchangeability" of PD-L1 immunohistochemistry assays: a meta-analysis of diagnostic accuracy. Mod Pathol 2020;33(1):4–17.

21. Marabelle A, Fakih M, Lopez J, et al. Association of tumour mutational burden with outcomes in patients with advanced solid tumours treated with pembrolizumab: prospective biomarker analysis of the multicohort, open-label, phase 2 KEYNOTE-158 study. Lancet Oncol 2020;21(10):1353–65.

22. Pepe F, Pisapia P, Gristina V, et al. Tumor mutational burden on cytological samples: a pilot study. Cancer Cytopathol 2021;129(6):460–7.

23. Stenzinger A, Allen JD, Maas J, et al. Tumor mutational burden standardization initiatives: Recommendations for consistent tumor mutational burden assessment in clinical samples to guide immunotherapy treatment decisions. Gene Chromosome Cancer 2019;58(8):578–88.

24. Ricciuti B, Wang X, Alessi JV, et al. Association of high tumor mutation burden in non-small cell lung cancers with increased immune infiltration and improved clinical outcomes of PD-L1 blockade across PD-L1 expression levels. JAMA Oncol 2022;8(8):1160–8.

25. Travis WD, Brambilla E, Noguchi M, et al. International Association for the Study of Lung Cancer/ American Thoracic Society/European Respiratory Society international multidisciplinary classification of lung adenocarcinoma. J Thorac Oncol 2011; 6(2):244–85.

26. Travis WD, Brambilla E, Nicholson AG, et al. The 2015 World Health Organization Classification of Lung Tumors: Impact of Genetic, Clinical and Radiologic Advances Since the 2004 Classification. J Thorac Oncol 2015;10(9):1243–60.

27. Nicholson AG, Tsao MS, Beasley MB, et al. The 2021 WHO Classification of Lung Tumors: Impact of Advances Since 2015. J Thorac Oncol 2022;17(3): 362–87.

28. Jain D, Nambirajan A, Chen G, et al. NSCLC Subtyping in Conventional Cytology: Results of the International Association for the Study of Lung Cancer Cytology Working Group Survey to Determine Specific Cytomorphologic Criteria for Adenocarcinoma and Squamous Cell Carcinoma. J Thorac Oncol 2022;17(6):793–805.

29. Layfield LJ, Baloch Z, Elsheikh T, et al. Standardized terminology and nomenclature for respiratory cytology: The Papanicolaou Society of Cytopathology guidelines. Diagn Cytopathol 2016;44(5):399–409.

30. Layfield LJ, Esebua M. A modified Papanicolaou Society of Cytopathology system for reporting respiratory cytology specimens: Implications for estimates of malignancy risk and diagnostic accuracy. Diagn Cytopathol 2021;49(11):1167–72.

31. Canberk S, Montezuma D, Aydın O, et al. The new guidelines of Papanicolaou Society of Cytopathology for respiratory specimens: Assessment of risk of malignancy and diagnostic yield in different cytological modalities. Diagn Cytopathol 2018;46(9): 725–9.

32. Hiroshima K, Yoshizawa A, Takenaka A, et al. Cytology Reporting System for Lung Cancer from the Japan Lung Cancer Society and Japanese Society of Clinical Cytology: An Interobserver Reproducibility Study and Risk of Malignancy Evaluation on Cytology Specimens. Acta Cytol 2020;64(5):452–62.

33. Schmitt FC, Bubendorf L, Canberk S, et al. The World Health Organization Reporting System for Lung Cytopathology. Acta Cytol 2023;67(1):80–91.

34. Canberk S, Field A, Bubendorf L, et al. A brief review of the WHO reporting system for lung cytopathology. J Am Soc Cytopathol 2023;12(4):251–7.

35. WHO Classification of Tumours of the Lung. Pleura, Thymus and Heart. World Health Organization classification of tumours. Lyon, France: International Agency for Research on Cancer; 2021.

36. Pinto D, Chandra A, Crothers BA, et al. The international system for reporting serous fluid cytopathology-diagnostic categories and clinical management. J Am Soc Cytopathol 2020;9(6):469–77.

37. VandenBussche CJ, Crothers B, Chandra A, et al. The international system for reporting serous fluid

cytopathology: The initial project survey. Cytopathology 2023;34(3):191–7.

38. Heymann JJ, Yoxtheimer LM, Park HJ, et al. Preanalytic variables in quality and quantity of nucleic acids extracted from FNA specimens of thyroid gland nodules collected in CytoLyt: Cellularity and storage time. Cancer Cytopathol 2020;128(9):656–72.

39. Levy EB, Fiel MI, Hamilton SR, et al. State of the art: toward improving outcomes of lung and liver tumor biopsies in clinical trials-a multidisciplinary approach. J Clin Oncol 2020;38(14):1633–40.

40. Roy-Chowdhuri S, Goswami RS, Chen H, et al. Factors affecting the success of next-generation sequencing in cytology specimens. Research Support, N.I.H., Extramural. Cancer Cytopathol 2015; 123(11):659–68.

41. Roy-Chowdhuri S, Stewart J. Preanalytic variables in cytology: lessons learned from next-generation sequencing-The MD Anderson experience. Arch Pathol Lab Med 2016;140(11):1191–9.

42. Roy-Chowdhuri S, Chen H, Singh RR, et al. Concurrent fine needle aspirations and core needle biopsies: a comparative study of substrates for next-generation sequencing in solid organ malignancies. Mod Pathol 2017;30(4):499–508.

43. Coley SM, Crapanzano JP, Saqi A. FNA, core biopsy, or both for the diagnosis of lung carcinoma: Obtaining sufficient tissue for a specific diagnosis and molecular testing. Comparative Study. Cancer Cytopathol 2015;123(5):318–26.

44. Ly A, Balassanian R, Alperstein S, et al. One procedure-one report: the Re-Imagine Cytopathology Task Force position paper on small tissue biopsy triage in anatomic pathology. J Am Soc Cytopathol 2023;12(6):395–406.

45. Gu P, Zhao YZ, Jiang LY, et al. Endobronchial ultrasound-guided transbronchial needle aspiration for staging of lung cancer: a systematic review and meta-analysis. Eur J Cancer 2009;45(8): 1389–96.

46. Makris D, Scherpereel A, Leroy S, et al. Electromagnetic navigation diagnostic bronchoscopy for small peripheral lung lesions. Eur Respir J 2007;29(6): 1187–92.

47. Pickering EM, Kalchiem-Dekel O, Sachdeva A. Electromagnetic navigation bronchoscopy: a comprehensive review. AME Medical Journal 2018;3.

48. Nishii Y, Nakamura Y, Fujiwara K, et al. Use of ultrathin bronchoscope on a need basis improves diagnostic yield of difficult-to-approach pulmonary lesions. Front Med 2020;7:588048.

49. Ost DE, Ernst A, Lei X, et al. Diagnostic yield and complications of bronchoscopy for peripheral lung lesions. Results of the AQuIRE Registry. Am J Respir Crit Care Med 2016;193(1):68–77.

50. Tanner NT, Yarmus L, Chen A, et al. Standard bronchoscopy with fluoroscopy vs thin bronchoscopy and radial endobronchial ultrasound for biopsy of pulmonary lesions: a multicenter, prospective, randomized trial. Chest 2018;154(5):1035–43.

51. Yarmus L, Akulian J, Wahidi M, et al. A prospective randomized comparative study of three guided bronchoscopic approaches for investigating pulmonary nodules: The PRECISION-1 Study. Chest 2020; 157(3):694–701.

52. Chen AC, Pastis NJ Jr, Mahajan AK, et al. Robotic bronchoscopy for peripheral pulmonary lesions: a multicenter pilot and feasibility study (BENEFIT). Chest 2021;159(2):845–52.

53. Ravikumar N, Ho E, Wagh A, et al. Advanced Imaging for Robotic Bronchoscopy: A Review. Diagnostics 2023;13(5).

54. Pritchett MA, Bhadra K, Calcutt M, et al. Virtual or reality: divergence between preprocedural computed tomography scans and lung anatomy during guided bronchoscopy. J Thorac Dis 2020;12(4):1595–611.

55. Chen A, Pastis N, Furukawa B, et al. The effect of respiratory motion on pulmonary nodule location during electromagnetic navigation bronchoscopy. Chest 2015;147(5):1275–81.

56. Cicenia J, Bhadra K, Sethi S, et al. Augmented Fluoroscopy: A New and Novel Navigation Platform for Peripheral Bronchoscopy. J Bronchology Interv Pulmonol 2021;28(2):116–23.

57. Pritchett MA, Schampaert S, de Groot JAH, et al. Cone-Beam CT with augmented fluoroscopy combined with electromagnetic navigation bronchoscopy for biopsy of pulmonary nodules. J Bronchology Interv Pulmonol 2018;25(4):274–82.

58. Pritchett MA. Prospective analysis of a novel endobronchial augmented fluoroscopic navigation system for diagnosis of peripheral pulmonary lesions. J Bronchology Interv Pulmonol 2021;28(2):107–15.

59. Kalchiem-Dekel O, Fuentes P, Bott MJ, et al. Multiplanar 3D fluoroscopy redefines tool-lesion relationship during robotic-assisted bronchoscopy. Respirology 2021;26(1):120–3.

60. Casal RF, Sarkiss M, Jones AK, et al. Cone beam computed tomography-guided thin/ultrathin bronchoscopy for diagnosis of peripheral lung nodules: a prospective pilot study. J Thorac Dis 2018; 10(12):6950–9.

61. DiBardino DM, Kim RY, Cao Y, et al. Diagnostic yield of cone-beam-derived augmented fluoroscopy and ultrathin bronchoscopy versus conventional navigational bronchoscopy techniques. J Bronchology Interv Pulmonol 2023;30(4):335–45.

62. Kalchiem-Dekel O, Connolly JG, Lin IH, et al. Shape-sensing robotic-assisted bronchoscopy in the diagnosis of pulmonary parenchymal lesions. Chest 2022;161(2):572–82.

63. Cho RJ, Senitko M, Wong J, et al. Feasibility of using the O-Arm imaging system during ENB-rEBUS-guided peripheral lung biopsy: a dual-center

experience. J Bronchology Interv Pulmonol 2021; 28(4):248–54.

64. Chhieng DC, Chen J, Connolly K, et al. High-risk HPV DNA detection rate in patients with atypical squamous cells and its relationship to the atypical squamous cell: squamous intraepithelial lesion ratio. Acta Cytol 2006;50(3):291–4.

65. Ko V, Nanji S, Tambouret RH, et al. Testing for HPV as an objective measure for quality assurance in gynecologic cytology: positive rates in equivocal and abnormal specimens and comparison with the ASCUS to SIL ratio. Cancer 2007;111(2):67–73.

66. Cibas ES, Zou KH, Crum CP, et al. Using the rate of positive high-risk HPV test results for ASC-US together with the ASC-US/SIL ratio in evaluating the performance of cytopathologists. Am J Clin Pathol 2008;129(1):97–101.

67. Chebib I, Rao RA, Wilbur DC, et al. Using the ASC:-SIL ratio, human papillomavirus, and interobserver variability to assess and monitor cytopathology fellow training performance. Cancer Cytopathol 2013;121(11):638–43.

68. Gokozan HN, Dilcher TL, Alperstein SA, et al. Combining molecular testing and the Bethesda category III:VI ratio for thyroid fine-needle aspirates: A quality-assurance metric for evaluating diagnostic performance in a cytopathology laboratory. Cancer Cytopathol 2022;130(4):259–74.

69. VanderLaan PA, Nishino M. Molecular testing results as a quality metric for evaluating cytopathologists' utilization of the atypia of undetermined significance category for thyroid nodule fine-needle aspirations. J Am Soc Cytopathol 2022;11(2):67–73.

70. VanderLaan PA, Roy-Chowdhuri S. Current and future trends in non-small cell lung cancer biomarker testing: The American experience. Cancer Cytopathol 2020;128(9):629–36.

71. Sung S, Heymann JJ, Crapanzano JP, et al. Lung cancer cytology and small biopsy specimens: diagnosis, predictive biomarker testing, acquisition, triage, and management. J Am Soc Cytopathol 2020;9(5):332–45.

72. VanderLaan PA, Roy-Chowdhuri S, Griffith CC, et al. Molecular testing of cytology specimens: overview of assay selection with focus on lung, salivary gland, and thyroid testing. J Am Soc Cytopathol 2022; 11(6):403–14.

73. Siegel RL, Miller KD, Wagle NS, et al. Cancer statistics, 2023. CA Cancer J Clin 2023;73(1):17–48.

74. Baum JE, Saqi A, Heymann JJ. Non-small cell lung carcinoma: molecular genetics with consideration of cytologic samples. Diagn Histopathol 2018; 24(10):388–96.

75. VanderLaan PA, Rangachari D, Costa DB. The rapidly evolving landscape of biomarker testing in non-small cell lung cancer. Cancer Cytopathol 2021;129(3):179–81.

76. Benci JL, Xu B, Qiu Y, et al. Tumor interferon signaling regulates a multigenic resistance program to immune checkpoint blockade. Cell 2016;167(6): 1540–54.e1512.

77. Benci JL, Johnson LR, Choa R, et al. Opposing functions of interferon coordinate adaptive and innate immune responses to cancer immune checkpoint blockade. Cell 2019;178(4):933–48.e914.

78. Yuan C, Chen H, Tu S, et al. A systematic dissection of the epigenomic heterogeneity of lung adenocarcinoma reveals two different subclasses with distinct prognosis and core regulatory networks. Genome Biol 2021;22(1):156.

79. Qiu J, Xu B, Ye D, et al. Cancer cells resistant to immune checkpoint blockade acquire interferon-associated epigenetic memory to sustain T cell dysfunction. Nat Cancer 2023;4(1):43–61.

80. DiBardino DM, Saqi A, Elvin JA, et al. Yield and clinical utility of next-generation sequencing in selected patients with lung adenocarcinoma. Clin Lung Cancer 2016;17(6):517–22.

81. Tian SK, Killian JK, Rekhtman N, et al. Optimizing workflows and processing of cytologic samples for comprehensive analysis by next-generation sequencing: Memorial Sloan Kettering Cancer Center experience. Arch Pathol Lab Med 2016;140(11):1200–5.

82. Zheng Z, Liebers M, Zhelyazkova B, et al. Anchored multiplex PCR for targeted next-generation sequencing. Nat Med 2014;20(12):1479–84.

83. De Luca C, Rappa AG, Gragnano G, et al. Idylla assay and next generation sequencing: an integrated EGFR mutational testing algorithm. J Clin Pathol 2018;71(8):745–50.

84. Roy-Chowdhuri S, Dacic S, Ghofrani M, et al. Collection and Handling of Thoracic Small Biopsy and Cytology Specimens for Ancillary Studies: Guideline From the College of American Pathologists in Collaboration With the American College of Chest Physicians, Association for Molecular Pathology, American Society of Cytopathology, American Thoracic Society, Pulmonary Pathology Society, Papanicolaou Society of Cytopathology, Society of Interventional Radiology, and Society of Thoracic Radiology. Arch Pathol Lab Med 2020. https://doi.org/10.5858/arpa.2020-0119-CP.

85. Baum JE, Zhang P, Hoda RS, et al. Accuracy of next-generation sequencing for the identification of clinically relevant variants in cytology smears in lung adenocarcinoma. Cancer Cytopathol 2017; 125(6):398–406.

86. Hwang DH, Garcia EP, Ducar MD, et al. Next-generation sequencing of cytologic preparations: An analysis of quality metrics. Comparative Study Evaluation Studies. Cancer Cytopathol 2017;125(10):786–94.

87. Kim D, Sundling KE, Virk R, et al. Digital cytology part 1: digital cytology implementation for practice: a concept paper with review and recommendations

from the American Society of Cytopathology Digital Cytology Task Force. J Am Soc Cytopathol 2023; 13(2):86–96.

88. Kim D, Sundling KE, Virk R, et al. Digital Cytology Part 2: Artificial Intelligence in Cytology A Concept Paper with Review and Recommendations from the American Society of Cytopathology Digital Cytology Task Force. J Am Soc Cytopathol 2023;13(2):97–110.

89. Reynolds JP, Zhou Y, Jakubowski MA, et al. Next-generation sequencing of liquid-based cytology non-small cell lung cancer samples. Cancer Cytopathol 2017;125(3):178–87.

90. Wei S, Lieberman D, Morrissette JJ, et al. Using "residual" FNA rinse and body fluid specimens for next-generation sequencing: An institutional experience. Cancer Cytopathol 2016;124(5):324–9.

91. Roy-Chowdhuri S, Mehrotra M, Bolivar AM, et al. Salvaging the supernatant: next generation cytopathology for solid tumor mutation profiling. Mod Pathol 2018;31(7):1036–45.

92. Janaki N, Harbhajanka A, Michael CW, et al. Comparison of cytocentrifugation supernatant fluid and formalin-fixed paraffin-embedded tissue for targeted next-generation sequencing. Cancer Cytopathol 2019;127(5):297–305.

93. Hannigan B, Ye W, Mehrotra M, et al. Liquid biopsy assay for lung carcinoma using centrifuged supernatants from fine-needle aspiration specimens. Ann Oncol 2019;30(6):963–9.

Pulmonary Cytopathology
Current and Future Impact of Microscopy and Immunohistochemistry

Niyati Desai, MD[a], Danielle D'Ambrosio, MD[b],
Katya S. Dombrowski, MD[c], Peter B. Illei, MD[c],
Jonas J. Heymann, MD[d],*

KEYWORDS

• Nonneoplastic lung disease • Lung cancer • Fine needle aspiration • Cytology • Cytopathology
• Small biopsy • pulmonary cytopathology

Key points:

• Cytopathologists should be familiar with the morphologic features of a wide range of lung diseases, both neoplastic and nonneoplastic and their differential diagnoses.

• Immunohistochemistry/immunocytochemistry plays a crucial role in ruling out possible diagnoses and reaching a final diagnosis of malignancy. A thorough understanding of this process is essential for cytopathologists.

ABSTRACT

With the advancement of tissue procurement techniques, in-depth knowledge of morphology is crucial for cytopathologists to diagnose neoplastic and nonneoplastic lung diseases optimally. Cytopathologists must also be well versed in immunohistochemistry/immunocytochemistry markers and their interpretation for an accurate diagnosis.

OVERVIEW

Per Global Health Metrics, globally in 2021, there were 2.28 million incident cases, 2.02 million deaths, and 46.5 million disability-adjusted life years lost to trachea, bronchus, and lung cancers, and trachea, bronchus, and lung cancers were the seventh-leading cause of death globally. Diagnostics, including cytopathology, will be required to prevent death from lung cancer, the number of which worldwide is estimated to increase by 67% by 2040.

Broadly, lung carcinomas are divided histologically into small cell (SCLCA, approximately 15% of cases) and non-small cell lung carcinoma (NSCLCA, approximately 85% of cases), with NSCLCA histologically subdivided into adenocarcinoma (ADCA), squamous cell carcinoma (SCCA), and large-cell carcinoma, with the presence of specific molecular alterations allowing for further molecular stratification. Metastatic carcinomas and noncarcinomatous neoplasms are less commonly encountered in biopsy series. Despite advances in molecular methodologies, morphologic examination and immunohistochemistry (IHC) still remain the first steps in diagnosis for all these neoplastic entities.

This review will focus on the enduring techniques of morphologic examination and IHC in

[a] Department of Pathology and Cell Biology, New York-Presbyterian Hospital-Columbia University Irving Medical Center, 630 West 168th Street, New York, NY 10032, USA; [b] Department of Pathology, New York University Grossman School of Medicine, 560 First Avenue, New York, NY 10016, USA; [c] Department of Pathology, The Johns Hopkins University School of Medicine, 600 North Wolfe St., Baltimore, MD 21287, USA; [d] Department of Pathology and Laboratory Medicine, New York-Presbyterian Hospital-Weill Cornell Medicine, 1300 York Avenue, New York, NY 10065, USA
* Corresponding author.
E-mail address: jjh7002@med.cornell.edu

Surgical Pathology 17 (2024) 411–429
https://doi.org/10.1016/j.path.2024.06.003

diagnosing lung diseases, particularly neoplastic lung diseases.

MICROSCOPY AND IMMUNOHISTOCHEMISTRY

INFLAMMATORY PROCESSES AND OTHER NONNEOPLASTIC LESIONS

Benign cells are seldom found as contaminants in fine needle aspiration (FNA) samples. Commonly found contaminants are reactive changes in squamous and bronchial cells, hyperplasia of bronchial reserve cell and type II pneumocytes, and mesothelial cells. It is pertinent to differentiate them from malignant cells and can be a diagnostic challenge.[1] Often noncellular elements like Curschmann's spirals, ferruginous bodies, Charcot–Leyden crystals, psammoma bodies, corpora amylacea, vegetable matter, pollen, and some pigmented fungus (eg, *Alternaria* spp) may be found that can be either contaminant or can point toward a chronic respiratory disease. Pleuropulmonary infections can be caused by a variety of microorganisms including viruses, bacteria, fungi, and parasites.[2] Granulomatous lesions, especially infectious necrotizing granulomas, commonly present clinically as tumors with persistent or interval growth, and they may be PET positive.[3] Cytology plays a crucial role in diagnosis of an array of lung infections, especially in immunocompromised patients, such as lung transplant recipients.

BENIGN NEOPLASTIC LESIONS

Although most lung neoplasms are malignant, there is a subset of true neoplasms that are benign. The spectrum of benign tumors of lung includes papilloma, sclerosing pneumocytoma, hamartoma, benign salivary gland neoplasms, PEComa, benign spindle cell tumors, meningiomas, and granular cell tumor. While establishing the final diagnosis, correlation of the cytopathology findings with the clinical and imaging findings is essential.[3] Knowledge of sclerosing pneumocytoma is particularly important due to its challenging differential diagnosis of bronchogenic carcinoma.[4–7] Cytologic diagnosis of sclerosing pneumocytoma requires the identification of its dual cell population, made up of cuboidal/surface cells and round/stromal cells, which may be more apparent in cell block sections than in direct smear or liquid-based preparations. The presence of large sheets and mucinous background are useful features variably present in carcinoma but uniformly absent in sclerosing pneumocytoma. It is important to re-

emphasize that not all thyroid transcription factor-1 (TTF-1) and napsin-A-positive lesions are lung ADCA. For sclerosing pneumocytoma, surface cells are positive for CK7, epithelial membrane antigen (EMA), TTF-1, and napsin A. Round cells are positive for TTF-1 and EMA and sometimes for smooth muscle actin (SMA) and progesterone receptor and are negative for napsin A and most keratins.[3,8] Detailed review of other benign lesions is beyond the scope of this review.

SPECIFIC MALIGNANT LESIONS

Non-small Cell Carcinomas

Adenocarcinoma

Microscopic features Eccentrically placed and enlarged nucleus with prominent nucleoli, finely textured chromatin, and translucent foamy cytoplasm with or without mucin vacuoles are characteristic of ADCA (**Fig. 1**). When well-differentiated, features may be more subtle and include

- High cellularity of the specimen with a large number of atypical tissue fragments.
- Clusters of cells with spherical, papillary, micropapillary, acinar, or sheet-like architecture with loss of polarity.
- Mild nuclear pleomorphism with indentations, grooves, and pseudoinclusions.[9,10]

Recent investigation has revealed significant divergence in the clinico-pathologic features of one specific subtype of primary pulmonary ADCA: mucinous ADCA.[11] Such tumors often present as synchronous or metachronous non-F-18-deoxyglucose avid radiographic lesions with the following morphologic features:

- Tightly cohesive clusters of cells with almost exclusive sheet-like architecture with only mild loss of polarity.
- Voluminous and widespread cytoplasmic mucin vacuoles.
- Mildly enlarged nuclei with minimally irregular contours and finely granular chromatin.

Differential diagnosis The differential diagnosis of ADCA primarily includes other carcinomas, particularly SCCA. Cohesive cells, more finely textured nuclear chromatin, and thin, vacuolated cytoplasm favors ADCA over SCCA. ADCAs of extrathoracic origin, as well as metastatic papillary thyroid carcinoma may also mimic primary lung ADCA. However, it is often virtually impossible to differentiate primary versus metastatic tumor, and IHC in addition to clinical and radiological correlation can be essential. The primary benign entity in the differential diagnosis of ADCA is sclerosing pneumocytoma. Identification

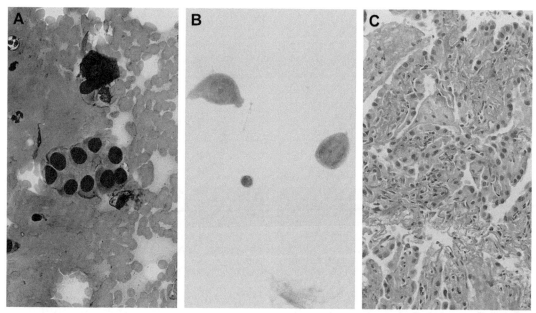

Fig. 1. Morphologic features of lepidic pattern pulmonary ADCA acquired by FNA (*A, B*) and core needle (*C*) biopsies. (*A*) A cluster in a direct smear preparation (Diff-Quik, 400×) contains cells with high N:C ratio and (*B*) finely textured chromatin and prominent nucleoli in a liquid-based (ThinPrep) preparation (Papanicolaou stain, 600×).[12,13] (*C*) Neoplastic cells grow along the surface of alveolar air spaces in corresponding core needle biopsy (H&E, 200×).

of bland appearing 2 cell population and round cells with a papillary architecture in a bloody background with hemosiderin-laden macrophages is suggestive of sclerosing pneumocytoma. Finally, preservation of cellular cohesion and nuclear polarity, macronucleoli without hyperchromasia and nuclear membrane irregularities, and denser cytoplasm in the presence of low number of atypical cells support a reactive process.

Immunohistochemistry In cases with diagnostic difficulty, ADCA can be separated from SCCA via special stains for mucin or with IHC in most cases. Napsin and TTF-1 (any amount of staining) are positive in the majority of primary lung ADCAs (**Fig. 2**).[12,13] If the differential diagnosis includes a metastasis or mesothelial lesion, a separate panel may be ordered (see "Diffuse Pleural Mesothelioma" section).[14,15] It is important to note that mucinous ADCA often does not express TTF-1 (up to 20% of cases); it may instead express CK20 and CDX-2. Additionally, p63 is positive in up to 20% to 30% of lung ADCAs; therefore, p40 is a preferred marker for squamous differentiation.[16]

SQUAMOUS CELL CARCINOMA

MICROSCOPIC FEATURES

The cytologic features of SCCA are variable depending on the degree of squamous

differentiation. Well-differentiated SCCA can appear as singly scattered cells or clusters of atypical cells in a background of necrotic debris and frequently anucleated cells. The cells are polymorphic and can have a variety of shapes (polygonal, rounded, spindle, and tadpole) with abundant smooth, dense cytoplasm filled with keratin (orangeophilic on Papanicolaou stain) with variable N:C ratio and pyknotic nuclei. Moderately and poorly differentiated SCCAs show cohesive aggregates with scant cytoplasm with less apparent keratinization. The nuclei are elongated with a small but conspicuous nucleolus and a highly irregular pattern of chromatin distribution.[17]

DIFFERENTIAL DIAGNOSIS

Depending on its differentiation, SCCA may be difficult to differentiate from ADCA, SCLCA, NUT carcinoma (NC), and SMARCA4-deficient thoracic undifferentiated tumor.[18] Many SCCA can be easily distinguished from ADCA based on the presence of keratinization, while the presence of glandular or papillary structures and intracellular or extracellular mucin favors a diagnosis of ADCA.[19] In cases with diagnostic difficulty, IHC for TTF-1 and p40 is recommended.[18] Distinguishing basaloid SCCA from high-grade neuroendocrine carcinomas, including SCLCA and large cell neuroendocrine carcinoma (LCNECA) can be challenging on lung cytology. Identification of

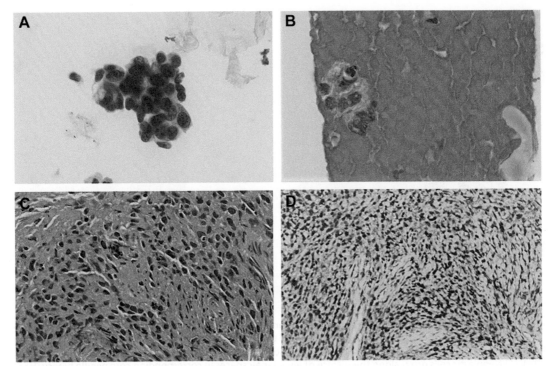

Fig. 2. Morphologic and immunohistochemical features of primary invasive pulmonary ADCA acquired by FNA (A, B) and core needle (C, D) biopsies. (A) Liquid-based (ThinPrep) preparation (Papanicolaou stain, 400×) and (B) formalin-fixed, paraffin-embedded cell block (H&E, 600×). (C) Corresponding core needle biopsy (H&E, 400×) with (D) coexpression of TTF-1 (brown) and Napsin (red, 200×).

predominantly dyscohesive cell pattern, extensive nuclear molding, salt-and-pepper finely granular chromatin, marked nuclear irregularity, chromatinic smearing, and apoptotic debris are supportive of SCLCA. The presence of larger cells with prominent nucleoli and more cytoplasm with focal rosette formation supports LCNECA over SCCA.[20] Occasional and abrupt squamous differentiation and basaloid appearance makes NC extremely difficult to differentiate from basaloid and poorly differentiated SCCA. NC should be suspected in tumors with primitive-appearing basaloid tumor cells with relatively monotonous, coarsely granular nuclei and conspicuous nucleoli. The diagnosis mandates molecular testing (MT) or IHC for NUT protein.[21]

NON-SMALL CELL CARCINOMA, NOS

MICROSCOPIC FEATURES

There are instances in which differentiation among all the entities that comprise NSCLCA is not possible based on a cytologic specimen. Cells may be either cohesive or dyscohesive with no definite cytoplasmic keratinization or vacuolization. When they are cohesive, cells may form syncytial clusters or demonstrate prominent cell borders. The background may be clean or demonstrate necrosis. Nuclei may demonstrate a broad range of morphologies, although NSCLCA, NOS is a difficult diagnosis to make in the absence of, at least, some degree of nuclear pleomorphism and alteration of the chromatin pattern.[22]

DIFFERENTIAL DIAGNOSIS

Final diagnoses made upon resection may include ADCA, SCCA, large cell carcinoma, other specific carcinoma, and neuroendocrine carcinoma (see later discussion), as well as secondary (metastatic) tumors.[23,24]

OTHER SPECIFIC CARCINOMAS

SALIVARY GLAND-TYPE CARCINOMAS

Salivary gland-type carcinoma (SGT) accounts for less than 1% of all lung tumors.[25,26] The 4 most common pulmonary SGTs are mucoepidermoid carcinoma (MEC), adenoid cystic carcinoma (AdCC), epithelial-myoepithelial carcinoma (EMC), and pleomorphic adenoma (PA).[27,28] Other pulmonary SGTs include hyalinizing clear cell carcinoma, mucous gland adenoma, acinic cell carcinoma, salivary gland duct-type carcinoma, and oncocytoma.[29]

Microscopic and Immunohistochemical Features

MEC is the most common pulmonary SGT.[30–33] It is composed of mucocytes, squamous cells, and intermediate-type cells, where mucocytes line cystic spaces and squamous and intermediate cells make up the solid component. Low-grade MEC has minimal cytologic atypia with few mitoses and lacks parenchymal invasion and necrosis. On smear, it has sheets of bland intermediate cells with admixed mucous cells. High-grade MEC is more solid with significant cytologic atypia, greater than 4 mitoses per 10 high power fields, and necrosis. On smear, it has a less apparent mucous component.[34,35] The tumor cells are variably positive for cytokeratin (CK) 7 and CK 5/6 with nuclear positivity for p40 and p63. A mucicarmine stain will highlight intracytoplasmic and extracellular mucin.[35]

AdCC is morphologically similar to its salivary gland counterpart. This neoplasm is cribriform, tubular, and/or solid, and there is associated myxoid and hyaline material, which is sharply demarcated from the neoplastic cells. The cells are arranged in clusters and are monotonous and small with bland hyperchromatic nuclei and scant cytoplasm.[35,36] AdCC is positive for CK7, p63, p40, S100, calponin, and CD117, with a unique p63 pattern of peripheral nuclear staining or nuclear staining of only the internal luminal cells.[35]

EMC is a biphasic tumor where an inner layer of cuboidal, columnar epithelial cells is surrounded by an outer layer of myoepithelial cells that can have a spindled, plasmacytoid, or clear appearance. The epithelial cells are positive for pan-CK, CK7, and CK5/6 while the myoepithelial cells are positive for S100, SMA, calponin, and p63.[35,37]

PA is composed of epithelial, myoepithelial, and stromal components. The cells are arranged in cords, tubules, ducts, or nests with an associated myxoid or chondromyxoid stroma. The myoepithelial cells can have a spindled, clear, or plasmacytoid appearance. Keratinization, secondary to squamous differentiation, can be present. The cells are positive for CK, p63, S100, GFAP, calponin, and SMA.[35]

Differential Diagnosis

When diagnosing pulmonary SGTs, metastatic SGTs need to be excluded, as do other morphologically similar neoplasms. MEC should be distinguished from adenosquamous carcinoma (ASC),

SCCA, and ADCA.[34,35] AdCC should be differentiated from neuroendocrine tumors (NETs), basaloid SCCA, and ADCA.[35,36] EMC should be differentiated from AdCC, PA, and other biphasic neoplasms.[35,37] PA should be differentiated from other SGTs, such as PA and AdCC, as well as hamartoma and SCCA.[35,38]

Molecular Pathology Features

MEC has been associated with mastermind-like gene 2 (MAML2) alterations. Most harbor a t(11;19) (q21;p13) translocation involving CREB-regulated transcription coactivator 1 (CRTC1), although a t(11;15) (q21;q26) CRTC3 fusion has been reported. AdCC has been associated with a v-myb avian MYB vial oncogene homology (MYB) gene rearrangement due to t(6;9) (q22-23;p23-24) chromosomal translocation. This results in MYB-NFIB (nuclear factor IB) gene fusion. Other cases of AdCC have been associated with a t(8;9) (q13;p22) chromosomal translocation, resulting in a MYBL1–NFIB gene fusion.[35] The molecular characteristics of EMC are largely unknown, but in some studies, it has been associated with overexpression of p53 and mutations in APC, HRAS, BCOR, TET2, DNMT3A, KDM5C, and STAT3.[37,39] PA is associated with gene rearrangement of pleomorphic adenoma gene 1 (PLAG1) at chromosome 8q12, leading to PLAG1 overexpression.[35]

ADENOSQUAMOUS CARCINOMA

MICROSCOPIC AND IMMUNOHISTOCHEMICAL FEATURES

ASC is an NSCLCA composed of both squamous and glandular components, with at least 10% of each component upon complete resection. For this reason, diagnosis may be suggested, but is not definitive, on small biopsies. It is rare, accounting for less than 4% of primary lung tumors. Cytologically, these tumors will have combined features of ADCA and SCCA, which can include cytoplasmic vacuolation, keratinization, and enlarged hyperchromatic nuclei with nucleoli. ASC can be positive or negative for p63 and thyroid TTF-1.[40,41]

DIFFERENTIAL DIAGNOSIS

The differential diagnosis of ASC includes ADCA, SCCA, and MEC. ASC may be misdiagnosed as ADCA or SCCA if the neoplasm is inadequately sampled. ASC can be differentiated from MEC as it lacks intermediate cells, while MEC lacks squamous pearls.[40,42]

MOLECULAR PATHOLOGY FEATURES

ASC has genetic abnormalities similar to those in ADCA, and no distinctive molecular profile has been identified.[42]

SARCOMATOID CARCINOMA

Sarcomatoid carcinoma is an umbrella term for the group of NSCLCAs that includes spindle cell carcinoma, giant cell carcinoma, pleomorphic carcinoma (PC), carcinosarcoma, and pulmonary blastoma (PB). These tumors have a worse prognosis than more well-differentiated NSCLCAs. Considerable overlap can exist between sarcomatoid carcinomas and metastases, sarcomas, and sarcomatoid mesothelioma, both morphologically and immunohistochemically. Thorough sampling, patient history, radiologic information, and molecular studies are useful in these settings.

PLEOMORPHIC CARCINOMA

MICROSCOPIC AND IMMUNOHISTOCHEMICAL FEATURES

PC is a rare, poorly differentiated NSCLCA composed of ADCA, SCCA, or undifferentiated NSCLCA with at least 10% spindle and/or neoplastic giant cells upon complete resection. The cells vary widely in size. They have abundant cytoplasm, which can appear vacuolated, and centrifugal, irregularly-shaped nuclei. They make small clusters or fascicles and have a background of mixed inflammatory cells.[43] The giant cell component of PC can be composed of syncytial-shaped multinucleated cells with smudged nuclei, coarsely dispersed chromatin, and nuclear molding or emperipoletic giant tumor cells. The cells in PC are usually positive for CK.[44]

DIFFERENTIAL DIAGNOSIS

The differential diagnosis of PC includes large cell carcinoma. PC should have more pleomorphic features than large cell carcinoma. If only the spindled portion is sampled, the differential diagnosis includes spindle cell sarcoma and sarcomatoid mesothelioma, the latter of which may express calretinin, podoplanin (D2-40), and WT-1 but not claudin-4, epithelial cell adhesion molecule (BerEP4/MOC-31), B72.3, carcinoembryonic antigen, or LeuM1 (CD15). If only the pleomorphic portion is sampled, the differential diagnosis primarily consists of pleomorphic sarcoma, which will lack expression of CK.[44,45]

MOLECULAR PATHOLOGY FEATURES

Similar to ADCA, PC may harbor *EGFR*, *KRAS*, and/or *TP53* mutations. PC may also be enriched in *MET* exon14-skipping alterations.[45,46] PCs frequently express programmed death ligand-1 (PD-L1) and PD-L2, particularly in the sarcomatoid component.[44]

PULMONARY BLASTOMA

MICROSCOPIC AND IMMUNOHISTOCHEMICAL FEATURES

PB is a rare neoplasm with a biphasic pattern of epithelial and primitive mesenchymal cells, with at least 10% sarcomatous elements upon complete resection (Fig. 3).[47–49] The epithelial component is composed of irregular branching glandular structures with pseudostratified columnar cells that have clear to finely vacuolated cytoplasm and hyperchromatic nuclei with minimal atypia. The mesenchymal cells are oval with high nuclear-to-cytoplasmic ratios and coarse chromatin.[48,49] The mesenchymal elements can be differentiated into osteosarcoma, chondrosarcoma, or rhabdomyosarcoma, although this is rare.[49] These tumors can be positive for β-catenin (nuclear), CK, α-fetoprotein, EMA, TTF-1, SMA, desmin, S100, calponin, CD56, and vimentin.[47]

DIFFERENTIAL DIAGNOSIS

PB should be distinguished from other sarcomatoid carcinomas of the lung, including carcinosarcoma, which does not have nuclear β-catenin staining. They must be distinguished from poorly differentiated carcinoma, primary biphenotypic synovial sarcoma, solitary fibrous tumor, and small round cell tumors, such as small cell neuroendocrine carcinoma, well-differentiated neuroendocrine ("carcinoid") tumor (NET), and basaloid SCCA.[49]

MOLECULAR PATHOLOGY FEATURES

PB is most frequently associated with mutations in *CTNNB1*. There have also been documented mutations in other genes, albeit sporadically.[48,50]

CARCINOSARCOMA

MICROSCOPIC AND IMMUNOHISTOCHEMICAL FEATURES

Pulmonary carcinosarcoma (PCS) is a rare NSCLCA. It is a biphasic tumor consisting of malignant epithelial and mesenchymal components

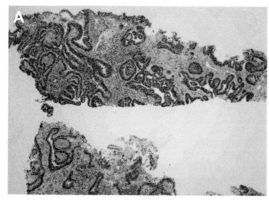
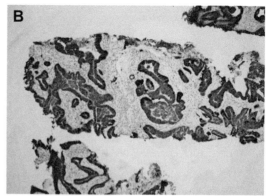
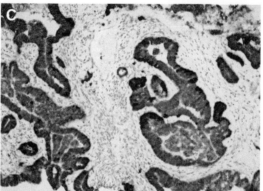

Fig. 3. Histomorphologic and immunohistochemical features of PB acquired by biopsy. (*A*) Formalin-fixed, paraffin-embedded tissue with branching structures (H&E, 100×). (*B, C*) Immunohistochemical analysis demonstrates cytoplasmic and focal nuclear β-catenin expression in the epithelial component and no staining of the mesenchymal component (100×).

(**Fig. 4**). The most common epithelial components are SCCA, ADCA, and large cell carcinoma, in descending order of frequency. The most common mesenchymal component is poorly differentiated spindle cell sarcoma although osteosarcoma, chondrosarcoma, and rhabdomyosarcoma have also been reported. These neoplasms can have abundant necrosis and tend to invade into adjacent structures.[51] The carcinomatous components can be positive for CK5/6, CK7, EMA, p63, CD56, chromogranin A, and synaptophysin, and the sarcomatous elements can be positive for SMA, desmin, and vimentin.[52]

DIFFERENTIAL DIAGNOSIS

PCS should be distinguished from other sarcomatoid carcinomas of the lung, such as PB, as well as primary or metastatic carcinomas or sarcomas.[49]

MOLECULAR PATHOLOGY FEATURES

PCS has been associated with elevated PD-L1 and KRAS expression.[51] Mutations in *TP53*,

CSMD3, *RYR3*, and *LYST* have also been identified.[52]

NUT CARCINOMA

MICROSCOPIC AND IMMUNOHISTOCHEMICAL FEATURES

NC is an aggressive neoplasm composed of nests and sheets of primitive, monotonous cells that have minimal cytoplasm and round-to-oval nuclei with varied chromatin patterns and, often, a distinct and small nucleolus (**Fig. 5**). Commonly, there is nuclear overlap and molding with bare nuclei and abrupt squamous differentiation and keratinization. Necrosis, karyorrhectic debris, and mixed inflammation are often identified. The mitotic rate is brisk with rare atypical figures. NC is positive for CK, p63, and p40 with speckled nuclear NUT1.[21]

DIFFERENTIAL DIAGNOSIS

The differential diagnosis for NC includes poorly differentiated SCCA, poorly differentiated ADCA,

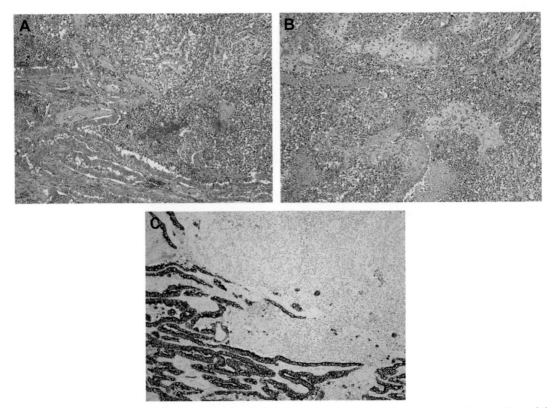

Fig. 4. Histomorphologic and immunohistochemical features of carcinosarcoma acquired by resection. (*A*) Formalin-fixed, paraffin-embedded tissue with malignant epithelial and mesenchymal components (H&E, 100×) and (*B*) a prominent myxoid matrix (H&E, 100×). (*C*) Immunohistochemical analysis demonstrates positive keratin staining in the carcinomatous component and negative staining in the sarcomatous component (pankeratin, 100×).

small cell carcinoma, thymic carcinoma, germ cell tumors, lymphoma, primitive neuroectodermal tumors, SMARCB1-deficient tumors, and SMARCA4-deficient tumors. These can be differentiated based on immunohistochemical stains, as NC would be positive for NUT1, while others are not.[21]

MOLECULAR PATHOLOGY FEATURES

These tumors have rearrangements of the NUT midline carcinoma family member 1 (*NUTM1*) gene on chromosome 15q14. The typical fusion partners are bromodomain-containing protein 4 (*BRD4*) on chromosome 19 and *BRD3*.[21]

SMARCA4-DEFICIENT UNDIFFERENTIATED TUMOR

MICROSCOPIC AND IMMUNOHISTOCHEMICAL FEATURES

SMARCA4-deficient undifferentiated tumors (SDUT) are aggressive neoplasms characterized by sheets of dyscohesive cells that are monomorphic and

round with prominent nucleoli and indistinct cell borders. Mitoses and necrosis are common and rhabdoid or hepatoid features may be present. However, gland formation, papillae, and keratinization are not seen. In a subset of cases (∼5%), they may be combined with a histologically conventional NSCLCA (ie, ADCA or less commonly SCCA). On IHC, these tumors may be positive for CD34, SALL4, HepPar1, synaptophysin, and SOX2 with complete loss or severe reduction of BRG1 (SMARCA4) or BRM (SMARCA2) and negative or focal CK, TTF-1, p40, and claudin-4.[53]

DIFFERENTIAL DIAGNOSIS

Although histogenetically related,[54] SDUTs and SMARCA4-deficient NSCLCAs should be differentiated from one another, as the former are associated with a worse prognosis. SMARCA4-deficient non-small cell lung carcinomas will have retained BRM, CK, and claudin 4 staining with negative CD34, SALL4, and SOX2. SDUT should also be differentiated from other poorly differentiated NSCLCAs without SMARCA4 loss, vascular

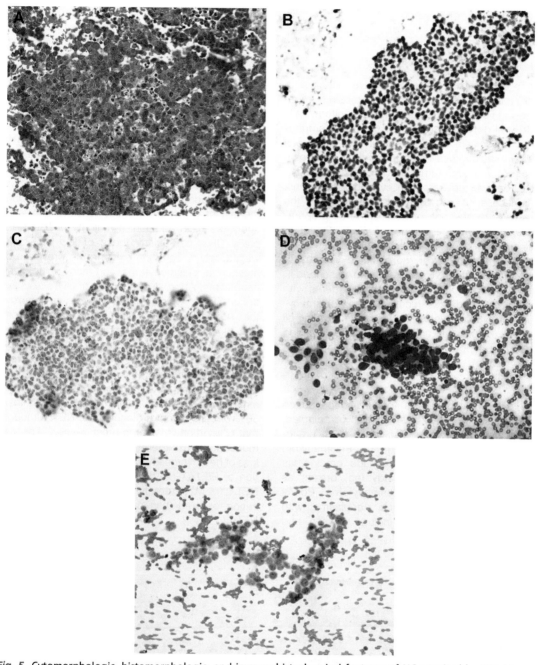

Fig. 5. Cytomorphologic, histomorphologic, and immunohistochemical features of NC acquired by FNA biopsy. (*A*) Formalin-fixed, paraffin-embedded cell block (H&E, 400×) with results of immunohistochemical analysis with expression of (*B*) p40 (400×) and (*C*) NUT (400×). (*D*) Primitive monotonous cells with minimal cytoplasm, nuclear overlap, and distinct nucleoli (Diff-Quik, 400×). (*E*) Tumor cells demonstrate varied chromatin patterns and a distinct nucleolus (Papanicolaou, 400×).

tumors, epithelioid sarcoma, melanoma, lymphoma, germ cell tumors, rhabdomyosarcoma, Ewing sarcoma, CIC-DUX4 sarcoma, and mesothelioma.[53]

MOLECULAR PATHOLOGY FEATURES

These tumors have a loss-of-function molecular alteration in SMARCA4, an ATPase subunit in the SWI/SNF chromatin modifying complex.[53]

NEUROENDOCRINE NEOPLASMS

NEUROENDOCRINE TUMORS

Microscopic Features

NETs demonstrate loosely cohesive cell clusters with focally branching or anastomosing transgressing vessels. Clusters consist of uniform cells with well-defined borders and granular, amphophilic cytoplasm in a background of numerous nuclei that have been stripped of their cytoplasm (**Fig. 6**A). Although tumor grade cannot be definitively determined based on cytology specimens, it is necessary for cytopathologists to report the presence or absence of necrosis in all preparations, as well as the number of mitotic figures in cell block sections (calculated per 2 mm²). An astonishing number of morphologic variants of well-differentiated NETs have been described.[55] However, a majority fall into 1 of 2 patterns with either round and eccentrically placed ("plasmacytoid") or oval-to-spindle shaped nuclei. Among all variants, nuclei are uniform with finely stippled ("salt-and-pepper") chromatin (**Fig. 6**B).

Differential Diagnosis

The differential diagnosis for NET depends on whether the cells are plasmacytoid or spindled, but in either case, it falls across 2 axes: provenance and differentiation (**Fig. 7**). Plasmacytoid cells of other provenance include carcinomas with plasmacytoid morphology (eg, breast) as well as melanoma and plasmacytoma. Poorly differentiated neuroendocrine neoplasms with plasmacytoid morphology include SCLCA and

LCNECA. Spindle cells of other provenance include a broad range of spindle cell neoplasms (eg, solitary fibrous tumor) as well as melanoma. It is unusual for poorly differentiated neuroendocrine neoplasms (carcinomas) to demonstrate spindle cell morphology.

Molecular Testing and Other Ancillary Studies

In order to determine the provenance of a suspected NET, multiple IHC markers of neuroendocrine differentiation are currently available, including insulinoma-associated protein 1 (INSM-1), chromogranin A, synaptophysin, and CD56, the last of which is the most sensitive and least specific.[13,56] In addition, a majority of NETs express CKs, particularly those of low molecular weight, which can help exclude the presence of melanoma, plasmacytoma, and many spindle cell neoplasms. Approximately 50% of NETs also express TTF-1, which, when present, can narrow the site of tumor origin to lung and thyroid (**Fig. 8**).[57,58] Note that this is not the case in neuroendocrine carcinomas (discussed in later section). Inversely, in order to establish the well-differentiated nature of a suspected NET, IHC and molecular markers are emerging but not yet established. Ki-67 expression by IHC in less than 30% of cells favors a diagnosis of NET, although that proportion is lower in most cases.[59] Low tumor mutation burden (TMB), mutation of *MEN1*, loss of heterozygosity at the *MEN1* locus, or mutation of *EIF1AX* may indicate the presence of an NET.[60–62] MT, currently, has no role in prognostication or prediction of response to therapy in NETs.

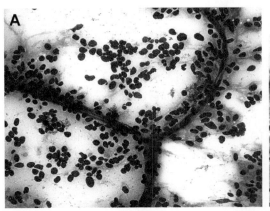
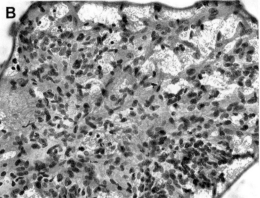

Fig. 6. Direct smear preparations of well-differentiated NET acquired by FNA biopsy. (*A*) Monotonous cells with oval nuclei, many of which have been stripped of their cytoplasm loosely adhere to branching, anastomosing capillaries (Diff-Quik stain, 400×). (*B*) Tumor cells demonstrate finely stippled ("salt-and-pepper") chromatin (Papanicolaou stain, 400×).

NEUROENDOCRINE CARCINOMAS: SMALL CELL LUNG CARCINOMA

MICROSCOPIC FEATURES

SCLCA has traditionally been considered a member of the "small, round, blue cell" tumors, and, as the name implies SCLCA cells are often, *but not always*, small and round. They may be medium-sized and/or polygonal or even spindled. (They do, however, universally demonstrate marked hyperchromasia.) They consist of loosely cohesive clusters of cells that contain amphophilic cytoplasm but demonstrate a markedly elevated nucleus-to-cytoplasm ratio (N:C, **Fig. 9A**). Nuclei are angulated with molding, finely granular chromatin with inconspicuous nucleoli and abundant karyorrhectic and karyolytic debris, which complements frank background necrosis/diathesis (**Fig. 9B**). Mitotic activity is easily discernible, even in alcohol-fixed cytologic preparations.

"Crush" artifact is conspicuous and may even limit cytomorphologic assessment.

DIFFERENTIAL DIAGNOSIS

The differential diagnosis for SCLCA falls across 3 axes: provenance, differentiation, and size (**Fig. 10**). Cells of other provenance that may mimic SCLCA include basaloid SCCA and, paradoxically, large cell lymphoma. Well-differentiated NETs may mimic SCLCA, especially those of high grade and in a necrotic background. Finally, one of the most difficult entities to differentiate from SCLCA is LCNECA, especially considering that both morphologies may be present in a given tumor.

MOLECULAR PATHOLOGY FEATURES

RB1 and *TP53* alterations are demonstrable in almost all SCLCs, either by MT or IHC.[63] Despite such genetic homogeneity, recent years have seen remarkable progress in elucidation of the

Fig. 7. Algorithm for differentiation of well-differentiated neuroendocrine tumor (WDNET) from entities with similar morphologic features depends on the presence of either plasmacytoid morphology (solid *arrows*) or spindle cell morphology (dashed *arrows*) followed by examination of chromatin pattern to determine appropriate immunohistochemical (IHC) workup, which, in most cases will include neuroendocrine markers. Note that the spectrum of spindle cell neoplasms is broad, ranging from benign (eg, solitary fibrous tumor) to malignant (eg, synovial sarcoma) entities. CK, cytokeratin; TTF1, thyroid transcription factor-1; MuM1, multiple myeloma-1; hi, high; Rb, retinoblastoma-1; WT, wild-type.

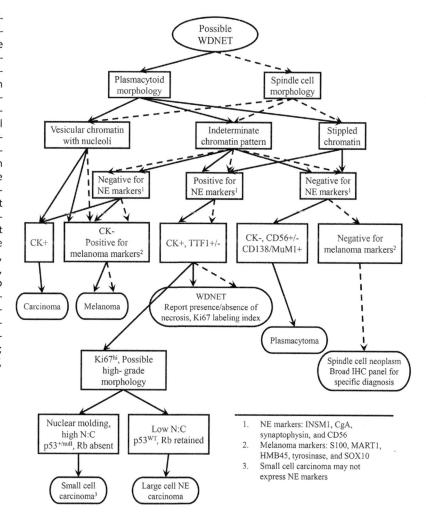

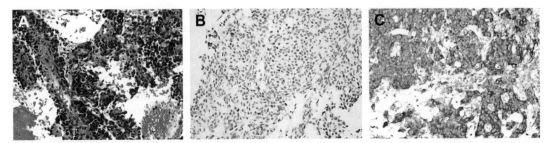

Fig. 8. Histomorphologic and immunohistochemical features of well-differentiated NET acquired by FNA biopsy. (*A*) Formalin-fixed, paraffin-embedded cell block (H&E, 400×) with results of immunohistochemical analysis for expression of (*B*) TTF-1 (400×) and (*C*) synaptophysin (400×).

spectrum of epigenetic and transcriptomic alterations among primary lung carcinomas with small cell morphology. Specifically, expression of lineage factors *ASCL1* and *NEUROD1* can define distinct subtypes. In addition, expression of *POU2F3*, which is mutually exclusive of *ASCL1* and *NEUROD1* defines a subtype of SCLCA for which the expression of neuroendocrine markers may be low or even absent.[64,65] The presence of high TMB also favors a diagnosis of neuroendocrine carcinoma, such as SCLC over well-differentiated NET.

ANCILLARY STUDIES, DIAGNOSTIC: IMMUNOHISTOCHEMISTRY

While the diagnosis of SCLCA is primarily based on microscopic features, IHC may be helpful in confirming a diagnosis in ambiguous cases, as follows (**Fig. 11**). Expression of CK, which may sporadically demonstrate a perinuclear, dot-like expression pattern (especially of low molecular weight keratins) is critical for differentiating SCLCA from large cell lymphoma. Expression of TTF-1 and neuroendocrine markers—INSM-1, synaptophysin, chromogranin (less sensitive), and CD56 (less specific)—may be absent, but when present will help differentiate SCLCA from basaloid

SCCA, which will instead express p40. TTF-1 positivity is not specific to small cell carcinomas of lung origin, so its positivity does not rule out metastasis.[66] In cases with elevated suspicion of SCLCA but lack of neuroendocrine marker expression, POU2F3 may help confirm a diagnosis.[65] In cases with poor cellular preservation, the expression of Ki-67 in greater than 30% of cells (usually >50%) will support a diagnosis of high-grade neuroendocrine carcinoma over well-differentiated NET.[59] Finally, the overexpression or complete absence of expression (null phenotype) of p53 combined with the absence of expression of Rb1 may help differentiate SCLCA from LCNECA. Caution is advised, however, as SCLCA may coexist with LCNECA or conventional NSCLCA in up to 10% of cases,[64] and SCLCA subsets exist that alternately express Rb1 despite molecular evidence of loss of function or maintain full Rb1 proficiency.[67]

NEUROENDOCRINE CARCINOMAS: LARGE CELL NEUROENDOCRINE CARCINOMA

MICROSCOPIC FEATURES

While histologic criteria for the diagnosis of LCNECA have been evaluated and evolved over

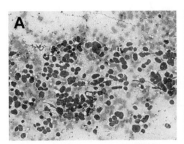
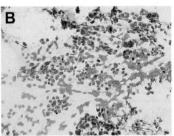
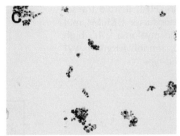

Fig. 9. Direct smear (*A*, *B*) and liquid-based (*C*) preparations of small cell carcinoma acquired by FNA biopsy. (*A*) Cells with high N:C ratio focally demonstrate nuclear molding and "crush" artifact (Diff-Quik stain, 400×). (*B*, *C*) Tumor cells demonstrate stippled chromatin as well as karyorrhectic and karyolytic debris (Papanicolaou stain, 400×).

Fig. 10. The differential diagnosis for small cell lung carcinoma falls across 3 axes depending on the morphologic features and results of immunohistochemical (IHC) analysis. SCCA, squamous cell carcinoma; Pos, positive; CK, cytokeratin; HMW, high molecular weight; TTF1, thyroid transcription factor-1; hi, high; NET, neuroendocrine tumor; lo, low; WT, wild-type.

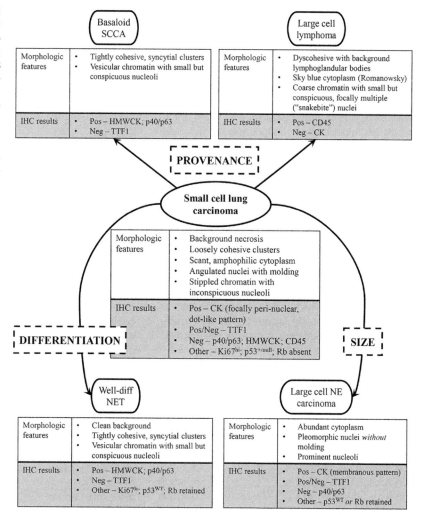

Basaloid SCCA

Morphologic features	• Tightly cohesive, syncytial clusters • Vesicular chromatin with small but conspicuous nucleoli
IHC results	• Pos – HMWCK; p40/p63 • Neg – TTF1

Large cell lymphoma

Morphologic features	• Dyscohesive with background lymphoglandular bodies • Sky blue cytoplasm (Romanowsky) • Coarse chromatin with small but conspicuous, focally multiple ("snakebite") nuclei
IHC results	• Pos – CD45 • Neg – CK

PROVENANCE

Small cell lung carcinoma

Morphologic features	• Background necrosis • Loosely cohesive clusters • Scant, amphophilic cytoplasm • Angulated nuclei with molding • Stippled chromatin with inconspicuous nucleoli
IHC results	• Pos – CK (focally peri-nuclear, dot-like pattern) • Pos/Neg – TTF1 • Neg – p40/p63; HMWCK; CD45 • Other – Ki67hi; p53+/null; Rb absent

DIFFERENTIATION   **SIZE**

Well-diff NET

Morphologic features	• Clean background • Tightly cohesive, syncytial clusters • Vesicular chromatin with small but conspicuous nucleoli
IHC results	• Pos – HMWCK; p40/p63 • Neg – TTF1 • Other – Ki67lo; p53WT; Rb retained

Large cell NE carcinoma

Morphologic features	• Abundant cytoplasm • Pleomorphic nuclei *without* molding • Prominent nucleoli
IHC results	• Pos – CK (membranous pattern) • Pos/Neg – TTF1 • Neg – p40/p63 • Other – p53WT *or* Rb retained

time,[12,68] the efficacy of previously proposed cytologic criteria have not been established in large-scale studies.[69] (A semiquantitative scoring system has been proposed for distinguishing LCNECA from other NSCLCAs in small histologic biopsies, but its use has not yet been extended to cytology specimens.)[70] For this reason, among others, The WHO System for Lung Cytopathology recommends utilizing the terminology "Non-small cell carcinoma with neuroendocrine morphology

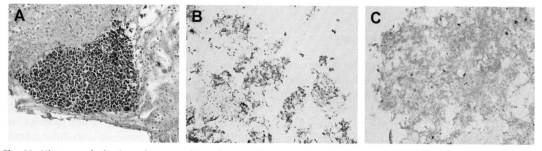

Fig. 11. Histomorphologic and immunohistochemical features of small cell carcinoma acquired by FNA biopsy. (*A*) Formalin-fixed, paraffin-embedded cell block (H&E, 400×). (*B*) Immunohistochemical analysis demonstrates focal perinuclear, dot-like tumor cell expression of CK (CAM5.2, 400×), (*C*) while expression of retinoblastoma (Rb-1, 400×) is absent in tumor cells and retained in incidentally sampled benign epithelial and inflammatory cells.

and positive neuroendocrine markers, possible large cell neuroendocrine carcinoma." Although a broad spectrum of morphologic features may be identified, typically loosely cohesive clusters of cells with abundant granular, amphophilic cytoplasm are identified in a background of abundant necrosis/diathesis. Although such clusters are often syncytial, careful examination may reveal focally prominent tumor cell borders. Nuclei are hyperchromatic and pleomorphic with irregular contours and coarsely granular chromatin with variably prominent nucleoli. Focal nuclear molding and "crush" artifact do not preclude a diagnosis of LCNECA.

DIFFERENTIAL DIAGNOSIS

The differential diagnosis for cases that ultimately turn out to be LCNECA falls into 1 of 3 categories, depending on the morphology. The most common scenario is that in which the "non-small" nature of the carcinoma is readily apparent, but the neuroendocrine differentiation is less easily discernible morphologically. The differential diagnosis of tumors in this category includes all subtypes of NSCLCA. MT and IHC may be very useful in such cases and may provide predictive and prognostic in addition to diagnostic information. A second and particularly difficult scenario is that in which the presence of a high-grade neuroendocrine carcinoma is evident, but of uncertain type. The differential diagnosis of tumors in this category consists primarily of SCLCA. Differentiation between LCNECA and SCLCA rests primarily on morphology, although MT and IHC may be useful in select cases. A third and, fortunately, uncommon scenario is that in which neoplastic neuroendocrine cells contain abundant cytoplasm, but their differentiation is uncertain. In most cases, the differential diagnosis in this scenario—atypical carcinoid—can be excluded by high mitotic activity (>10 mitoses per 2 mm^2) or high Ki67 proliferative index (>30%). Furthermore, MT may also be diagnostically valuable.

MOLECULAR PATHOLOGY FEATURES

Although integrative molecular profiling has uncovered a broad range of recurrent genetic and genomic changes in LCNECA, they generally fall into 2 categories: those that share genomic features of SCLCA ("SCLCA-like") and those that share genomic features of ADCA ("NSCLCA-like").[71] A majority of the former harbor loss-of-function TP53 alterations, and a subset of those also harbor loss-of-function RB1 mutations. They are also enriched in MYCL1 and NKX2-1

amplifications.[72] The latter are also enriched in loss-of-function TP53 alterations, as well as STK11, KEAP1, KRAS, and NOTCH alterations, and they have higher median TMB than other NSCLCAs. Both are enriched in transversion mutations, typical of tobacco-induced carcinogenesis. Neither harbor alterations in MEN1 or ARID1A. As NSCLCA-like LCNECA may harbor targetable genetic or genomic alterations (including high TMB), it is advisable to submit LCNECA samples for comprehensive genetic profiling to direct therapy.

ANCILLARY STUDIES, DIAGNOSTIC: IMMUNOHISTOCHEMISTRY

Unlike SCLCA, expression of at least one neuroendocrine IHC marker is required for a diagnosis of LCNECA. It should be noted that neuroendocrine markers should only be performed in the presence of neuroendocrine morphology on hematoxylin–eosin (H&E). An IHC panel consisting of napsin A, which will be absent in SCLCA[73] and one or more keratins (including those of low molecular weight) to identify perinuclear, dot-like expression, as well as p53 and Rb1 may be helpful to differentiate LCNECA from SCLCA. However, neither napsin A nor CK IHC have demonstrated high sensitivity, while p53 and Rb1 IHC is not entirely specific. Ki-67 IHC may also be helpful in differentiating LCNECA from well-differentiated NETs, particularly atypical carcinoids. Although MT has revealed overlap in a small proportion of cases, the expression of Ki-67 in greater than 30% of tumor cells favors a diagnosis of LCNECA.[74]

OTHER MALIGNANCIES

LANGERHANS CELL HISTIOCYTOSIS

Per the WHO Reporting System, pulmonary Langerhans cell histiocytosis falls within the broader category of lymphoproliferative diseases. Langerhans cell histiocytosis is a neoplasm of dendritic cells expressing a Langerhans cell phenotype. It occurs in the lung interstitium and is commonly seen in smokers.[75] The tumor is of moderate-to-high cellularity, with characteristic Langerhans cells showing enlarged, deeply indented and convoluted nuclei with fine chromatin, and indistinct nucleoli. The cytoplasm is abundant and finely granular. The tumor background has plentiful eosinophils occasionally admixed with other inflammatory cells. Langerhans cells are characterized by the expression of CD1a, CD207 (langerin), and S100 by IHC and Birbeck granules by electron microscopy, as well as the presence of BRAF

V600 E mutation via IHC or MT in a majority of cases.[75]

Other lymphoproliferative disorders of the lung are most likely to represent secondary involvement of lymph nodes or, less commonly, the lung parenchyma. Diffuse large B-cell lymphoma, extranodal marginal zone lymphoma of the mucosa-associated lymphoid tissue, and Erdheim–Chester disease may present as primary neoplasms of the lung and are similar to their non-pulmonary counterparts.[12]

SPINDLE CELL TUMORS

Spindle cell lesions of the lung comprise of a wide variety of benign and malignant conditions. They are all difficult to diagnose based on cytomorphology alone, requiring IHC and/or MT, if sufficient material is available.

Pulmonary artery intimal sarcoma is a rare intraluminal tumor that is often clinically misdiagnosed as recurrent pulmonary embolism.[76] The cytology is composed of pleomorphic malignant spindled and epithelioid cells arranged in loosely cohesive clusters. The size of the tumor nuclei varies with irregular nuclear membranes, coarse chromatin, and prominent nucleoli. Occasional binucleated and multinucleated cells may be observed. The tumor cells exhibit varying amounts of cytoplasm and ill-defined cell borders.[77,78]

Leiomyosarcoma cells demonstrate high nuclear grade, and specimens are typically hypercellular. The cytoplasm is pale to eosinophilic with moderately pleomorphic plump nuclei with blunt ends. As leiomyosarcoma in the lung is most commonly metastatic, particularly from the gynecologic tract (myometrium), diagnosis of a primary lung leiomyosarcoma should be made with caution.

Synovial sarcomas are classified into 2 subtypes: monophasic spindle cell and biphasic.[79] The characteristic t(X: 18) (p11:q11) reciprocal translocation is identified in greater than 90% of biphasic and monophasic tumors.[80] Regardless of the subtype, the predominant cytology pattern is a mixture of cell-tight tumor tissue fragments with irregular borders and dispersed cells. Monophasic synovial sarcoma displays monomorphic, delicate, relatively uniform and small spindle cells with a high N:C ratio. The cytoplasm is sparse with ovoid or bipolar and hyperchromatic nuclei with inconspicuous nucleoli. Biphasic synovial sarcoma has epithelial and spindle cell components in varying proportions with varying proportion of tubule or gland like structures.[81] SSX IHC has recently been shown to be an effective diagnostic alternative to polymerase chain reaction

and in situ hybridization.[82] Other IHC is nonspecific but useful in the initial phases of a workup to support the nature of the tumor and suggest evaluation for the characteristic translocation. Synovial sarcomas demonstrate keratin, EMA, calretinin, and TLE1 staining, but these are not specific.

Solitary fibrous tumors are mesenchymal tumors arising from within the lung or more commonly the visceral pleura. They have a characteristic appearance of uniform fibroblastic spindle cells arranged in a "patternless" pattern, with staghorn-shaped branching vessels. Cellularity and mitotic activity vary between tumors, with an increasing aggressiveness associated with an increased mitotic activity.[12] SFTs harbor a characteristic and diagnostic NAB2-STAT6 fusion, which results in high nuclear expression of a fusion protein. They are positive for CD34, and the STAT6 fusion product can very reliably be detected by IHC for STAT6.[83]

DIFFUSE PLEURAL MESOTHELIOMA

When cytopathologists are called upon to make a diagnosis of malignant epithelioid mesothelioma, it is usually in the context of exfoliative effusion fluid cytology, which is beyond the scope of this review. However, mesothelioma may uncommonly present as a lung mass or large pleural mass and be diagnosed on FNA. In such instances, differentiation between malignant and benign mesothelial proliferations can be challenging as many of the cytologic features, including scalloped borders of cell clumps, intercellular windows with lighter, dense cytoplasm edges, and low N:C ratio are shared between reactive and malignant epithelioid mesothelial cells.[84] Localized pleural mesothelioma is microscopically identical to diffuse malignant pleural mesothelioma, aside from its solitary nature and a stalk-like attachment to the pleura.[85] On cytology, one can observe an abundance of large, cohesive tissue fragments, which often take on a morular, papillary, or tubular form. The cytoplasm is 2 toned, imparting a "lacy skirt" appearance, and the nuclei contain prominent, centrally located nucleoli. Extracellular proteinaceous background material may be present in both cell blocks and direct smears. Care must be taken not to confuse it with chondromyxoid matrix or true mucin. To establish a diagnosis of malignant mesothelioma, IHC with or without MT is usually necessary.[84]

Sarcomatoid mesothelioma is characterized by spindle cells arranged in fascicles or haphazard patterns. The spindle cells are long and tapered with atypical nuclei ranging from bland to pleomorphic.[86] Unlike its epithelioid counterpart, sarcomatoid mesothelioma often demonstrates loss of high molecular weight CK, homozygous deletion of CDKN2A/p16, and retained BAP1 expression.

IHC may be used to first confirm the mesothelial nature of the tissue when the possibility exists of a primary lung or metastatic tumor. Epithelioid mesothelioma may mimic primary lung or metastastic ADCA, while sarcomatoid/desmoplastic mesothelioma may mimic sarcomas sarcomatoid carcinomas. The International Mesothelioma Interest Group recommends the use of 1 CK, 2 carcinoma, and 2 mesothelioma markers as a panel for this distinction and has published several helpful tables.[84]

Once cells are confirmed to be mesothelial, a different set of immunohistochemical stains combined with MT can help determine their benign or malignant nature. In small specimens and particularly in cytologic preparations, evidence of invasion of adjacent structures is likely to be lacking. Many IHC markers have been proposed to distinguish benign, reactive mesothelial proliferations from mesothelioma (EMA, p53, IMP3, CD16, GLUT-1, and others); however, they do not reliably do so on an individual patient basis.[87] Homozygous deletion of CDKN2A/p16, and methyladenosine phosphorylase (MTAP) or BAP-1 loss by IHC are specific markers of malignancy, but they are only seen in 60% to 70% of epithelioid mesothelial proliferations, while homozygous deletion of CDKN2A/p16 and MTAP loss are seen in a majority of sarcomatoid mesotheliomas.[87] BAP-1 loss, on the other hand, is rare in sarcomatoid mesotheliomas. IHC for MTAP may be used as a surrogate marker for homozygous CDKN2A/p16 deletion as the 2 genes are often (~90%) codeleted in mesotheliomas. Retained expression may be seen in both benign and malignant mesothelial proliferations and, therefore, is not helpful in making a diagnosis of malignant mesothelioma. IHC for p16 cannot be used to assess p16 loss, as the protein is not expressed at detectable levels in benign mesothelial cells. Additional markers continue to be studied for their utility in this specific scenario.

DISCLOSURE

The authors have nothing to disclose.

REFERENCES

1. Saad RS, Silverman JF. Respiratory cytology: differential diagnosis and pitfalls. Diagn Cytopathol 2010;38(4):297–307.
2. Magda G. Opportunistic Infections Post-Lung Transplantation: Viral, Fungal, and Mycobacterial. Clin Chest Med 2023;44(1):159–77.
3. Borczuk AC. Neoplastic and nonneoplastic benign mass lesions of the lung. Arch Pathol Lab Med 2012;136(10):1227–33.
4. Dettrick A, Meikle A, Fong KM. Fine-needle aspiration diagnosis of sclerosing hemangioma (pneumocytoma): report of a case and review of the literature. Diagn Cytopathol 2014;42(3):242–6.
5. Zeng J, Zhou F, Wei XJ, et al. Sclerosing hemangioma: A diagnostic dilemma in fine needle aspiration cytology. CytoJournal 2016;13:9.
6. Hissong E, Rao R. Pneumocytoma (sclerosing hemangioma), a potential pitfall. Diagn Cytopathol 2017; 45(8):744–9.
7. Maleki Z, Muller S, Layfield L, et al. Pulmonary sclerosing pneumocytoma: Cytomorphology and immunoprofile. Cancer Cytopathol 2020;128(6):414–23.
8. Devouassoux-Shisheboran M, Hayashi T, Linnoila RI, et al. A clinicopathologic study of 100 cases of pulmonary sclerosing hemangioma with immunohistochemical studies: TTF-1 is expressed in both round and surface cells, suggesting an origin from primitive respiratory epithelium. Am J Surg Pathol 2000; 24(7):906–16.
9. Schmitt FC, Bubendorf L, Canberk S, et al. The World Health Organization Reporting System for Lung Cytopathology. Acta Cytol 2023;67(1):80–91.
10. Canberk S, Field A, Bubendorf L, et al. A brief review of the WHO reporting system for lung cytopathology. J Am Soc Cytopathol 2023;12(4):251–7.
11. Yang SR, Chang JC, Leduc C, et al. Invasive Mucinous Adenocarcinomas With Spatially Separate Lung Lesions: Analysis of Clonal Relationship by Comparative Molecular Profiling. J Thorac Oncol 2021;16(7):1188–99.
12. WHO Classification of Tumours of the Lung. Pleura, Thymus and Heart. World Health Organization Classification of Tumours. International Agency for Research on Cancer; 2021.
13. Yatabe Y, Dacic S, Borczuk AC, et al. Best practices recommendations for diagnostic immunohistochemistry in lung cancer. J Thorac Oncol 2019;14(3): 377–407.
14. Layfield LJ, Baloch Z, Elsheikh T, et al. Standardized terminology and nomenclature for respiratory cytology: The Papanicolaou Society of Cytopathology guidelines. Diagn Cytopathol 2016;44(5): 399–409.
15. Roh MH. The utilization of cytologic and small biopsy samples for ancillary molecular testing. Mod Pathol 2019;32(Suppl 1):77–85.
16. Bishop JA, Teruya-Feldstein J, Westra WH, et al. p40 (ΔNp63) is superior to p63 for the diagnosis of pulmonary squamous cell carcinoma. Mod Pathol 2012;25(3):405–15.
17. Idowu MO, Powers CN. Lung cancer cytology: potential pitfalls and mimics - a review. Int J Clin Exp Pathol 2010;3(4):367–85.

18. Travis WD, Brambilla E, Noguchi M, et al. International association for the study of lung cancer/american thoracic society/european respiratory society international multidisciplinary classification of lung adenocarcinoma. J Thorac Oncol 2011;6(2):244–85.

19. Witt BL, Wallander ML, Layfield LJ, et al. Respiratory cytology in the era of molecular diagnostics: a review. Diagn Cytopathol 2012;40(6):556–63.

20. Maleki Z. Diagnostic issues with cytopathologic interpretation of lung neoplasms displaying high-grade basaloid or neuroendocrine morphology. Diagn Cytopathol 2011;39(3):159–67.

21. Dutta R, Nambirajan A, Mittal S, et al. Cytomorphology of primary pulmonary NUT carcinoma in different cytology preparations. Cancer Cytopathol 2021;129(1):53–61.

22. Travis WD, Rekhtman N. Pathological diagnosis and classification of lung cancer in small biopsies and cytology: strategic management of tissue for molecular testing. Semin Respir Crit Care Med 2011;32(1):22–31.

23. Borczuk AC. Uncommon types of lung carcinoma with mixed histology: sarcomatoid carcinoma, adenosquamous carcinoma, and mucoepidermoid carcinoma. Arch Pathol Lab Med 2018;142(8):914–21.

24. Jain D, Nambirajan A, Chen G, et al. NSCLC Subtyping in Conventional Cytology: Results of the International Association for the Study of Lung Cancer Cytology Working Group Survey to Determine Specific Cytomorphologic Criteria for Adenocarcinoma and Squamous Cell Carcinoma. J Thorac Oncol 2022;17(6):793–805.

25. Heitmiller RF, Mathisen DJ, Ferry JA, et al. Mucoepidermoid lung tumors. Ann Thorac Surg 1989;47(3):394–9.

26. Kang DY, Yoon YS, Kim HK, et al. Primary salivary gland-type lung cancer: surgical outcomes. Lung Cancer 2011;72(2):250–4.

27. Travis WD, Brambilla E, Burke AP, et al. Introduction to The 2015 World Health Organization Classification of Tumors of the Lung, Pleura, Thymus, and Heart. J Thorac Oncol 2015;10(9):1240–2.

28. Moran CA. Primary salivary gland-type tumors of the lung. Semin Diagn Pathol 1995;12(2):106–22.

29. Falk N, Weissferdt A, Kalhor N, et al. Primary pulmonary salivary gland-type tumors: a review and update. Adv Anat Pathol 2016;23(1):13–23.

30. Turnbull AD, Huvos AG, Goodner JT, et al. Mucoepidermoid tumors of bronchial glands. Cancer 1971;28(3):539–44.

31. Limaiem F, Lekkala MR, Sharma S. Mucoepidermoid lung tumor. StatPearls. StatPearls publishing Copyright © 2023. StatPearls Publishing LLC.; 2023.

32. Welsh JH, Maxson T, Jaksic T, et al. Tracheobronchial mucoepidermoid carcinoma in childhood and adolescence: case report and review of the literature. Int J Pediatr Otorhinolaryngol 1998;45(3):265–73.

33. Rojas Y, Shi YX, Zhang W, et al. Primary malignant pulmonary tumors in children: a review of the national cancer data base. J Pediatr Surg 2015;50(6):1004–8.

34. Puzyrenko A, Shponka V, Sheinin Y, et al. Primary pulmonary mucoepidermoid carcinoma: Cyto-histologic correlation and review of the literature. Ann Diagn Pathol 2021;51:151698.

35. Wang M, Gilani S, Xu H, et al. Salivary Gland-type Tumors of the Lung. Arch Pathol Lab Med 2021;145(11):1379–86.

36. Qiu S, Nampoothiri MM, Zaharopoulos P, et al. Primary pulmonary adenoid cystic carcinoma: report of a case diagnosed by fine-needle aspiration cytology. Diagn Cytopathol 2004;30(1):51–6.

37. Chen L, Fan Y, Lu H. Pulmonary Epithelial-Myoepithelial Carcinoma. J Oncol 2022;2022:4559550.

38. Zhu Z, Lian X, Yang D. Right main bronchial pleomorphic adenoma: A case report and literature review. Medicine (Baltim) 2018;97(42):e12648.

39. Charles R, Murray S, Gray E, et al. Pulmonary epithelial-myoepithelial carcinoma (P-EMC) with focal high grade transformation: Molecular and cytologic findings. Diagn Cytopathol 2022;50(6):E156–62.

40. Li C, Lu H. Adenosquamous carcinoma of the lung. OncoTargets Ther 2018;11:4829–35.

41. Shelton DA, Rana DN, Holbrook M, et al. Adenosquamous carcinoma of the lung diagnosed by cytology?: a diagnostic dilemma. Diagn Cytopathol 2012;40(9):830–3.

42. White VA, Hyrcza MD, Lennerz JK, et al. Mucoepidermoid carcinoma (MEC) and adenosquamous carcinoma (ASC), the same or different entities? Mod Pathol 2022;35(10):1484–93.

43. Hiroshima K, Dosaka-Akita H, Usuda K, et al. Cytological characteristics of pulmonary pleomorphic and giant cell carcinomas. Acta Cytol 2011;55(2):173–9.

44. Jeong JH, Seo HJ, Yoon SH, et al. Pulmonary pleomorphic carcinoma presenting as undifferentiated non-small cell carcinoma with giant cells: A case report and review of literature. Respir Med Case Rep 2020;31:101225.

45. Chen Z, Liu J, Min L. Clinicopathological characteristics, survival outcomes and prognostic factors in pleomorphic carcinoma: a SEER population-based study. BMC Pulm Med 2022;22(1):116.

46. Nagano M, Kohsaka S, Hayashi T, et al. Comprehensive molecular profiling of pulmonary pleomorphic carcinoma. npj Precis Oncol 2021;5(1):57.

47. Luo Z, Cao C, Xu N, et al. Classic biphasic pulmonary blastoma: a case report and review of the literature. J Int Med Res 2020;48(10), 300060520962394.

48. Tsamis I, Chachali SP, Gomatou G, et al. Pulmonary blastoma: a comprehensive overview of a rare entity. Adv Respir Med 2021;89(5):511–9.

49. Shastri M, Kundu R. Scalp metastasis of pulmonary blastoma-a rare entity: Cytomorphology with differential diagnoses. Cytopathology 2023;34(3):259–63.

50. Xie Y, Su N, Li C, et al. Pulmonary blastoma treatment response to anti-PD-1 therapy: a rare case report and literature review. Front Oncol 2023;13: 1146204.

51. Mekheal E, Kapoor A, Roman S, et al. Pulmonary carcinosarcoma: a rare disease with challenging diagnosis and treatment. Cureus 2022;14(7):e26901.

52. Li F, Hu S, Kong K, et al. Next-generation sequencing analysis identified genomic alterations in pathological morphologies of 3 cases of pulmonary carcinosarcoma. OncoTargets Ther 2020;13:7963–72.

53. Kezlarian B, Montecalvo J, Bodd FM, et al. Diagnosis of thoracic SMARCA4-deficient undifferentiated tumor in cytology. Cancer Cytopathol 2023; 131(8):526–34.

54. Rekhtman N, Montecalvo J, Chang JC, et al. SMARCA4-deficient thoracic sarcomatoid tumors represent primarily smoking-related undifferentiated carcinomas rather than primary thoracic sarcomas. J Thorac Oncol 2020;15(2):231–47.

55. Rekhtman N. Neuroendocrine tumors of the lung: an update. Arch Pathol Lab Med 2010;134(11):1628–38.

56. Viswanathan K, Siddiqui MT, Borczuk AC. Insulinoma-associated protein 1 is a sensitive and specific marker for lung neuroendocrine tumors in cytologic and surgical specimens. J Am Soc Cytopathol 2019;8(6):299–308.

57. Zhang C, Schmidt LA, Hatanaka K, et al. Evaluation of napsin A, TTF-1, p63, p40, and CK5/6 immunohistochemical stains in pulmonary neuroendocrine tumors. Am J Clin Pathol 2014;142(3):320–4.

58. Papaxoinis G, Lamarca A, Quinn AM, et al. Clinical and pathologic characteristics of pulmonary carcinoid tumors in central and peripheral locations. Endocr Pathol 2018;29(3):259–68.

59. Pelosi G, Rodriguez J, Viale G, et al. Typical and atypical pulmonary carcinoid tumor overdiagnosed as small-cell carcinoma on biopsy specimens: a major pitfall in the management of lung cancer patients. Am J Surg Pathol 2005;29(2):179–87.

60. Fernandez-Cuesta L, Peifer M, Lu X, et al. Frequent mutations in chromatin-remodelling genes in pulmonary carcinoids. Nat Commun 2014;5:3518.

61. Alcala N, Leblay N, Gabriel AAG, et al. Integrative and comparative genomic analyses identify clinically relevant pulmonary carcinoid groups and unveil the supra-carcinoids. Nat Commun 2019;10(1):3407.

62. Laddha SV, da Silva EM, Robzyk K, et al. Integrative genomic characterization identifies molecular subtypes of lung carcinoids. Cancer Res 2019;79(17): 4339–47.

63. George J, Lim JS, Jang SJ, et al. Comprehensive genomic profiles of small cell lung cancer. Nature 2015;524(7563):47–53.

64. Baine MK, Hsieh MS, Lai WV, et al. SCLC Subtypes Defined by ASCL1, NEUROD1, POU2F3, and YAP1: A Comprehensive Immunohistochemical and Histopathologic Characterization. J Thorac Oncol 2020; 15(12):1823–35.

65. Baine MK, Febres-Aldana CA, Chang JC, et al. POU2F3 in SCLC: clinicopathologic and genomic analysis with a focus on its diagnostic utility in neuroendocrine-Low SCLC. J Thorac Oncol 2022; 17(9):1109–21.

66. Agoff SN, Lamps LW, Philip AT, et al. Thyroid transcription factor-1 is expressed in extrapulmonary small cell carcinomas but not in other extrapulmonary neuroendocrine tumors. Mod Pathol 2000;13(3):238–42.

67. Febres-Aldana CA, Chang JC, Ptashkin R, et al. Rb tumor suppressor in small cell lung cancer: combined genomic and IHC analysis with a description of a distinct Rb-proficient subset. Clin Cancer Res 2022;28(21):4702–13.

68. Travis WD, Brambilla E, Nicholson AG, et al. The 2015 World Health Organization Classification of Lung Tumors: Impact of Genetic, Clinical and Radiologic Advances Since the 2004 Classification. J Thorac Oncol 2015;10(9):1243–60.

69. Wiatrowska BA, Krol J, Zakowski MF. Large-cell neuroendocrine carcinoma of the lung: proposed criteria for cytologic diagnosis. Diagn Cytopathol 2001;24(1): 58–64.

70. Baine MK, Sinard JH, Cai G, et al. A semiquantitative scoring system may allow biopsy diagnosis of pulmonary large cell neuroendocrine carcinoma. Am J Clin Pathol 2020;153(2):165–74.

71. Rekhtman N, Pietanza MC, Hellmann MD, et al. Next-generation sequencing of pulmonary large cell neuroendocrine carcinoma reveals small cell carcinoma-like and non-small cell carcinoma-like subsets. Clin Cancer Res 2016;22(14):3618–29.

72. George J, Walter V, Peifer M, et al. Integrative genomic profiling of large-cell neuroendocrine carcinomas reveals distinct subtypes of high-grade neuroendocrine lung tumors. Nat Commun 2018;9(1):1048.

73. Rekhtman N, Pietanza CM, Sabari J, et al. Pulmonary large cell neuroendocrine carcinoma with adenocarcinoma-like features: napsin A expression and genomic alterations. Mod Pathol 2018;31(1): 111–21.

74. Pelosi G, Rindi G, Travis WD, et al. Ki-67 antigen in lung neuroendocrine tumors: unraveling a role in clinical practice. J Thorac Oncol 2014;9(3):273–84.

75. Vassallo R, Harari S, Tazi A. Current understanding and management of pulmonary Langerhans cell histiocytosis. Thorax 2017;72(10):937–45.

76. Tavora F, Miettinen M, Fanburg-Smith J, et al. Pulmonary artery sarcoma: a histologic and follow-up study with emphasis on a subset of low-grade myofibroblastic sarcomas with a good long-term follow-up. Am J Surg Pathol 2008;32(12):1751–61.

77. Harbhajanka A, Dahoud W, Michael CW, et al. Cytohistological correlation, immunohistochemistry and Murine Double Minute Clone 2 amplification of pulmonary artery intimal sarcoma: A case report with review of literature. Diagn Cytopathol 2019;47(5):494–7.

78. Caraway NP, Salina D, Deavers MT, et al. Pulmonary artery intimal sarcoma diagnosed using endobronchial ultrasound-guided transbronchial needle aspiration. CytoJournal 2015;12:3.

79. Akerman M, Ryd W, Skytting B. Fine-needle aspiration of synovial sarcoma: criteria for diagnosis: retrospective reexamination of 37 cases, including ancillary diagnostics. A Scandinavian Sarcoma Group study. Diagn Cytopathol 2003;28(5):232–8.

80. Srinivasan R, Gautam U, Gupta R, et al. Synovial sarcoma: diagnosis on fine-needle aspiration by morphology and molecular analysis. Cancer 2009; 117(2):128–36.

81. Zhang Y, Wessman S, Wejde J, et al. Diagnosing synovial sarcoma by fine-needle aspiration cytology and molecular techniques 2019;30(5):504–9.

82. Baranov E, McBride MJ, Bellizzi AM, et al. A novel SS18-SSX fusion-specific antibody for the diagnosis of synovial sarcoma. Am J Surg Pathol 2020;44(7): 922–33.

83. Doyle LA, Vivero M, Fletcher CD, et al. Nuclear expression of STAT6 distinguishes solitary fibrous tumor from histologic mimics. Mod Pathol 2014;27(3): 390–5.

84. Husain AN, Colby TV, Ordóñez NG, et al. Guidelines for pathologic diagnosis of malignant mesothelioma 2017 update of the consensus statement from the international mesothelioma interest group. Arch Pathol Lab Med 2018;142(1):89–108.

85. Hung YP, Dong F, Dubuc AM, et al. Molecular characterization of localized pleural mesothelioma. Mod Pathol 2020;33(2):271–80.

86. Shaker N, Wu D, Abid AM. Cytology of malignant pleural mesothelioma: Diagnostic criteria, WHO classification updates, and immunohistochemical staining markers diagnostic value. Diagn Cytopathol 2022;50(11):532–7.

87. Churg A, Sheffield BS, Galateau-Salle F. New markers for separating benign from malignant mesothelial proliferations: are we there yet? Arch Pathol Lab Med 2016;140(4):318–21.

Cervical Human Papillomavirus Testing
Current and Future Impact on Patient Care

Carol N. Rizkalla, MB BCh, BAO[a], Eric C. Huang, MD, PhD[b],*

KEYWORDS

• Human papillomavirus • FDA • Molecular • Cervical cancer • Self-collection

---

Key points

- *Human papillomavirus* (HPV) is the main etiologic agent that causes most cervical cancers, and this understanding has led to the development and adaptation of HPV molecular diagnostics as part of cervical cancer screening and prevention.

- Currently there are six Food and Drug Administration (FDA)-approved HPV tests with three of them approved for primary HPV screening.

- HPV testing is more sensitive but less specific than cytology for the detection of high-risk cervical lesions.

- HPV vaccination has transformed the landscape of HPV prevention and may shift the prevalence of HPV genotypes and alter future testing strategies.

- HPV self-collection methods have shown comparable accuracy to clinician-collected samples and have the potential to increase screening rates and accessibility.

ABSTRACT

Cervical cancer is the fourth most common malignancy in women worldwide. The identification of *human papillomavirus* (HPV) as the main etiologic cause of cervical cancer has led to the development and adaptation of HPV molecular diagnostics as a cervical cancer screening and prevention tool. This article highlights six Food and Drug Administration-approved HPV molecular platforms, each with unique advantages and disadvantages. In addition, HPV vaccination and the emergence of HPV self-collection as an alternative testing strategy are discussed.

OVERVIEW

Cervical cancer is the fourth most common cancer affecting women worldwide, with an estimated 604,000 new cases and 343,000 deaths.[1] Nearly 85% of the tumor burden occurs in developing countries, particularly in low-income and middle-income populations, where universal screening programs are lacking. With the introduction of cervical cytology (Papanicolaou test) and the implementation of cervical cancer screening programs, the incidence of cervical

---

[a] Department of Laboratory Medicine and Pathology, University of Washington School of Medicine, 1959 NE Pacific Street, Box 357470, Seattle, WA 98195, USA; [b] Department of Laboratory Medicine and Pathology, University of Washington School of Medicine, Harborview Medical Center, 325 9th Avenue, Box 359791, Seattle, WA 98104, USA

* Corresponding author. Department of Laboratory Medicine and Pathology, University of Washington School of Medicine, Harborview Medical Center, 325 9th Avenue, Box 359791, Seattle, WA 98104.
E-mail address: ecchuang@uw.edu
Twitter: @Carol2Path (C.N.R.)

Surgical Pathology 17 (2024) 431–439
https://doi.org/10.1016/j.path.2024.04.006
1875-9181/24/© 2024 Elsevier Inc. All rights reserved.

cancer deaths in the United States has reduced dramatically by over 80% from 1930 to 2012.[2] It was later discovered that *human papillomavirus* (HPV) is the main etiologic agent causing cervical cancers. This discovery has enabled the development of HPV detection as a screening tool for cervical cancer. With persistent infection, precancerous lesions can undergo malignant transformation, leading to cancer of the cervix and other lower anogenital and oropharyngeal regions. It is important to note that HPV are generally classified as oncogenic low-risk or high-risk genotypes, with the latter accounting for the majority of cervical cancer cases.[3,4] This underscores the importance of early detection and management.

In the era of genomic medicine, there are widespread applications of molecular diagnostics for the detection of HPV infection in gynecologic cytology specimens. The US Food and Drug Administration (FDA) has approved six HPV testing modalities that have resulted in a shift from cytologic testing alone to a combination of cytology and HPV molecular testing (cotesting) or primary HPV molecular testing alone.[5,6] While HPV molecular testing has a higher sensitivity for detecting precancerous high-grade squamous intraepithelial lesions or worse (cervical intraepithelial neoplasia grade 2 [CIN2]+), cytology remains more specific as it can evaluate for cytologic evidence of dysplasia or malignancy, which the HPV test alone cannot.[7–9] In fact, cotesting has the highest sensitivity for cervical cancer screening compared to either test used alone.[10–13] In this review article, we delve into the molecular pathogenesis of HPV, explore available molecular platforms for detecting HPV, and discuss potential developments in future HPV testing methods.

HUMAN PAPILLOMAVIRUS GENOMICS AND MECHANISM OF TRANSFORMATION TO NEOPLASM

HPV is a small, non-enveloped, double-stranded circular DNA virus with over 200 identified genotypes.[14] Based on its association with cervical cancer and precursor lesions, HPV is generally grouped into low-risk and high-risk. The most prevalent low-risk HPV types are 6 and 11, which have been associated with genital warts. The 14 most clinically relevant high-risk HPV (hrHPV) types are 16, 18, 31, 33, 35, 39, 45, 51, 52, 56, 58, 59, 66, and 68.[5] Although the expression of these types alone does not cause cancer progression, it is primarily oncoproteins E6 and E7 that

interfere with the function of tumor suppressor p53 and retinoblastoma (Rb) protein, respectively, which contribute to HPV-related diseases. Under normal conditions, p53 regulates the cell cycle, activates DNA repair, and initiates apoptosis, whereas Rb protein inhibits the cell cycle progression and suppresses DNA synthesis. When their functions are dysregulated, there is a delay in host keratinocyte differentiation and prolonged proliferation, which provides a suitable environment for viral replication. It is a persistent infection with these oncoproteins that can lead to the accumulation of cellular mutations.[15–17] The failure of the immune system to clear the persistent HPV can lead to invasive carcinoma after several decades[18,19]; thus, immunocompromised individuals are at a higher risk of developing HPV-associated cancers.[20,21] Fortunately, HPV infection found in the female genital tract tends to be transient in nature and often resolves spontaneously without the development of carcinoma.[22]

MOLECULAR TESTING PLATFORMS FOR HUMAN PAPILLOMAVIRUS

Currently, six FDA-approved molecular tests are available for HPV detection using three main methods: nucleic acid hybridization, signal amplification, and nucleic acid amplification (summarized in **Table 1**). All six tests utilize a liquid-based cytology method that preserves cervical cell samples in liquid medium. This method offers several advantages over conventional Papanicolaou smears, such as preservation of nucleic acids within cells and elimination of potential contaminants, thereby enhancing the accuracy of hrHPV detection and improving the effectiveness of cervical cancer screening.

Notably, the accuracy of HPV molecular tests can be compromised by external factors, leading to false-negative results. These variables include the use of contraceptive jelly, antifungal cream, vaginal discharge, and lubricants, among others. Some molecular tests lack an internal control to detect such interference; hence, these false-negative results can be mistakenly reported as negative test results rather than test failures.[5] In addition, many of these platforms exhibit cross-reactivity to low-risk HPV subtypes, leading to false-positive molecular test results and unnecessary colposcopy and possible biopsy. It is also worth noting that most of these platforms have not been FDA-approved for specimen types beyond the cervix, a circumstance that is unfortunate given the prevalence of HPV at noncervical sites.

Table 1
Summary of the six Food and Drug Administration-approved human papillomavirus tests[5,8]

Instrument	HC2	Cervista	Aptima	Cobas	Onclarity	Alinity
Manufacturer	Qiagen (formerly Digene)	Hologic	Gen Probe (acquired by Hologic)	Roche	Becton Dickinson (BD)	Abbott
Year FDA-approved	2003	2009	2011	2011	2018	2023
Approved for primary screening	No	No	No	Yes (2014)	Yes (2018)	Yes (2023)
Nucleic acid targeted	DNA	DNA	RNA	DNA	DNA	DNA
PCR-based assay	No	No	Yes	Yes	Yes	Yes
Gene targeted	Whole viral genome	L1/E6/E7	E6/E7	L1	E6/E7	L1
Test principle	Nucleic acid hybridization followed by signal amplification	Signal amplification	Target capture, target amplification, and detection by hybridization	Target amplification followed by fluorescently labeled detection	Target amplification followed by fluorescently labeled detection	Target amplification followed by fluorescently labeled detection
Genotypes detected	16, 18, 31, 33, 35, 39, 45, 51, 52, 56, 58, 59, and 68	16, 18, 31, 33, 35, 39, 45, 51, 52, 56, 58, 59, 66, and 68	16, 18, 31, 33, 35, 39, 45, 51, 52, 56, 58, 59, 66, and 68	16, 18, 31, 33, 35, 39, 45, 51, 52, 56, 58, 59, 66, and 68	16, 18, 31, 33, 35, 39, 45, 51, 52, 56, 58, 59, 66, and 68	16, 18, 31, 33, 35, 39, 45, 51, 52, 56, 58, 59, 66, and 68
Separate genotyping	No	Yes 16, 18 on a separate assay	Yes 16, 18/45 (combined) on a separate assay	Yes 16, 18	Yes 16, 18, 31, 45, 51, 52 Combined: 33/58, 35/39/68, and 56/59/66	Yes 16, 18, 45 Combined: 31/33/52/58 and 35/39/51/56/59/66/68
Internal control for human genes	No	Yes (histone 2)	No	Yes (β-globin)	Yes (β-globin)	Yes (β-globin)
Clinical trial	ASC-US/LSIL Triage Study	Cervista HPV HR	CLEAR	ATHENA, IMPACT	Onclarity	Alinity m HR HPV

FOOD AND DRUG ADMINISTRATION-APPROVED MOLECULAR HUMAN PAPILLOMAVIRUS TESTING PLATFORMS

HYBRID CAPTURE 2

Hybrid Capture 2 (HC2) by Qiagen (formerly Digene) was the first FDA-approved molecular testing platform for detecting HPV infection in 2003. It utilizes solution hybridization followed by signal amplification and chemiluminescence. This platform has been extensively employed in clinical practice and research for over two decades. The mechanism underlying HC2 involves the utilization of specific RNA probes with a mixture of sequences complementary to the viral DNA of 13 hrHPV subtypes, including HPV 16, 18, 31, 33, 35, 39, 45, 51, 52, 56, 58, 59, and 68. The resulting RNA:DNA hybridizations are captured and subsequently identified through conjugate of antihybrid antibodies, yielding a light signal intensity proportional to the viral load.[8]

The drawback associated with HC2 is cross-reactivity with numerous low-risk HPV subtypes, leading to false-positive outcomes.[5,23] Another disadvantage is the potential false-negative results caused by some antifungal creams and contraceptive jelly.[5] It is noteworthy that a positive HC2 HPV result, prompting colposcopy, resulting in findings less than CIN2, is associated with a cross-reactivity rate of approximately 25%. This percentage varies depending on the specific region and the population under examination.[24]

CERVISTA

The FDA approved Cervista by Hologic in 2009. It is based on solution hybridization by utilizing signal amplification for the detection of nucleic acid sequences targeting L1, E6, and E7 genes.[5] While the Cervista HPV HR platform has the capability to simultaneously assess 14 distinct hrHPV subtypes, it is not possible to ascertain the precise HPV type that is present.[5] However, a separate Cervista HPV 16/18 assay contains oligonucleotides complementary to HPV 16 and 18. The advantages of Cervista are that it requires lower sample volume and it includes an internal control. The disadvantages include cross-reactivity with HPV types 67 and 70 (indeterminate-risk) and the potential for false negatives caused by contraceptive gels and antifungal creams.

APTIMA

The Aptima by Gen-Probe (later acquired by Hologic) gained FDA approval in 2011 and has two variants: Aptima HPV and Aptima 16 18/45. Aptima HPV uses nucleic acid amplification for the qualitative detection of E6/E7 messenger RNA (mRNA) expression of 14 hrHPV types, while Aptima 16 18/45 detects the 3 specific genotypes. The main advantage of targeting mRNA instead of DNA is that it can detect transcriptionally active viruses. Therefore, a positive test result would better reflect the presence of precancer than latent HPV infections. The sensitivity of Aptima is comparable to HC2, but it is more specific at detecting CIN2+.[16,25]

The Aptima test has garnered increasing support as a primary cervical cancer screening tool, primarily due to its heightened sensitivity and specificity in identifying CIN2+.[16,26] This assay has been effectively employed in triaging Aptima HPV and HC2 hrHPV-positive cases, showing significantly increased specificity, positive predictive value, and comparable sensitivity for identifying CIN2+.[16,27] The disadvantage is cross-reactivity with low-risk HPV subtypes 26, 61, 62, 67, 70, 82, and 83, leading to false-positive results.[24] Additionally, there is about a 20% colposcopy referral rate associated with results below CIN2, suggesting a potential for over-referral in certain cases.

PRIMARY HUMAN PAPILLOMAVIRUS TESTING PLATFORMS

The concept of primary HPV molecular screening, employed as a standalone approach for cervical cancer detection, has attracted significant attention and has been embraced by countries, such as Australia and the Netherlands. This approach aims to streamline resource utilization by eliminating cytology while maintaining a robust level of sensitivity.[28] The heightened sensitivity translates to earlier detection of CIN2+ for treatment; however, it can also lead to higher rate of colposcopy and overtreatment of CIN2 that can often regress in young patients.[29,30]

Of the six FDA-approved molecular test platforms for HPV detection, Roche cobas, Becton Dickinson (BD) Onclarity, and Abbott Alinity have been approved for primary HPV screening in women aged 25 to 65 years in the United States.[31–34]

COBAS

The cobas HPV test by Roche is a qualitative in vitro test for the detection of 14 hrHPV types. It employs polymerase chain reaction (PCR) and nucleic acid hybridization to amplify the sequence of approximately 200 nucleotides of the targeted

L1 protein, which can identify hrHPV types 16 and 18 separately, as well as 12 other clinically relevant hrHPV types. The advantage of cobas is that in addition to being approved for routine HPV testing in 2011, it is the first platform to receive FDA approval for primary HPV screening in 2014. Nevertheless, certain limitations were observed in the cobas test. A retrospective study reported that 8.7% of CIN2+ lesions identified during col-poscopy were preceded by HPV-negative results from the cobas method, signaling false-negative outcomes.[10] Given the most recent American Cancer Society recommendation of primary HPV testing as the preferred method in cervical cancer screening, the significance of false-negative outcomes cannot be underestimated. Another study highlighted the cross-reactivity of the assay with low-risk HPV subtypes, leading to false-positive results.[24] Furthermore, the presence of inflammatory cells in a sample can lead to a false-positive control due to a lack of specificity for epithelial cells in the β-globin internal control.[5] In view of these discoveries and constraints, a comprehensive grasp of the cobas' strengths and challenges underscores the ongoing necessity of refining its integration into cervical cancer screening protocols.

ONCLARITY

The Onclarity HPV Assay by BD was FDA-approved for primary HPV screening in 2018. This method offers a sophisticated and comprehensive approach to detect 14 hrHPV types by targeting hrHPV DNA amplification using real-time PCR and nucleic acid hybridization. In addition to the detection of HPV 16 and 18, Onclarity provides extended genotyping for HPV 31, 45, 51, and 52.[35] The inclusion of additional hrHPV genotyping is particularly important for triaging and management decisions. The ability to identify specific subtypes enables more precise risk stratification and the determination of appropriate clinical actions. In a vaccinated population, Onclarity has demonstrated lower sensitivity, but higher specificity when compared to unvaccinated individuals.[35] Unlike other systems, BD claimed that Onclarity has no cross-reactivity with other HPV genotypes. When using mucin, acyclovir, and clindamycin, it is possible to obtain false-negative results.[36]

ALINITY

The Alinity by Abbott is the newest HPV molecular diagnostic tool, having gained FDA approval for cotesting and primary testing in 2023.[37] This system operates as a fully automated platform, conducting DNA extraction, amplification, and result analysis.[38] Employing a qualitative multiplex real-time PCR assay, it hones in on a conserved sequence within the L1 gene of 14 hrHPV subtypes 16, 18, 31, 33, 35, 39, 45, 51, 52, 56, 58, 59, 66, and 68.[34] A feature of the Alinity that is analogous to Onclarity is its capacity to individually identify genotypes 16, 18, and 45, a capability that holds significant value in patient risk stratification.[34,39] Furthermore, it proficiently identifies additional 11 high-risk genotypes. These genotypes are categorized into group A, encompassing the 4 most carcinogenic types (31, 33, 52, and 58) and group B, comprising the remaining 7 types (35, 39, 51, 56, 59, 66, and 68).[38,39] Together, with the 3 separately identified genotypes and the group A genotypes, this molecular test encompasses the hrHPV subtypes contained within the 9 valent vaccine, Gardasil 9.[40,41]

Comparative studies have shown Alinity performance to be comparable to cobas and HC2, including its ability to identify hrHPV genotypes 16/18.[34,38] Moreover, it has exhibited notable sensitivity akin to clinician-collected samples when used for patient self-collected samples, like vaginal self-samples and first-void urine.[34]

HUMAN PAPILLOMAVIRUS VACCINATION FOR CERVICAL CANCER PREVENTION

The landscape of cervical cancer prevention has undergone a significant transformation with the introduction of HPV vaccines. Guidelines recommend that two doses of HPV vaccine should be administered starting at the age of 9 years and prior to 15 years of age, with the second dose administered 6 to 12 months after the initial dose.[42,43] A third dose may be required for patients who received two doses less than 5 months apart, started the vaccine after the age of 15 years, or are immunocompromised. Vaccination is not recommended for anyone aged older than 26 years; although some patients aged 27 to 45 years may benefit from the vaccine based on discussion with their clinician. For the best results, the HPV vaccine should be inoculated prior to any HPV exposure.

There are three FDA-approved HPV vaccines in the United States: Gardasil, Cervarix, and Gardasil 9. Gardasil is a quadrivalent vaccine targeting HPV types 6, 11, 16, and 18, whereas Cervarix is a bivalent vaccine that protects against HPV types 16 and 18. Perhaps the most remarkable addition to the armamentarium is Gardasil 9; a 9 valent vaccine that extends its protective umbrella to encompass a broader range of HPV types, including both low-risk and high-risk subtypes 6, 11, 16, 18, 31, 33, 45, 52, and 58.[44] This expanded coverage has proven to be pivotal in the ongoing battle against HPV-related diseases. As of late 2016, Gardasil 9 has become the only HPV vaccine distributed in the United States. The vaccines' effective targeting of hrHPV types, notably HPV 16 and 18, is expected to lead to a reduction in their prevalence across the population.[45–47] Consequently, this shift may result in an increased detection of diseases caused by other hrHPV subtypes not covered by the vaccines.[48–50] As these vaccines continue to gain broader acceptance, the landscape of molecular HPV testing must adapt to the anticipated changes in HPV epidemiology.[51] Continuous monitoring and in-depth research are of paramount importance to keep a vigilant eye on HPV infection trends and their potential impact on cervical disease, fostering ongoing evolution and refinement in the field.

HUMAN PAPILLOMAVIRUS SELF-COLLECTION AS AN EMERGING METHOD FOR CERVICAL CANCER SCREENING

Cervical cancer screening is undergoing a revolutionary shift with the emergence of self-collection methods for HPV testing, an innovative approach that allows individuals to collect their own samples at clinics or home using vaginal swabs or urine samples. This approach addresses several barriers that hinder regular screening such as discomfort, embarrassment, and logistical challenges. It empowers individuals who might otherwise avoid or delay screening due to these barriers to actively engage in their own health care.[52] Moreover, self-collection has the potential to reach underserved populations, including those with limited access to health care facilities, remote areas, or cultural barriers that affect their willingness to undergo traditional screening methods.[53] During prolonged coronavirus 2019 pandemic, HPV self-collection would have allowed the continual cervical cancer screening without interruption due to shutdown of the clinics. By enabling women to take control of the screening process, self-collection reduces the dependence on clinic visits and health care professionals, making screening more accessible to a broader demographic.[54]

Several studies have demonstrated the effectiveness of self-collected samples in detecting hrHPV, with results comparable to those of clinician-collected samples.[55–58] The accuracy of self-collection indicates its potential as a reliable primary screening method, further reinforcing its potential for widespread adoption. Despite its numerous benefits, the implementation of self-collection does present challenges. Ensuring proper sample collection and preventing contamination are key considerations.[53] Education and clear instructions are essential to ensure that individuals collect and handle adequate samples appropriately. Additionally, integrating self-collection into existing health care systems and ensuring follow-up for positive results require careful planning.[52,53]

SUMMARY

HPV molecular testing have changed the landscape of cervical cancer screening and prevention. The higher sensitivity in detecting CIN2+ with HPV molecular tests has allowed the American Cancer Society to initiate a seismic change in cervical cancer screening by recommending primary HPV as the preferred screening method.[6,28,59] Although primary HPV screening holds allure, it comes with challenges, such as false HPV-negative results.[10] While the majority of cervical carcinomas are associated with hrHPV, low-risk HPV and HPV-negative causing cancers have been reported.[60,61] In fact, approximately 20% of cervical adenocarcinomas are independent from HPV.[61] This is where cytologic evaluation of the cervix with the Papanicolaou test still has the highest specificity in detecting early precancer and should not be underappreciated.[9,62–64] The combination of cytology and HPV testing provides the highest protection against cervical cancer.

In conclusion, HPV molecular testing is a valuable tool for cervical cancer screening and management programs. Although these molecular platforms provide higher sensitivity for CIN2+ detection when compared to cytologic screening alone, challenges such as false-negative HPV results, detection of low-risk HPV, and HPV-independent cervical lesions still need to be addressed. These false reassurances are of particular concern as cervical cancer screening is shifting from cotesting to primary HPV screening. The Papanicolaou test has higher specificity than the HPV test, and the ability of cytology to identify hrHPV-negative lesions should not be ignored. As more people receive HPV vaccines to protect against the nine most common types of HPV, how this will affect the prevalence of clinically relevant HPV types remains uncertain. The future of HPV molecular testing is moving toward self-collection methods, which holds great promise for revolutionizing cervical cancer screening as they can overcome screening barriers and increase accessibility. As primary HPV screening with self-collection becomes more widely adopted, it can increase screening rates, reach underserved populations, and ultimately contribute to earlier detection and improved outcomes in the fight against cervical cancer. Evolving strategies, guided by risk-based management, have the potential to transform cervical cancer detection and prevention efforts, and improve precision and resource efficiency in safeguarding women's health.

CLINICS CARE POINTS

- Cotesting with cytology and HPV molecular testing optimizes sensitivity and specificity in cervical cancer screening.
- HPV vaccination alters HPV genotype prevalence in the long-term; clinicians ought to follow the evolving epidemiology for appropriate screening.
- Self-collection methods are a useful tool for increasing access to screening, particularly for underserved groups.

DISCLOSURE

The authors declare no conflicts of interest.

REFERENCES

1. Singh D, Vignat J, Lorenzoni V, et al. Global estimates of incidence and mortality of cervical cancer in 2020: a baseline analysis of the WHO Global Cervical Cancer Elimination Initiative. Lancet Glob Health 2023;11(2):e197–206.
2. Lees BF, Erickson BK, Huh WK. Cervical cancer screening: evidence behind the guidelines. Am J Obstet Gynecol 2016;214(4):438–43.
3. Graham SV. The human papillomavirus replication cycle, and its links to cancer progression: a comprehensive review. Clin Sci 2017;131(17):2201–21.
4. Walboomers JM, Jacobs MV, Manos MM, et al. Human papillomavirus is a necessary cause of invasive cervical cancer worldwide. J Pathol 1999;189(1):12–9.
5. Salazar KL, Duhon DJ, Olsen R, et al. A review of the FDA-approved molecular testing platforms for human papillomavirus. J Am Soc Cytopathol 2019; 8(5):284–92.
6. Fontham ETH, Wolf AMD, Church TR, et al. Cervical cancer screening for individuals at average risk: 2020 guideline update from the American Cancer Society. CA Cancer J Clin 2020;70(5):321–46.
7. Perkins RB, Guido RS, Castle PE, et al. 2019 ASCCP Risk-Based Management Consensus Guidelines for Abnormal Cervical Cancer Screening Tests and Cancer Precursors. J Low Genit Tract Dis 2020; 24(2):102–31.
8. Arbyn M, Snijders PJF, Meijer CJLM, et al. Which high-risk HPV assays fulfil criteria for use in primary cervical cancer screening? Clin Microbiol Infect 2015;21(9):817–26.
9. Kang M, Ha SY, Cho HY, et al. Comparison of papanicolaou smear and human papillomavirus (HPV) test as cervical screening tools: can we rely on HPV test alone as a screening method? An 11-year retrospective experience at a single institution. J Pathol Transl Med 2020;54(1):112–8.
10. Zhou H, Mody RR, Luna E, et al. Clinical performance of the Food and Drug Administration-Approved high-risk HPV test for the detection of high-grade cervicovaginal lesions. Cancer Cytopathol 2016;124(5):317–23.
11. Austin RM, Onisko A, Zhao C. Enhanced detection of cervical cancer and precancer through use of imaged liquid-based cytology in routine cytology and HPV cotesting. Am J Clin Pathol 2018;150(5): 385–92.
12. Blatt AJ, Kennedy R, Luff RD, et al. Comparison of cervical cancer screening results among 256,648 women in multiple clinical practices. Cancer Cytopathol 2015;123(5):282–8.
13. Kaufman HW, Alagia DP, Chen Z, et al. Contributions of Liquid-Based (Papanicolaou) Cytology and Human Papillomavirus Testing in Cotesting for Detection of Cervical Cancer and Precancer in the United States. Am J Clin Pathol 2020;154(4): 510–6.
14. Bernard HU, Burk RD, Chen Z, et al. Classification of papillomaviruses (PVs) based on 189 PV types and proposal of taxonomic amendments. Virology 2010; 401(1):70 9.
15. Scarth JA, Patterson MR, Morgan EL, et al. The human papillomavirus oncoproteins: a review of the host pathways targeted on the road to transformation. J Gen Virol 2021;102(3). https://doi.org/10. 1099/jgv.0.001540.
16. Wang J, Du Y, Dong J, et al. Clinical significance of genotyping for human papillomavirus (HPV) 16 18/ 45 combined with cytology in cervical exfoliated cells in HPV oncogenic mRNA-positive women. Gynecol Oncol 2019;153(1):34–40.
17. Duensing S, Münger K. Mechanisms of genomic instability in human cancer: insights from studies with human papillomavirus oncoproteins. Int J Cancer 2004;109(2):157–62.
18. zur Hausen H. Papillomaviruses and cancer: from basic studies to clinical application. Nat Rev Cancer 2002;2(5):342–50.
19. Kjær SK, Frederiksen K, Munk C, et al. Long-term absolute risk of cervical intraepithelial neoplasia grade 3 or worse following human papillomavirus

infection: role of persistence. J Natl Cancer Inst 2010;102(19):1478–88.

20. Denny LA, Franceschi S, de Sanjosé S, et al. Human papillomavirus, human immunodeficiency virus and immunosuppression. Vaccine 2012;30(Suppl 5): F168–74.

21. Wieland U, Kreuter A, Pfister H. Human papilloma-virus and immunosuppression. Curr Probl Dermatol 2014;45:154–65.

22. Tainio K, Athanasiou A, Tikkinen KAO, et al. Clinical course of untreated cervical intraepithelial neoplasia grade 2 under active surveillance: systematic review and meta-analysis. BMJ 2018;k499. https://doi.org/10.1136/bmj.k499. Published online February 27.

23. Peyton CL, Schiffman M, Lörincz AT, et al. Compar-ison of PCR- and hybrid capture-based human papillomavirus detection systems using multiple cer-vical specimen collection strategies. J Clin Microbiol 1998;36(11):3248–54.

24. Preisler S, Rebolj M, Ejegod DM, et al. Cross-reac-tivity profiles of hybrid capture II, cobas, and AP-TIMA human papillomavirus assays: split-sample study. BMC Cancer 2016;16:510.

25. Ratnam S, Coutlee F, Fontaine D, et al. Aptima HPV E6/E7 mRNA test is as sensitive as Hybrid Capture 2 Assay but more specific at detecting cervical pre-cancer and cancer. J Clin Microbiol 2011;49(2): 557–64.

26. Nieves L, Enerson CL, Belinson S, et al. Primary cer-vical cancer screening and triage using an mRNA human papillomavirus assay and visual inspection. Int J Gynecol Cancer 2013;23(3):513–8.

27. Guo YL, You K, Geng L, et al. Clinical Performance of APTIMA Human Papillomavirus (HPV) 16 18/45 mRNA Genotyping Testing for the Detection of Cer-vical Intraepithelial Neoplasia 3 (CIN3) or Cancer in a Select Group of Chinese Women. Pathol Oncol Res 2016;22(3):549–54.

28. Ronco G, Dillner J, Elfström KM, et al. Efficacy of HPV-based screening for prevention of invasive cer-vical cancer: follow-up of four European randomised controlled trials. Lancet 2014;383(9916):524–32.

29. Ronco G, Giorgi-Rossi P, Carozzi F, et al. Efficacy of human papillomavirus testing for the detection of invasive cervical cancers and cervical intraepithelial neoplasia: a randomised controlled trial. Lancet On-col 2010;11(3):249–57.

30. Bergengren L, Ryen L, Flodström C, et al. Effective-ness and costs of an implemented primary HPV cer-vical screening programme in Sweden - A population based cohort study. Prev Med Rep 2022;25:101675.

31. Wright TC, Stoler MH, Behrens CM, et al. Primary cervical cancer screening with human papilloma-virus: End of study results from the ATHENA study using HPV as the first-line screening test. Gynecol Oncol 2015;136(2):189–97.

32. Stoler MH, Wright TC, Parvu V, et al. The Onclarity Human Papillomavirus Trial: Design, methods, and baseline results. Gynecol Oncol 2018;149(3): 498–505.

33. Meijer CJLM, Berkhof J, Castle PE, et al. Guidelines for human papillomavirus DNA test requirements for primary cervical cancer screening in women 30 years and older. Int J Cancer 2009;124(3):516–20.

34. Latsuzbaia A, Van Keer S, Vanden Broeck D, et al. Clinical Accuracy of Alinity m HR HPV Assay on Self- versus Clinician-Taken Samples Using the VAL-HUDES Protocol. J Mol Diagn JMD 2023;25(12): 957–66.

35. Becton Dickinson (BD) Onclarity HPV Assay. Avail-able at: https://static.bd.com/documents/eifu/8089899_ZMG_J_SD_8089899.pdf. [Accessed 2 February 2024].

36. U.S. Food and Drug Administration. BD Onclarity™ HPV Assay. Available at: https://www.accessdata.fda.gov/cdrh_docs/pdf16/P160037C.pdf. [Accessed 11 October 2023].

37. Abbott Receives FDA Approval for HPV Test to Run on Alinity m, Offering Primary HPV Screening and Assessment of High-Risk Cancer-Causing Types of HPV. Abbott MediaRoom. Available at: https://abbott.mediaroom.com/2023-11-02-Abbott-Receives-FDA-Approval-for-HPV-Test-to-Run-on-Alinity-m,-Offeri ng-Primary-HPV-Screening-and-Assessment-of-High -Risk-Cancer-Causing-Types-of-HPV. [Accessed 2 February 2024].

38. Jang D, Ratnam S, Smieja M, et al. Comparison of Alinity m HPV and cobas HPV assays on cervical specimens in diverse storage media. Tumour Virus Res 2021;12:200224.

39. Dhillon SK, Oštrbenk Valenčak A, Xu L, et al. Clinical and Analytical Evaluation of the Alinity m HR HPV Assay within the VALGENT-3 Framework. J Clin Mi-crobiol 2021;59(6). https://doi.org/10.1128/jcm.00286-21.

40. Oštrbenk Valenčak A, Šterbenc A, Seme K, et al. Alinity m HR HPV assay fulfills criteria for human papillomavirus test requirements in cervical cancer screening settings. J Clin Microbiol 2019;58(1). https://doi.org/10.1128/jcm.01120-19.

41. Oštrbenk Valenčak A, Bertram A, Gröning A, et al. Comparison of the clinical and analytical perfor-mance of Alinity m HR HPV and cobas 4800 HPV as-says in a population-based screening setting. J Clin Virol 2021;140:104851.

42. Markowitz LE, Dunne EF, Saraiya M, et al. Human papillomavirus vaccination: recommendations of the Advisory Committee on Immunization Practices (ACIP). MMWR Recomm Rep Morb Mortal Wkly Rep Recomm Rep 2014;63(RR-05):1–30.

43. Meites E, Szilagyi PG, Chesson HW, et al. Human papillomavirus vaccination for adults: updated rec-ommendations of the advisory committee on

immunization practices. MMWR Morb Mortal Wkly Rep 2019;68(32):698–702.

44. Illah O, Olaitan A. Updates on HPV Vaccination. Diagnostics 2023;13(2):243.

45. Karube A, Saito F, Nakamura E, et al. Reduction in HPV 16/18 prevalence among young women following HPV vaccine introduction in a highly vaccinated district, Japan, 2008-2017. J Rural Med JRM 2019;14(1):48–57.

46. Hariri S, Unger ER, Schafer S, et al. HPV type attribution in high-grade cervical lesions: assessing the potential benefits of vaccines in a population-based evaluation in the United States. Cancer Epidemiol Biomarkers Prev 2015;24(2):393–9.

47. Jeannot E, Viviano M, de Pree C, et al. Prevalence of vaccine type infections in vaccinated and non-vaccinated young women: HPV-IMPACT, a self-sampling study. Int J Environ Res Public Health 2018;15(7):1447.

48. Rideg O, Dergez T, Farkas K, et al. High prevalence of non-vaccinated oncogenic human papillomavirus genotypes in high-grade squamous intraepithelial lesions of the cervix: thought-provoking results of a detailed hpv genotype analysis. Vaccines 2022; 10(5):748.

49. Enerly E, Flingtorp R, Christiansen IK, et al. An observational study comparing HPV prevalence and type distribution between HPV-vaccinated and -unvaccinated girls after introduction of school-based HPV vaccination in Norway. PLoS One 2019;14(10):e0223612.

50. Guo F, Hirth JM, Berenson AB. Comparison of HPV prevalence between HPV-vaccinated and non-vaccinated young adult women (20-26 years). Hum Vaccines Immunother 2015;11(10):2337–44.

51. Zhu Y, Wang Y, Hirschhorn J, et al. Human Papillomavirus and Its Testing Assays, Cervical Cancer Screening, and Vaccination. Adv Clin Chem 2017; 81:135–92.

52. Hawkes D, Keung MHT, Huang Y, et al. Self-Collection for Cervical Screening Programs: From Research to Reality. Cancers 2020;12(4):1053.

53. Daponte N, Valasoulis G, Michail G, et al. HPV-Based Self-Sampling in Cervical Cancer Screening: An Updated Review of the Current Evidence in the Literature. Cancers 2023;15(6):1669.

54. Camara H, Zhang Y, Lafferty L, et al. Self-collection for HPV-based cervical screening: a qualitative evidence meta-synthesis. BMC Publ Health 2021; 21(1):1503.

55. Polman NJ, Ebisch RMF, Heideman DAM, et al. Performance of human papillomavirus testing on self-collected versus clinician-collected samples for the detection of cervical intraepithelial neoplasia of grade 2 or worse: a randomised, paired screen-positive, non-inferiority trial. Lancet Oncol 2019; 20(2):229–38.

56. Arbyn M, Smith SB, Temin S, et al, Collaboration on Self-Sampling and HPV Testing. Collaboration on self-sampling and HPV testing. detecting cervical precancer and reaching underscreened women by using HPV testing on self samples: updated meta-analyses. BMJ 2018;363:k4823.

57. Arbyn M, Castle PE, Schiffman M, et al. Meta-analysis of agreement/concordance statistics in studies comparing self- vs clinician-collected samples for HPV testing in cervical cancer screening. Int J Cancer 2022;151(2):308–12.

58. Cho HW, Shim SR, Lee JK, et al. Accuracy of human papillomavirus tests on self-collected urine versus clinician-collected samples for the detection of cervical precancer: a systematic review and meta-analysis. J Gynecol Oncol 2022;33(1):e4.

59. Cuzick J, Cadman L, Mesher D, et al. Comparing the performance of six human papillomavirus tests in a screening population. Br J Cancer 2013;108(4):908–13.

60. Liu MZ, Hung YP, Huang EC, et al. HPV 6-associated HSIL/Squamous Carcinoma in the Anogenital Tract. Int J Gynecol 2019;38(5):493–7.

61. Nicolás I, Marimon L, Barnadas E, et al. HPV-negative tumors of the uterine cervix. Mod 2019;32(8):1189–96.

62. Ashman D, Zhang H, Li J, et al. HPV detection rates and histopathologic follow-up of patients with HSIL cytology in a large academic women's hospital laboratory. J Am Soc Cytopathol 2020;9(6):550–5.

63. Agoff SN, Brockmeyer AD, Barrie AM, et al. High-grade squamous intraepithelial lesion cervicovaginal paps with negative high-risk HPV testing, a prospective study with histological follow-up. Diagn Cytopathol 2023;51(8):475–9.

64. Ge Y, Mody RR, Olsen RJ, et al. HPV status in women with high-grade dysplasia on cervical biopsy and preceding negative HPV tests. J Am Soc Cytopathol 2019;8(3):149–56.

Pancreas Fine Needle Aspiration
Current and Future Impact on Patient Care

Melanie C. Kwan, MD[a,b], M. Lisa Zhang, MD[a,b],*

KEYWORDS

- Fine needle aspiration • Pancreatic neoplasms • Pancreatic cytology • Cytology • Cytopathology
- Pancreatic cyst fluid • Pancreatic cystic lesion • Cyst fluid triage

Key Points

- Minimally invasive fine needle aspiration of solid and cystic pancreatic lesions can provide essential diagnostic material from an anatomically challenging site and preclude the need for more invasive and costly procedures.

- For solid lesions, particularly non-ductal neoplasms, immunohistochemical studies performed on small core biopsy/cell block specimens aid in rendering a definitive diagnosis.

- For cystic lesions, optimal handling of pancreatic cyst fluid is essential to ensure that the limited diagnostic material is appropriately utilized for cytologic evaluation, biochemical studies, and molecular testing.

- Accurate preoperative diagnosis provides clinically actionable information and helps to inform patient management and outcomes, particularly in the evolving landscape of personalized care and targeted therapies.

ABSTRACT

Pancreatic lesions can be solid or cystic and comprise a wide range of benign, premalignant, and malignant entities. Endoscopic ultrasound–guided fine needle aspiration (EUS-FNA) is the current primary sampling method for the preoperative diagnosis of pancreatic lesions. Optimal handling of cytology/small tissue specimens is critical to ensure that the often-scant diagnostic material is appropriately utilized for ancillary and/or molecular studies when appropriate. Ultimately, evaluation of EUS-FNA cytology and small biopsy material can provide accurate and timely diagnoses to guide patient management and triage them to surveillance or surgical intervention.

OVERVIEW

Pancreatic lesions can be solid or cystic and encompass a wide range of benign, premalignant, and malignant entities. Currently, endoscopic ultrasound–guided fine needle aspiration (EUS-FNA) is the primary modality for the preoperative sampling and diagnosis of pancreatic lesions, as other methods to sample the pancreas (ie, large biopsy or resection) incur high morbidity and mortality. EUS-FNA is minimally invasive and has proven to be effective in obtaining diagnostic material from both solid and cystic pancreatic lesions. For solid lesions, cytology has a relatively high sensitivity (73%–97%) and specificity (72%–100%) for diagnosing pancreatic ductal

[a] Department of Pathology, Massachusetts General Hospital, Boston, MA, USA; [b] Harvard Medical School, Boston, MA, USA

* Corresponding author. Department of Pathology, Massachusetts General Hospital, 55 Fruit Street, Boston, MA 02114.
E-mail address: mlzhang@mgh.harvard.edu
Twitter: @melaniekwan (M.C.K.); @MLisaZhang (M.L.Z.)

Surgical Pathology 17 (2024) 441–452
https://doi.org/10.1016/j.path.2024.04.007
1875-9181/24/© 2024 Elsevier Inc. All rights reserved.

adenocarcinoma (PDAC), which is the most common pancreatic neoplasm.[1–4] Cytology and cyst fluid analysis also play an important role in the preoperative management of cystic lesions, including the ability to identify molecular alterations associated with neoplastic mucinous cysts and high-risk cysts.[5–7] An accurate and timely diagnosis is essential in order to appropriately triage patients to surgery or surveillance.

SOLID PANCREATIC LESIONS

TISSUE MANAGEMENT

Imaging by computerized tomography (CT) and magnetic resonance imaging (MRI) are the main modalities used to characterize pancreatic lesions in determining their location, distribution, and if the lesion is cystic or solid. If there are imaging features that warrant sampling of an identified lesion, EUS-FNA would be the next step.[8] Samples from solid pancreatic lesions can be evaluated for adequacy by rapid on-site evaluation (ROSE), and the material obtained can be made into Papanicolaou-stained smears for cytologic evaluation with possible additional cell block and/or small core biopsies. In the setting of a solid lesion, ROSE is a useful procedure to determine the adequacy of a sample and thereby triage the available tissue for optimal diagnostic yield. Ancillary studies—such as immunohistochemistry, flow cytometry, molecular testing—may be performed on cell blocks or core biopsies obtained by EUS-FNA. Though molecular testing does not currently play a major role in the diagnosis or prognostication of solid pancreatic lesions, certain molecular findings can inform more specific treatments (eg, immunotherapy, poly ADP ribose polymerase [PARP] inhibitors, platinum-based chemotherapy agents) in a small percentage of cases.[9,10]

Pancreatic Ductal Adenocarcinoma

PDAC is the most common malignancy of the pancreas comprising nearly 85% to 90% of adult pancreatic neoplasms,[11,12] and should be the primary consideration in the differential diagnosis when encountering a solid pancreatic mass. The median age of diagnosis in the United States is 70 years. PDAC arises in males and females equally, most commonly in the head of the pancreas.[11,13]

PDAC is an invasive epithelial tumor with glandular (ductal) differentiation and ranges from well to poorly differentiated; most tumors demonstrate appreciable glandular morphology and are typically associated with dense fibrotic stroma (as the tumor elicits a desmoplastic stromal response).[11,14] Diagnosing well-differentiated PDAC can be challenging, as the epithelial atypia may appear relatively bland and difficult to distinguish from benign/reactive ductal epithelium.[11,13] Cytologic features of PDAC seen in pancreatic FNA specimens include highly cellular smears, marked anisonucleosis (>4:1), irregular nuclear spacing/crowding with loss of polarity (drunken honeycomb architecture), varying hypochromatic to hyperchromatic nuclei with irregular nuclear contours, and mucinous cytoplasm (sometimes voluminous).[15] Single atypical cells and background necrosis can be helpful features in higher grade tumors. Particularly for well-differentiated adenocarcinoma, the differential diagnosis includes benign gastrointestinal contamination, chronic pancreatitis, or autoimmune pancreatitis.[16] For example, chronic pancreatitis is also associated with fibrotic stroma and can demonstrate reactive epithelial atypia, but lacks significant cytologic atypia and evidence of stromal infiltration (as well as perineural or vascular invasion) by irregular/abortive glands and single malignant cells.

Select ancillary immunohistochemistry can help distinguish benign from malignant ductal epithelium (Fig. 1). Immunohistochemistry for SMAD4 and p53 can be used as surrogate markers of mutations in their respective genes. Loss of SMAD4 expression (at least nuclear but ideally nuclear and cytoplasmic) (see Fig. 1B) is seen in 50% to 55% of PDAC while abnormal p53 expression (diffuse nuclear overexpression of complete loss of nuclear expression) (see Fig. 1C) has been reported in 50% to 75% of PDACs.[5,17] S100P is another marker that demonstrates strong diffuse nuclear and cytoplasmic expression in greater than 90% of PDACs but not in benign ductal epithelium.[18] Most recently, complete loss of nuclear and cytoplasmic methylthioadenosine phosphorylase (MTAP) (see Fig. 1D), which is a surrogate marker for the MTAP gene that is frequently co-deleted with CDKN2A due to proximity on the same chromosome, has been reported in ~30% of PDACs (and not in benign pancreatic tissues) in EUS-FNA small biopsy specimens, offering yet another highly specific genetically based marker to support the diagnosis of PDAC.[19]

Though routine molecular testing does not yet play a major role in the diagnosis of PDAC, the detection of classic PDAC mutations (ie, KRAS, CDKN2A, TP53, SMAD4) in very poorly differentiated or undifferentiated carcinomas can support a diagnosis of PDAC.[4] Furthermore, the identification of certain mutations can have implications for therapy. Mismatch repair testing (either

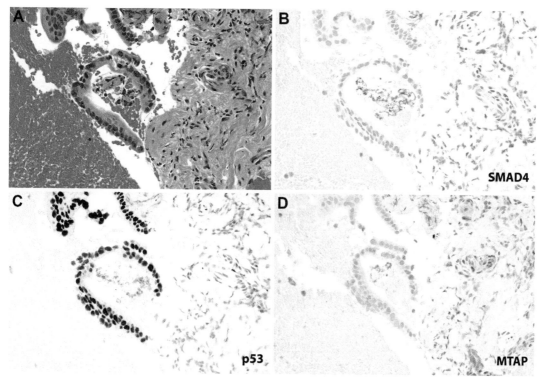

Fig. 1. Pancreatic ductal adenocarcinoma on core biopsy. (*A*) Strips of atypical epithelium showing irregular nuclear contours, and irregular nuclear spacing/crowding (hematoxylin and eosin [H&E], 400x). (*B*) Immunostain for SMAD4 shows complete loss of nuclear and cytoplasmic staining (400x). (*C*) Immunostain for p53 demonstrates abnormal diffuse nuclear overexpression (400x). (*D*) Immunostain for methylthioadenosine phosphorylase (MTAP) shows complete loss of nuclear and cytoplasmic staining (400x).

immunohistochemistry or polymerase chain reaction [PCR] testing) can be performed to screen for the approximately 1% of microsatellite-unstable cases that are associated with germline mutations in mismatch repair genes, which can potentially be used to predict a favorable response to checkpoint inhibition.[20] In FNA specimens that yield limited tissue for adequate evaluation of the 4 mismatch repair protein immunostains, PCR testing may be a potential alternative.[21] Additionally, pancreatic cancers with *BRCA1/2* mutations (~2.5%) can be treated with PARP inhibitors such as olaparib, as can those with defects in DNA repair genes (may also be effectively treated with platinum-based agents).[9,10]

Pancreatic Neuroendocrine Neoplasm (Neuroendocrine Tumor and Neuroendocrine Carcinoma)

Pancreatic neuroendocrine neoplasms (NENs) comprise 2% to 5% of pancreatic tumors and are epithelial lesions with neuroendocrine differentiation. Pancreatic NENs include well-differentiated neuroendocrine tumors (PanNETs) and poorly

differentiated neuroendocrine carcinomas (PanNECs).[22] PanNETs are typically found incidentally as they are indolent and slow-growing but are still malignant in nature and can metastasize.[23] Compared to PDACs, PanNETs are stroma-poor and tend to be more well circumscribed.

On EUS-FNA cytology specimens, PanNETs typically produce cellular smears composed of singly dispersed and loosely cohesive epithelioid or plasmacytoid cells containing monotonous round to ovoid nuclei with smooth nuclear membranes and coarse chromatin.[23] As the differential diagnosis of this cytomorphologic pattern includes acinar cell carcinoma, solid pseudopapillary neoplasm (SPN), and rarely pancreatoblastoma, the diagnosis is ideally confirmed using immunohistochemistry on a cell block or core biopsy. PanNETs express the neuroendocrine markers chromogranin, synaptophysin, and insulinoma-associated protein 1 (nuclear positivity). Grading of PanNETs using Ki-67 proliferation index on cell blocks/small biopsies should be approached with caution, as a significant proportion of grade 2 tumors may be under-graded.[24,25] In a recent large multi-institutional study, only 60% of

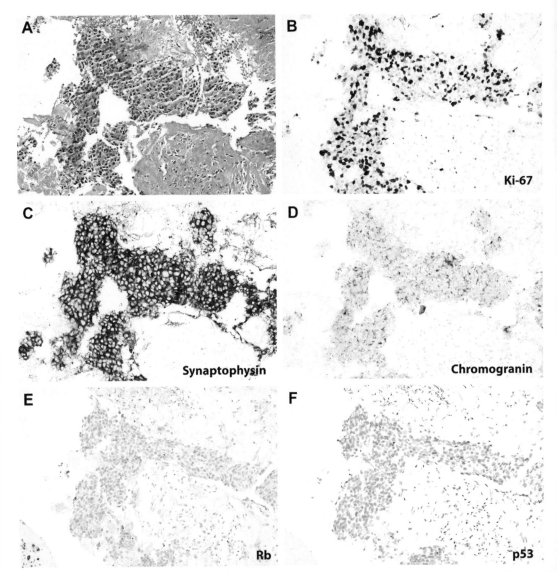

Fig. 2. Pancreatic neuroendocrine carcinoma on core biopsy showing (*A*) epithelioid cells with round to oval nuclei, minimal pleomorphism, a solid growth pattern (200x), and a (*B*) markedly elevated Ki-67 proliferation index (200x). The tumor cells are diffusely positive for (*C*) synaptophysin and (*D*) chromogranin (200x, respectively). (*E*) Immunohistochemistry Rb shows loss of nuclear staining, and immunohistochemistry for (*F*) for p53 shows an aberrant null expression pattern (negative nuclear staining, mutant phenotype) (200x, respectively).

EUS-FNA cases diagnostic of PanNETs were graded, and of those, there was 80% concordance between the FNA specimen and the subsequent resection; however, among small tumors less than 2 cm, the concordance rose to 98%.[26]

Like PDACs, molecular testing does not play a major role in the diagnosis or prognostication of PanNETs, except to aid in the distinction between grade 3 PanNETs and PanNECs (**Fig. 2**A–D). PanNETs are associated with genetic alterations in *MEN1*, *ATRX*, *DAXX*, which are not found in PanNECs.[23,27] In contrast, PanNECs can have genetic alterations in *RB1*, *TP53*, and *SMAD4*. A recent study proposed using a panel of immunohistochemical stains (ATRX, p53, Rb, p16) as surrogate markers for their gene mutations to arrive at an "integrated diagnosis" of grade 3 PanNET or PanNEC.[28] Of those markers, loss of nuclear Rb expression (**Fig. 2**E) and diffuse p16 expression in PanNECs, and loss of nuclear ATRX expression in PanNETs were entirely specific, while mutant p53 expression patterns (**Fig. 2**F) were seen in 24% of grade 3 PanNETs and 71% of PanNECs.

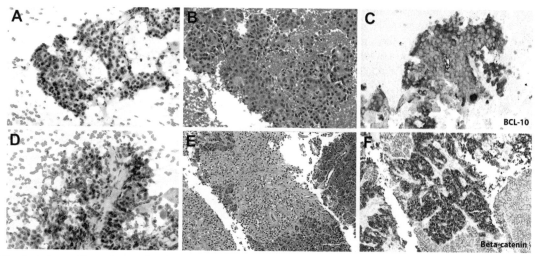

Fig. 3. Acinar cell carcinoma (*A–C*). (*A*) Cytology shows a loosely cohesive acinar/trabecular configuration of epithelioid cells with abundant granular cytoplasm and large nuclei with prominent nucleoli (Papanicolaou stain, 400x). (*B*) Cell block preparation shows epithelioid cells with granular cytoplasm in a mixed acinar and solid pattern (hematoxylin and eosin[H&E], 400x). (*C*) An immunostain for BCL10 shows diffuse positive granular cytoplasmic staining, confirming acinar differentiation (400x). Solid pseudopapillary neoplasm (*D–F*) can demonstrate morphologic overlap with acinar cell carcinoma. (*D*) Cytology shows monomorphic cells falling off the edge of a characteristic papillarylike branching vessel (Papanicolaou stain, 400x). (*E*) Core biopsy shows papillary-like structures surrounded by myxoid stroma with an outer layer of neoplastic cells (H&E, 200x). (*F*) Immunohistochemistry for beta-catenin demonstrates diffuse nuclear staining (200x).

Acinar Cell Carcinoma

Acinar cell carcinoma is a malignant epithelial neoplasm of the pancreas with acinar cell differentiation and comprises 1% of all pancreatic tumors in adults.[29] On imaging, acinar cell carcinoma typically presents as a large, circumscribed mass with a slight predilection for the pancreatic head. Like pancreatic NENs, acinar cell carcinomas are stroma-poor cellular lesions.

Cytology of acinar cell carcinoma shows hypercellular smears composed of dispersed, loosely cohesive, and sometimes acinar configurations of epithelioid tumor cells with abundant granular cytoplasm (**Fig. 3**A). A granular background can also be appreciated in smears and is attributed to zymogen granules released from the cytoplasm of disrupted tumor cells.[29] Compared to benign acinar cells, malignant acinar cells lose the organized "grapes on a vine" architecture and instead appear more dispersed; individual tumor cells have large nuclei with coarse chromatin and prominent nucleoli, and mitoses can be readily identified. In small tissue fragments, the tumor cells can have mixed solid and acinar growth patterns (**Fig.** 3B).

Immunohistochemistry for BCL10 (**Fig.** 3C), trypsin, and chymotrypsin showing granular cytoplasmic expression are helpful to confirm acinar differentiation. Acinar cell carcinomas can also show focal synaptophysin or chromogranin expression. A subset of cases harbor *CTNNB1* and *APC* mutations.[29] *BRAF* and *RAF1* fusions occur in a quarter of cases and can be detected by fluorescence in situ hybridization.[29]

Solid Pseudopapillary Neoplasm

SPN is a low-grade malignant epithelial neoplasm of the pancreas comprising 0.9% to 2.7% of all exocrine pancreatic neoplasms.[30] SPNs occurs mostly in younger women (90%) and tend to have a diagnostic solid/cystic appearance on imaging, often not necessitating preoperative diagnosis.[30]

On cytology, SPNs show highly cellular smears with discohesive, monomorphic cells, sometimes with nuclear grooves or cytoplasmic vacuoles/globules. In addition, some specimens will demonstrate characteristic papillary-like branching vessels with myxoid stroma and an outer layer of neoplastic cells (**Fig.** 3D-E).[30] Again, within the same cytomorphological pattern, SPNs can demonstrate morphologic overlap with PanNET, acinar cell carcinoma, pancreatoblastoma, and some metastatic malignancies.

Diffuse nuclear staining with beta-catenin immunohistochemistry confirms this diagnosis and reflects the underlying *CTNNB1* mutations characteristic of SPN (see **Fig.** 3F). Of note, some acinar cell carcinomas and PanNETs also have mutations in *CTNNB1*. However, SPN is essentially negative for the neuroendocrine markers synaptophysin (sometimes focal positivity) and chromogranin, as well as acinar markers.

Pitfalls
SOLID PANCREATIC LESIONS

! In the differential between reactive ductal epithelium and well-differentiated ductal adenocarcinoma, select immunohistochemical stains (ie, SMAD4, p53, MTAP, S100P) may be helpful in making the distinction.

! PanNETs, acinar cell carcinoma, and SPNs can demonstrate cytomorphologic overlap, and the diagnosis should be confirmed with lineage-defining immunohistochemistry when possible.

! Though most pancreatic lesions are primary, metastatic tumors are occasionally encountered and should be considered especially if there is pertinent patient history.

CYSTIC PANCREATIC LESIONS

TISSUE MANAGEMENT

Analogous to solid pancreatic lesions, CT and MRI imaging are used to characterize cystic pancreatic lesions, including the identification of any concerning features. Pancreatic cysts are often found incidentally, particularly in the aging patient population.[31] EUS can discern lesions a few millimeters in diameter, along with the presence of internal septa or mural nodules, which cannot be detected on CT or MRI.[32] Unlike solid pancreatic lesions, samples of cystic lesions obtained by EUS-FNA are often paucicellular and do not contain tissue for histologic examination. Next-generation small forceps biopsies have been successfully used to sample the cyst wall and provide tissue to aid in making a more specific diagnosis.[2]

Notably, ROSE is not recommended on cyst fluid specimens, as it does not contribute to patient management and is a waste of the scant fluid that should be allocated for cytologic examination, biochemical testing (carcinoembryonic antigen [CEA], amylase), and molecular studies (**Fig. 4**). The handling of pancreatic cyst fluid is unique in that fresh, unfixed, and undiluted pancreatic cyst fluid is recommended for evaluation, as fixing or diluting cyst fluid precludes the ability to perform accurate biochemical analysis.[32] In contrast to the evaluation of solid pancreatic lesions, molecular testing can provide important diagnostic and prognostic information in cystic pancreatic lesions.

Neoplastic Mucinous Cysts

Cystic lesions of the pancreas can be broadly categorized into mucinous and non-mucinous cysts. This distinction is important because mucinous pancreatic cysts are considered premalignant lesions requiring closer surveillance and potentially surgery. Intraductal papillary mucinous neoplasm (IPMN) and mucinous cystic neoplasm (MCN) are the 2 types of neoplastic mucinous cysts and cannot be distinguished from one another on cytology alone, as the diagnosis of MCN requires the identification of subepithelial ovarian-type stroma on histology. The prevalence of IPMNs is reported to range from 1.7% to 6.7%, increasing with age with the highest prevalence in the eighth decade of life.[31,33] Clinically, IPMNs present with vague, nonspecific symptoms, such as abdominal pain, and up to 40% of patients are asymptomatic.[34] The classification of IPMNs into main duct, branch duct, and mixed types can be determined by imaging.[34] As MCNs are typically found in the pancreatic tail in younger women, the preferred management is curative surgical resection (ie, distal pancreatectomy) to avoid the need for lifelong surveillance. In contrast, low-risk IPMNs can be monitored with serial imaging and usually do not require surgical intervention.

Multiple modalities can help determine that a cyst is mucinous: cytology (thick colloid-like extracellular mucin and/or neoplastic mucinous epithelium), elevated CEA ($\geq$ 192/250 ng/mL),[35] and molecular testing. Cytologic examination of mucinous epithelium is important for the determination of cytologic grade (**Fig. 5**A, B), as high-grade atypia is associated with increased risk of histologic high-grade dysplasia or invasive carcinoma,[36,37] which are the most important factors contributing to poor patient outcomes and warrant resection in appropriate surgical candidates.

The ability to use fresh cyst fluid from the EUS-FNA procedure for next-generation sequencing (NGS) offers useful additional information.[6,7] Detection of *KRAS*, *GNAS*, or *RNF43* mutations support a mucinous cyst, with *GNAS* being specific for IPMN over MCN. In addition, NGS can provide evidence for a high-risk mucinous cyst by detection of late mutations in the development of carcinoma, including mutations in *TP53*, *SMAD4*, and *CDKN2A* (p16).[5] Molecular analysis is

Fig. 4. Pancreatic cyst fluid triage. CEA, carcinoembryonic antigen. (*From* Zhang ML, Pitman MB. Practical Applications of Molecular Testing in the Cytologic Diagnosis of Pancreatic Cysts. *J Mol Pathol.* 2021;2(1):11-22; with permission. (Figure 1 in original).)

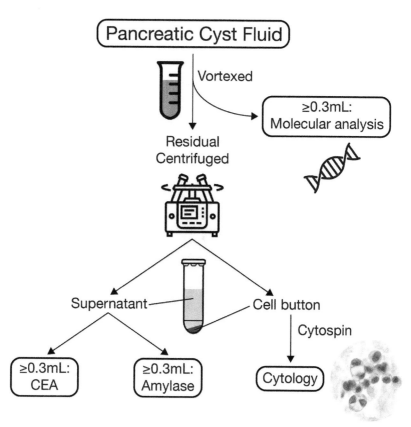

especially informative when neither cytology nor CEA are diagnostic of a mucinous cyst.

Non-Neoplastic Cystic Lesions

Serous cystadenoma

Serous cystadenoma of the pancreas is a benign non-mucinous epithelial neoplasm and is the most common benign pancreatic cystic neoplasm.[38,39] The clinical presentation of serous cystadenomas, like other pancreatic cystic lesions, is variable (such as nonspecific abdominal pain), or they can be asymptomatic and found incidentally on imaging studies.[40] Preoperative identification of serous cystadenomas help triage patients to a conservative approach rather than surgical resection (as these cysts are benign), and often the diagnosis can be made or suggested on imaging (characteristic multicystic, lobulated mass). On EUS-FNA specimens, serous cystadenomas are often paucicellular and nondiagnostic.[41] If cyst lining epithelium is available for evaluation, the cells are bland, cuboidal, and non-mucinous, often with clear glycogen-rich cytoplasm on histology (**Fig. 5**C). Hemosiderin-laden macrophages can be present and associated with a bloody background, which is suggestive of the diagnosis in the context of supporting imaging findings. Serous cystadenomas typically have low CEA (<5 ng/mL) and low amylase levels. Traditionally, periodic acid-Schiff (PAS) (positive) and PAS-diastase (negative) stains were used to support the presence of cytoplasmic glycogen and the diagnosis of serous cystadenoma. In practice, particularly on small tissue samples, immunohistochemistry is preferred: the neoplastic serous cells are positive for inhibin (**Fig. 5**D), GLUT1, and carbonic anhydrase IX. Detection of mutations in *VHL* by molecular testing supports a diagnosis of serous cystadenoma. However, cystic PanNETs can also harbor *VHL* mutations.

Pseudocyst

Pancreatic pseudocysts are the most commonly encountered pancreatic cyst in clinical practice, but are less frequently sampled as the diagnosis can usually be made based on association with recent pancreatitis or trauma (causing autolysis of pancreatic parenchyma) and imaging finding a thick-walled cyst with internal debris.[42] EUS-FNA specimens will not contain lining epithelial cells, as pseudocysts do not have a true epithelial lining

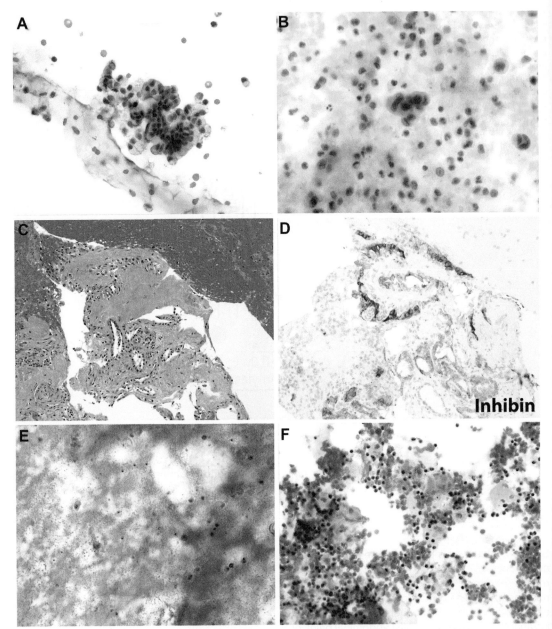

Fig. 5. Cystic pancreatic lesions. Neoplastic mucinous cysts on cytology show mucinous epithelium with (*A*) low-grade atypia: abundant apical cytoplasmic mucin with mildly atypical basally oriented nuclei (Papanicolaou stain, 600x), and (*B*) high-grade atypia: nuclear crowding, increased nuclear to cytoplasmic ratios, and background necrosis (Papanicolaou stain, 600x). (*C*) Serous cystadenoma on biopsy shows round, uniform, cuboidal, non-mucinous epithelial cells (hematoxylin and eosin [H&E], 100x). (*D*) Immunohistochemistry for inhibin shows positive staining in the cytoplasm of the cuboidal epithelial cells (100x). (*E*) Cytology of pseudocyst shows a lack of epithelial cells and background inflammation, histiocytes, and hematoidin-like pigment (Papanicolaou stain, 100x). (*F*) Cytology of lymphoepithelial cyst shows nucleated and anucleated squamous cells and admixed small lymphocytes (Papanicolaou stain, 200x).

(but can contain gastrointestinal contamination), and typically show a proteinaceous background with inflammation, necrosis, and sometimes hematoidin-like pigment (**Fig.** 5E). Biochemical cyst fluid analysis has utility in diagnosing

pseudocysts as the cyst fluid will have a markedly elevated amylase (>250 U/L) due to the pancreatic enzymes in the cyst fluid from auto-digestion (and low CEA). Molecular alterations are absent in pseudocysts.

Lymphoepithelial cyst

Lymphoepithelial cysts are benign non-mucinous cysts of the pancreas lined by squamous epithelium overlying benign lymphoid tissue with germinal center formation. Cytology specimens show variable proportions of the squamous and lymphoid components, which include nucleated and anucleated squamous cells, keratinaceous debris, polymorphous lymphocytes, and cholesterol crystals (**Fig. 5**F). A known phenomenon is that these cysts can have markedly elevated CEA levels, representing a potential pitfall that can lead to misclassification as a mucinous cyst. Molecular alterations are absent in lymphoepithelial cysts.

Pitfalls
CYSTIC PANCREATIC LESIONS

! ROSE is not recommended for pancreatic cysts, which produce paucicellular cyst fluid specimens. Instead, fresh cyst fluid should be sent for liquid-based cytology, biochemical testing, and molecular studies, if possible.

! In cases where no neoplastic mucinous epithelium is identified on cytology, elevated CEA and molecular mutations (*KRAS, GNAS, RNF43*) can be helpful to classify cysts as mucinous.

! Lymphoepithelial cysts can have markedly elevated CEA levels and should not be misclassified as mucinous cysts.

MISCELLANEOUS ENTITIES/ EXTRAPANCREATIC LESIONS

Although metastases to the pancreas are uncommon and represent only 2% to 5% of pancreatic malignancies, more common primary sites include the kidney, lung, breast, and colon.[43,44] Renal cell carcinoma is the most common malignancy to metastasize to the pancreas and can mimic a primary pancreatic lesion.[11,43–45] As with primary pancreatic lesions, EUS-FNA is the primary method to sample and diagnose metastatic lesions to the pancreas, which will usually involve an immunohistochemical workup.[44,45]

Ectopic splenic tissue can present as a well-circumscribed, vascular nodule in the pancreatic tail, mimicking a PanNET on imaging.[45] FNA specimens of ectopic splenic tissue show numerous lymphocytes and lymphoid aggregates, and the diagnosis can be confirmed by performing CD8 on a cell block or small core biopsy, which

highlights the splenic littoral cells lining vascular spaces in the splenic red pulp.[45] As ectopic splenic tissue could be concerning for a low-grade lymphoma, making the correct diagnosis is essential to prevent unnecessary treatment.

When an FNA procedure does not target a true pancreatic mass (but rather adjacent tissues), adrenal cortical tissue sampling may occur and potentially mimic a PanNET.[16] Other diagnostic considerations for non-epithelial spindled/epithelioid neoplasms seen on pancreatic/peripancreatic FNA include gastrointestinal stromal tumor, schwannoma, paraganglioma, and others.[16] Immunohistochemistry would be helpful in classifying these less common entities which can occur in close proximity to the pancreas.

SUMMARY

Minimally invasive FNA of the pancreas is a useful and timely procedure which can readily deliver a diagnosis while simultaneously providing information for personalized patient management through allocating diagnostic material for ancillary/molecular studies, when applicable. FNA sampling is useful in the diagnosis of solid, cystic, and metastatic lesions in the pancreas, and can reduce the number of more costly and invasive procedures. Knowledge of and familiarity with the optimal handling of cytology/small tissue specimens, particularly in the evaluation of pancreatic cysts, are critical to ensure that the often-scant diagnostic material is appropriately utilized. Most solid pancreatic lesions will require surgical excision following a diagnosis of malignancy, whereas for pancreatic cystic lesions, the preoperative diagnosis is important to triage patients to interval surveillance versus surgical intervention. In summary, FNA specimens can provide essential diagnostic material from this anatomically challenging site, leading to clinically actionable information to inform patient management and outcomes.

CLINICS CARE POINTS

- FNA of pancreatic lesions can provide diagnostic material for cytologic and histologic (cell block, small core biopsy) evaluation.

- For solid lesions, particularly non-ductal neoplasms, prioritizing material for immunohistochemical studies aids in making a definitive diagnosis.

- For cystic lesions, optimal handling of pancreatic cyst fluid is essential to ensure that the limited diagnostic material is appropriately utilized for cytologic evaluation, biochemical studies, and molecular testing.
- Accurate preoperative diagnosis informs patient management and helps to triage patients to surgical intervention or surveillance.

DISCLOSURE

The authors have nothing to disclose.

REFERENCES

1. Banafea O, Mghanga FP, Zhao J, et al. Endoscopic ultrasonography with fine-needle aspiration for histological diagnosis of solid pancreatic masses: a meta-analysis of diagnostic accuracy studies. BMC Gastroenterol 2016;16(1):108.
2. Zhang ML, Arpin RN, Brugge WR, et al. Moray micro forceps biopsy improves the diagnosis of specific pancreatic cysts. Cancer Cytopathol 2018;126(6): 414–20.
3. Fitzpatrick MJ, Hernandez-Barco YG, Krishnan K, et al. Diagnostic yield of the SharkCore EUS-guided fine-needle biopsy. J Am Soc Cytopathol 2019;8(4):212–9.
4. Zhang ML, Sabatino ME, Castillo CFD, et al. Cytologic, histologic, and molecular features of pancreatic sarcomatoid undifferentiated carcinoma with heterologous osteosarcomatous transformation. Diagn Cytopathol 2023;51(5):E164–9.
5. Zhang ML, Pitman MB. Practical Applications of Molecular Testing in the Cytologic Diagnosis of Pancreatic Cysts. J Mol Pathol 2021;2(1):11–22.
6. Rosenbaum MW, Jones M, Dudley JC, et al. Next-generation sequencing adds value to the preoperative diagnosis of pancreatic cysts. Cancer Cytopathol 2017;125(1):41–7.
7. Jones M, Zheng Z, Wang J, et al. Impact of next-generation sequencing on the clinical diagnosis of pancreatic cysts. Gastrointest Endosc 2016;83(1): 140–8.
8. Krishnan K, Policarpio Nicolas ML, Itoi T, et al. FNAB techniques and specimen management for solid pancreatic masses. In: International Academy of Cytology – International Agency for Research on Cancer – World Health Organization Joint Editorial Board, ed. WHO reporting System for Pancreaticobiliary Cytopathology. 1st edition. (IAC-IARC-WHO Cytopathology reporting Systems, vol 2). Lyon: International Agency for Research on Cancer; 2022. Available at: https://publications.iarc.fr/621.
9. Brown TJ, Reiss KA. PARP Inhibitors in Pancreatic Cancer. Cancer J 2021;27(6):465.
10. Sahin IH, Lowery MA, Stadler ZK, et al. Genomic instability in pancreatic adenocarcinoma: a new step towards precision medicine and novel therapeutic approaches. Expert Rev Gastroenterol Hepatol 2016;10(8):893–905.
11. Wang Q, Reid MD. Cytopathology of solid pancreatic neoplasms: An algorithmic approach to diagnosis. Cancer Cytopathol 2022;130(7):491–510.
12. Klimstra DS, Gill AJ, Washington MK. Tumours of the pancreas: Introduction. In: WHO Classification of Tumours Editorial Board, editor. Digestive System Tumours. 5th ed. (World Health Organization classification of Tumours, vol 1). Lyon: International Agency for Research on Cancer; 2019. Available at: https://publications.iarc.fr/579.
13. Hruban RH, Adsay N, Esposito I, et al. Pancreatic ductal adenocarcinoma. In: WHO Classification of Tumours Editorial Board, editor. Digestive System Tumours. 5th ed. (World Health Organization classification of Tumours, vol 1). Lyon: International Agency for Research on Cancer; 2019. Available at: https://publications.iarc.fr/579.
14. Hruban RH, Pitman MB, Klimstra DS. Tumors of the pancreas. Washington, DC: Armed Forces Institute of Pathology; 2007.
15. Weynand B, Pitman MB, Kumarasinghe P, et al. Pancreatic ductal adenocarcinoma. In: International Academy of Cytology – International Agency for Research on Cancer – World Health Organization Joint Editorial Board. In: WHO reporting System for Pancreaticobiliary Cytopathology. 1st ed. (IAC-IARC-WHO Cytopathology reporting Systems, vol 2). Lyon: International Agency for Research on Cancer; 2022. Available at: https://publications.iarc.fr/621.
16. Thompson ED, Zhang ML, VandenBussche CJ. The Diagnostic Challenge of Evaluating Small Biopsies from the Pancreatobiliary System. Surg Pathol Clin. 2022;15(3):435–53.
17. Chen ZE, Lin F. Application of immunohistochemistry in gastrointestinal and liver neoplasms: new markers and evolving practice. Arch Pathol Lab Med 2015; 139(1):14–23.
18. Sweeney J, Rao R, Margolskee E, et al. Immunohistochemical staining for S100P, SMAD4, and IMP3 on cell block preparations is sensitive and highly specific for pancreatic ductal adenocarcinoma. J Am Soc Cytopathol 2018;7(6):318–23.
19. Yu S, Doyle LA, Hornick JL, et al. The Diagnostic Utility of MTAP Immunohistochemistry for Pancreatic Ductal Adenocarcinoma in Fine Needle Aspiration and Small Biopsy Specimens. Cancer Cytopathol 2024;132(2):87–95.
20. Hu ZI, Shia J, Stadler ZK, et al. Evaluating Mismatch Repair Deficiency in Pancreatic Adenocarcinoma: Challenges and Recommendations. Clin Cancer Res Off J Am Assoc Cancer Res 2018;24(6): 1326–36.

21. Gheonea DI, Ciurea ME, Săftoiu A, et al. Quantitative RT-PCR analysis of MMR genes on EUS-guided FNA samples from focal pancreatic lesions. Hepato-Gastroenterology 2012;59(115):916–20.

22. Kloppel G, Klimstra DS, Singhi AD, et al. Pancreatic neuroendocrine neoplasms: Introduction. In: WHO classification of Tumours Editorial board, ed. Digestive System Tumours. 5th ed. (World Health Organization classification of Tumours, vol 1). Lyon: International Agency for Research on Cancer; 2019. Available at: https://publications.iarc.fr/579.

23. Weynand B, Reid M, Sigel C. Neuroendocrine tumour. In: International Academy of Cytology – International Agency for Research on Cancer – World Health Organization Joint Editorial Board. In: WHO reporting System for Pancreaticobiliary Cytopathology. 1st ed. (IAC-IARC-WHO Cytopathology reporting Systems, vol 2). Lyon: International Agency for Research on Cancer; 2022. Available at: https://publications.iarc.fr/621.

24. Jin M, Roth R, Gayetsky V, et al. Grading pancreatic neuroendocrine neoplasms by Ki-67 staining on cytology cell blocks: manual count and digital image analysis of 58 cases. J Am Soc Cytopathol 2016; 5(5):286–95.

25. Abi-Raad R, Lavik JP, Barbieri AL, et al. Grading Pancreatic Neuroendocrine Tumors by Ki-67 Index Evaluated on Fine-Needle Aspiration Cell Block Material. Am J Clin Pathol 2020;153(1):74–81.

26. Javed AA, Pulvirenti A, Razi S, et al. Grading Pancreatic Neuroendocrine Tumors via Endoscopic Ultrasound-guided Fine Needle Aspiration: A Multi-Institutional Study. Ann Surg 2022. https://doi.org/10.1097/SLA.0000000000005390.

27. Marinoni I, Kurrer AS, Vassella E, et al. Loss of DAXX and ATRX are associated with chromosome instability and reduced survival of patients with pancreatic neuroendocrine tumors. Gastroenterology 2014;146(2):453–60.e5.

28. Umetsu SE, Kakar S, Basturk O, et al. Integrated Genomic and Clinicopathologic Approach Distinguishes Pancreatic Grade 3 Neuroendocrine Tumor From Neuroendocrine Carcinoma and Identifies a Subset With Molecular Overlap. Mod Pathol Off J U S Can Acad Pathol Inc. 2023;36(3):100065.

29. Sigel C, Stelow EB. Pancreatic acinar cell carcinoma. In: International Academy of Cytology – International Agency for Research on Cancer – World Health Organization Joint Editorial Board, editor. WHO reporting System for Pancreaticobiliary Cytopathology. 1st ed. (IAC-IARC-WHO Cytopathology reporting Systems, vol 2). Lyon: International Agency for Research on Cancer; 2022. Available at: https://publications.iarc.fr/621.

30. Kloppel G, Klimstra DS, Lam AK yin, et al. Solid pseudopapillary neoplasm of the pancreas. In: WHO Classification of Tumours Editorial Board, editor. Digestive System Tumours. 5th ed. (World Health Organization classification of Tumours, vol 1). Lyon: International Agency for Research on Cancer; 2019. Available at: https://publications.iarc.fr/579.

31. Laffan TA, Horton KM, Klein AP, et al. Prevalence of Unsuspected Pancreatic Cysts on MDCT. Am J Roentgenol 2008;191(3):802–7.

32. Itoi T, Pereira SP, Yoon WJ, et al. FNAB techniques and specimen management for pancreatic cysts. In: International Academy of Cytology – International Agency for Research on Cancer – World Health Organization Joint Editorial Board, editor. WHO reporting System for Pancreaticobiliary Cytopathology. 1st ed. (IAC-IARC-WHO Cytopathology reporting Systems, vol 2). Lyon: International Agency for Research on Cancer; 2022. Available at: https://publications.iarc.fr/621.

33. Chang YR, Park JK, Jang JY, et al. Incidental pancreatic cystic neoplasms in an asymptomatic healthy population of 21,745 individuals: Large-scale, single-center cohort study. Medicine (Baltim) 2016;95(51):e5535.

34. Sahani DV, Lin DJ, Venkatesan AM, et al. Multidisciplinary Approach to Diagnosis and Management of Intraductal Papillary Mucinous Neoplasms of the Pancreas. Clin Gastroenterol Hepatol 2009;7(3):259–69.

35. Kwan MC, Pitman MB, Fernandez-Del Castillo C, Zhang ML. Revisiting the performance of cyst fluid carcinoembryonic antigen as a diagnostic marker for pancreatic mucinous cysts: a comprehensive 20-year institutional review. Gut 2024;73(4):629–38.

36. Pitman MB, Centeno BA, Daglilar ES, et al. Cytological criteria of high-grade epithelial atypia in the cyst fluid of pancreatic intraductal papillary mucinous neoplasms. Cancer Cytopathol 2014;122(1):40–7.

37. Valsangkar NP, Morales-Oyarvide V, Thayer SP, et al. 851 resected cystic tumors of the pancreas: a 33-year experience at the Massachusetts General Hospital. Surgery 2012;152(3 Suppl 1):S4–12.

38. Zhang ML, Kwan MC, Pitman MB. Grading Cytological Epithelial Atypia in Pancreatic Mucinous Cysts Predicts Patient Survival: Correlation with Histological. Molecular, and Clinical Follow-Up. Mod Pathol 2024;100510.

39. Kosmahl M, Pauser U, Peters K, et al. Cystic neoplasms of the pancreas and tumor-like lesions with cystic features: a review of 418 cases and a classification proposal. Virchows Arch Int J Pathol 2004; 445(2):168–78.

40. Colonna J, Plaza JA, Frankel WL, et al. Serous Cystadenoma of the Pancreas: Clinical and Pathological Features in 33 Patients. Pancreatology 2008;8(2):135–41.

41. Lilo MT, VandenBussche CJ, Allison DB, et al. Serous Cystadenoma of the Pancreas: Potentials and

Pitfalls of a Preoperative Cytopathologic Diagnosis. Acta Cytol 2017;61(1):27–33.

42. Layfield L, Centeno BA. Pseudocysts. In: International Academy of Cytology – International Agency for Research on Cancer – World Health Organization Joint Editorial Board, editor. WHO reporting System for Pancreaticobiliary Cytopathology. 1st ed. (IAC-IARC-WHO Cytopathology reporting Systems, vol 2). Lyon: International Agency for Research on Cancer; 2022. Available at: https://publications.iarc.fr/621.

43. Alzahrani MA, Schmulewitz N, Grewal S, et al. Metastases to the pancreas: The experience of a high volume center and a review of the literature. J Surg Oncol 2012;105(2):156–61.

44. Hou T, Stewart JM, Lee JH, et al. Solid Tumor Metastases to the Pancreas Diagnosed Using Fine-Needle Aspiration. Am J Clin Pathol 2020;154(5):692–9.

45. Pitman MB. Pancreas and Biliary Tree. In: Cibas ES, Ducatman BS, editors. Cytology: diagnostic Principles and clinical Correlates. Fifth edition. Philadelphia: Elsevier; 2021. p. 451–75.

Minimally Invasive, Maximally Effective
The Power of Precision Cytoanalysis on Effusion Samples—A Comprehensive Exploration from Traditional Methods to Innovative Approaches

Ricella Souza da Silva, MD, PhD[a],
Fernando Schmitt, MD, PhD, FIAC[a,b,c,*]

KEYWORDS

- Effusion • Cytology • Ancillary test • Molecular alterations • Actionable therapeutic targets
- Precision cytopathology

Key points

- Effusion cytology plays multiple roles in the management of benign and malignant disease, from primary diagnosis to tissue allocation for ancillary diagnostics and theranostic studies.
- Standardized cytologic effusion processing allows genetic material extraction, and under these criteria, a tissue sample should not be preferred over a cytologic sample with high cellularity.
- Effusions, analyzed through traditional or innovative methods like supernatants and cell-free DNA, offer valuable insights via molecular testing for precision therapies.
- Effusion cytologic analysis complements plasma and biopsy methods, offering a comprehensive approach to tumor genotyping, early disease detection, tumor progression assessment, and therapeutic response monitoring.

ABSTRACT

Precision medicine translates through molecular assays and in minimally invasive diagnosis, evident in analyses of effusions that serve therapeutic and diagnostic purposes. This cost-effective and low-risk approach provides advantages, playing a pivotal role in late-stage oncology and frequently standing as the primary resource for cancer diagnosis and treatment pathways. This article outlines the workflow for managing serous fluid and explores how cytology effusion analysis extends beyond immunocytological diagnosis. Combined with current molecular tests it showcases the potential to be a skillful tool in precision cytopathology.

OVERVIEW

Effusions occur in up to 15% of all cancer patients.[1] They are amenable to various investigations, encompassing chemical analysis, cultures, cell counting, microscopy, and assessments for biomarkers.[2] The immunohistochemistry remains

---

[a] IPATIMUP Diagnostics, IPATIMUP—Institute of Molecular Pathology and Immunology of Porto University, Porto, 4200-135, Portugal; [b] Faculty of Medicine of the University of Porto, Porto, 4200-319, Portugal; [c] CINTESIS@RISE (Health Research Network), Porto, 4200-319, Portugal
* Corresponding author.
E-mail address: fschmitt@ipatimup.pt

Surgical Pathology 17 (2024) 453–481
https://doi.org/10.1016/j.path.2024.04.008
1875-9181/24/© 2024 Elsevier Inc. All rights reserved.

the predominant technique employed.[3] Nonetheless, a diverse array of innovate techniques for measuring nucleic acids, proteins, and other molecules may be applied in the evaluation of serous effusions, particularly in the context of cancer.[4–7]

Centesis and aspiration of such fluids are performed for therapeutic reasons; it is frequently the initial diagnostic procedure that triggers subsequent management plan and may represent the only available material.[8] This non-invasive approach offers several advantages, including the ability to obtain samples easily and repeatedly, low cost, minimizing patient discomfort, and reducing the need for more invasive procedures.[9]

Cavity effusion represents a late stage of the oncology disease, upstages cancer diagnosis, and alters the disease trajectory and treatment pathway in many cancer types.[10] Due to their optimal suitability for molecular testing, serous effusions have assumed a central role in recent years as specimens that provide critical insights for predicting outcomes in the context of targeted therapy and prognostic considerations.

This article outlines the workflow for managing pleural, peritoneal, and pericardial serous fluid and how effusion cytology, combined with current ancillary tests, can collaborate in advancing of personalized medicine. Apart from distinguishing between benign and malignant processes and determination of the origin of malignant cells, the identification of genetic alterations has transformed the analysis of effusion samples into a skillful tool in precision cytopathology.

PRE-ANALYTICAL

Good performance of the pre-analytic steps is fundamental for successful cytologic analyses and implementation of ancillary studies. Specially because there are more pre-analytical variables in cytology specimens compared to routine formalin-fixed paraffin-embedded (FFPE) tissue samples.[11] The first steps in the management of cytologic effusion samples include the fluid acquisition procedure, through collection, preservation, and processing.

Fluid body cavity for cytologic analysis can be obtained by thoracentesis, paracentesis, pericardiocentesis with aspiration of fresh fluid into a syringe or vial, by drainage via flexible tubes into a collection container, and by intraoperative washing with NaCl 0.9% or balanced electrolyte solutions.[12] The ideal quality of cell preservation is observed in samples freshly obtained through centesis procedures. In contrast, the drainage fluid collected in a container typically exhibits pronounced degenerative alterations. Additionally, degeneration is a remarkable concern in washings, where the morphology of mesothelial cells can be significantly altered compared to naturally accumulated effusion fluid.[13]

Effusion fluid is inherently nutrient-rich, eliminating the need for the addition of preservatives. To maintain sample integrity, refrigeration at temperatures between 4°C and 8°C is recommended when immediate processing is not possible. The studies have demonstrated that refrigerated storage preserves morphologic details and immunoreactions for several days to even weeks, whether stored at either 4°C or room temperature from day 0 to day 4, with immunostaining remained consistent until day 4[14]; however, storage conditions had a detrimental impact on certain lymphocyte markers[15]; even stored at 4°C from day 0 to day 14 with both the morphology, immunocytochemical profiles, and amplifiable DNA were effectively preserved during this extended storage period.[16]

In cases where ideal storage conditions cannot be upheld and delays in processing are anticipated, the use of alcohol-based preservatives becomes a viable option for pre-fixation. A practical method involves the addition of an equal volume of 50% ethanol to the sample. Additionally, commercially available solutions such as CytoLyt and CytoRich, which are based on methanol and ethanol, respectively, offer valuable alternatives. These specified media are basic components in the routine processing of samples when employing liquid-based cytology techniques like SurePath or ThinPrep for the ultimate sample preparation.[12]

The international system for reporting serous fluid cytopathology recommends submitting at least 50 to 75 mL of serous fluid to decrease false-negative results.[17] There is a significant relationship between fluid volume, adequacy, and detection of malignancy in serous effusion cytopathology. The malignancy fraction increases with larger fluid volumes but at least 75 to 100 mL of fluid should be submitted for optimal diagnosis of malignancy in pleural and peritoneal fluids.[18] A specimen volume of ≥ 80 mL improves cytologic sensitivity for malignant ascites, and minimizes the influence of specimen size on diagnostic adequacy in paracentesis specimens.[19] For pericardial fluids, a volume of more than 60 mL should be submitted to cytology to ensure adequate diagnosis.[20] Processing volumes of 20 to 30 mL of serous fluids containing cells is feasible, but it may result in suboptimal cytology preparation, potentially affecting the ability to create cell blocks.[21] The yield from sending additional pleural fluid samples is low; cytology is positive in an additional

27% from a second specimen and 5% from a third specimen.[22]

The fluid should be grossly evaluated, and the volume and gross characteristics should be documented, such as color, clarity, and any unusual features such as viscosity.[2] Effusion fluids can undergo various processing techniques, including a DQ-stained direct smear from an unconcentrated effusion specimen, a DQ-stained Cytospin smear using the concentrated cell pellet, PAP-stained SurePath preparation, PAP-stained ThinPrep preparation, and PAP-stained direct smears. Furthermore, the residual effusion fluid can be utilized for cell block preparation in hematoxylin and eosin (HE)-stained sections, as well as for elective immunocytochemistry.[17]

CLASSIFICATION

Cytologic effusion samples must be classified into 5 categories according to The International System for Reporting Serous Fluid Cytology (TIS)—Nondiagnostic (ND); Negative for malignancy (NFM); atypia of unknown significance (AUS); Suspicious for malignancy (SFM); malignant (MAL).[17] TIS is a valuable classification with widespread acceptance and utility contributing to optimal patient care and facilitating clinical research interpretation.[23]

Recent literature review of 25 studies by Mikou and colleagues[24] describe the risk of malignancy (ROM) for each diagnostic category, separately for pleural, peritoneal, and pericardial effusions. For pleural effusions, the estimated ROM for each category was ND, 0% to 57.1%; NFM, 1.8% to 29.8%; AUS, 33.3% to 62.3%; SFM, 76.2% to 99.3%; and MAL, 90.2% to 100%. Peritoneal effusion data showed ROM for each category: ND, 0% to 100%; NFM, 1.8% to 27.5%; AUS, 22.2% to 62.5%; SFM, 80% to 100%; MAL, 100%. SFM and MAL categories encompassed 8.79% to 68.9%. In pericardial effusions, the estimated ROM for each category was ND, 0% to 100%; NFM, 1.3% to 17.4%; AUS, 0% to 35%; SFM, 57.1% to 100%; MAL, 89.3% to 100%. Using the current classification system, the authors have reported high cytohistological correlations in effusion fluids, with similar values, ranging from 60.29% to 66.9% for sensitivity and 98.4% to 98.56% for specificity.[25,26]

In this classification, special section on pelvic and peritoneal washings seems necessary due to diagnostic challenges. The morphologic features of peritoneal and pelvic washings, conducted intraoperatively for staging, may share similarities with effusions, but pose distinct diagnostic challenges, reflecting the serosal surface's status in diverse circumstances.[21] Noteworthy features in peritoneal washings include benign elements like mesothelial cells and collagen balls, diagnosed as NFM; acellular mucin, diagnosed as NFM; psammoma bodies with atypical cells, diagnosed as AUS; pseudomyxoma peritonei with variable epithelial cells, diagnosed as SFM; and fluids with overtly malignant features, diagnosed as malignant.[27]

In specific cases, ancillary testing is crucial, especially for specimens categorized as atypical or suspicious. Gokozan and colleagues[28] showed a root cause analysis on atypia or suspicious for malignancy diagnoses, identifying low cellularity and volume as the primary contributing factors, emphasizing the significance of thorough sample collection.

DIAGNOSIS

Cytologic examination of the effusion fluid provides valuable information regarding the presence of malignancy. At times, it is challenging to diagnose malignant cells in serous effusion.[7] The morphologic features of most of the cancer cells in effusion smears are different from those seen in exfoliative, brushing, and fine-needle aspiration cytology.[21]

The cytomorphological diagnosis of pleural, pericardial, and peritoneal effusion samples, can be structured into the following keys steps: identifying any additional cellular population beyond mesothelial and inflammatory cells; analyzing the nuclear features of this additional cellular population; evaluation of the mesothelial cells (individually scattered vs groups of 3-dimensional [3D]); certification of the additional cellular population; and differential diagnosis for determining their primary neoplasm by ancillary tests, including immunostaining, as specified.

Outstanding to the cytomorphologic similarities between reactive mesothelial cells and malignant cells, conventional cytologic criteria for diagnosing malignancy in isolated cells are often not applicable in most effusion specimens. Neoplastic cells in effusions typically present in 3D clusters, with monolayers being uncommon. Interpreters must be cognizant of the diverse cytomorphologic variations exhibited by reactive mesothelial cells in effusion fluids.[21] Within malignant effusions, adenocarcinomas stand out as the predominant source of metastatic cancers. However, virtually any malignancy, encompassing melanomas, hematopoietic neoplasms, sarcomas, and mesotheliomas, has the potential to affect serous cavities. Frequently opting for cell block preparations, cytopathologists commonly utilize ancillary studies.[23]

Immunohistochemical staining plays an essential role in diagnosing cytologic samples from effusions, confirming malignancy, and determining the primary site. Distinct applications of immuno-histochemistry (IHC) involve determining the mesothelial or epithelial origin of isolated atypical cells and cell clusters, as well as indicative the primary site of malignancy. Additionally, it assists in evaluating prognostic markers such as for human epidermal growth factor receptors-2 (Her-2), estrogen receptors (ER), and programmed death-ligand 1 (PD-L1).

Cytomorphology, prevalence, differential diagnosis, immunohistochemical profile, and genetic markers of malignancies seen in serous effusions are summarized in **Table 1**.

ANCILLARY STUDIES, PREDICTIVE

IMMUNOHISTOCHEMISTRY BIOMARKERS

Targeted immunotherapies (based on PD-L1 status) have become an integral part of treating advanced-stage cancers such as non-small cell lung cancer (NSCLC), melanoma, pancreas, and triple-negative breast carcinomas.[46] Studies have shown good agreement with corresponding histology for PD-L1 testing in cytology specimens from the lung, head and neck, and melanomas.[47] For cytologic samples, microscopic criteria of adequacy and scoring systems include greater than 100 assessable tumor cells and partial or complete linear membrane staining in tumor cells considered positive at $\geq 1\%$, greater than 5%, greater than 10%, and greater than 50% cutoff levels.[48]

Different works have supported the feasibility of effusions cytologic material for PD-L1 IHC analysis. Song and colleagues[49] showed PD-L1 expression with 86.2% concordance between tumor tissue and malignant pleural effusion samples, while Hagmeyer and colleagues[50] demonstrated that PD-L1 testing with $\geq 50\%$ expression exhibited 100% sensitivity from pleural effusion. In 2 studies, Mansour and colleagues revealed that malignant mesothelioma (MM) effusions are suitable for PD-L1 assessment with results comparable to those reported in histologic studies.[51] The PD-L1 expression in paired effusion and biopsy samples showed 69% and 84% overall agreement at $\geq 1\%$ and greater than 50% cutoffs, respectively. The concordance between cytology and histology tended to be higher for epithelioid MM versus nonepithelioid MM at a $\geq 1\%$ cutoff.[52]

MOLECULAR TESTING

Currently, effusion samples are increasingly utilized for molecular tests, offering not just malignancy diagnosis but essential information for personalized therapy, management, and prognosis. Therefore, when faced with a malignant effusion, particularly in the context of lung and breast carcinomas, one must consider whether additional theranostic or diagnostic tests might be necessary using this sample.

The effusion is rich in cells and cell-free fluid that contains free DNA, cytokines, and extracellular vesicles, and allows for the detection of specific gene mutations, rearrangements, or amplifications associated with certain cancers. Effusion cytology, with its high sensitivity and abundance of material, shows adequate for molecular testing, as efficacious as FFPE tissue. Various molecular techniques exhibit similar effectiveness in serous effusions compared to tissue biopsies, highlighting the pivotal role of sample adequacy irrespective of the sample type.

MOLECULAR PRE-ANALYTICAL

Any cytology sample, with adequate cellularity and preservation, may be used for molecular testing[53,54] and all molecular tests can be done on routine preparations of effusion samples.[12] The choice of cytologic sample preparation method should be made with careful consideration of the specific diagnostic requirements, the unique characteristics of each method, and the advantages and challenges of each approach. See **Table 2**.

SAMPLE QUALITY AND QUANTITY

One of the greatest barriers to obtaining molecular results using cytology specimens is the low cellularity. However, cytologic samples provide a higher quality of nucleic acids with higher purity, higher cellular yield, and better tumor fraction for molecular testing.[57] When submitting material for molecular testing, it is important to consider various factors such as total cellularity, the extent of necrosis, and the tumor content in the specimen.[11] The presence of reactive mesothelial cells and inflammatory cells in the sample can impact the proportion of tumor cells, potentially leading to contamination. The configuration of tumor cells whether found singly or in dense complexes with nuclei overlapping does not interfere with the process. Nevertheless, it is advisable to concentrate them with minimal inclusion of benign cells.[7] Increased levels of necrosis can elevate the presence of low-quality nucleic acids and impede optimal amplification. The preferred scenario is to obtain a sample with less than 20% necrosis.[11] Ensuring the submission of specimens with the highest cellular content is the aim for accurate molecular testing.

Table 1
Cytomorphology, prevalence, differential diagnosis, immunohistochemical profile, and genetic markers of malignancies seen in serous effusions

Malignant Effusion[29]	Diagnosis	Prevalence[30-32]	Cytomorphology[17,30,33-36]	Differential Diagnosis	IHC Profile[17,37-43]	Actionable Genomic Alterations or Pathogenic Alterations Related (Prevalence)[34,35,44,45]
Epithelial: Carcinoma Intercellular cohesion, forming cohesive clusters	Lung Adenocarcinoma	PE: 29%-37% PerE: 1% PCE: 33%-50%	• Architecture: clusters, papillary micropapillae, single cells • Nuclear pleomorphism • Nucleoli, rounded	Breast, gastric, colon, mesothelioma	Ber-EP4; MOC31; Claudin-4 + CK7 +/CK20 - WT-1 -; Calretinin - TTF-1 + (74%-99%) Napsin A+ (65%-83%)	EGFR (12%-31%); MET (3%); ALK (5-7%); RET (1-2%); ROS1 (1-2%); NTRK (0.23%-3%); BRAF V600E (2%) — ESCAT I HER2 (2-5%); KRAS (12%) — ESCAT II
	Breast Carcinoma, NOS	PE: 8%-40% PerE: 13% PCE: 18%	• Architecture: cannonball pattern, branched clusters, 3-dimensional tightly cohesive cell clusters • Nuclear pleomorphism • Nucleoli rounded	Lung, mesothelioma	Ber-EP4; MOC31; Claudin-4 + CK7 +, CK20 - WT-1 -; Calretinin - GATA 3 + (94%-100%) TRPS-1 + (95%-100%) Mammaglobin + (22%-87%) ER + (86%); PR + (80%) HER2 + (13%-15%)	ERBB2 amplification (15%-20%); NTRK fusions (1%); PIK3CA (30%-40%); BRCA1/2 germline (4%) — ESCAT I BRCA1/2 somatic (3%); ERBB2 mutation (4%); ESR1 (30-40%); PTEN (6%-7%); AKT1 (5%) — ESCAT II PALB2 germline (1%) — ESCAT III
	Breast Carcinoma, Lobular		• Architecture: single file pattern • Cellular features: signet ring cells, small cells • Intracytoplasmic vacuoles, low to moderate N/C ratio	Mesothelial cells, histiocytes, mesothelioma, melanoma	Ber-EP4; MOC31; Claudin-4 + CK7 +, CK20 -, E-cadherin - WT-1 -; Calretinin - GATA 3 + (100%) TRPS-1 + (95%-100%) ER/PR + (>95%) HER2 + (<5%); SOX 10 +	CDH1 (12%-83%) — ESCAT I
	Ovarian carcinoma, high-grade serous	PE: 18%-23% PerE: 27%	• Architecture: papillary formation and/or psammoma bodies, cannonball pattern • Cellular features: signet ring cells • High N/C ratio • Prominent nucleoli	Mesothelioma, Mullerian clear cell carcinoma, endometrioid adenocarcinoma	Ber-EP4; MOC31; Claudin-4 + CK7 +, CK20 - WT-1 + (80%-97%); Calretinin - PAX 8 + (>95%) ER + (97%-100%) Napsin A+	BRCA1/2 germline (15-17%); BRCA1/2 somatic (5%-7%); HRD (50%) — ESCAT I TP53 (63%-95%); ARID1A, PTEN, PIK3CA, BRAF, HER2 — Pathogenic

(continued on next page)

Table 1
(continued)

Malignant Effusion[29]	Diagnosis	Prevalence[30-32]	Cytomorphology[17,30,33-36]	Differential Diagnosis	IHC Profile[17,37-43]	Actionable Genomic Alterations or Pathogenic Alterations Related (Prevalence)[34,35,44,45]	
	Gastric Adenocarcinoma	PE: 2% PerE: 14%	• Architecture: single cells or clusters • Cellular features: signet ring cells or intestinal morphology	Breast carcinoma (lobular), lung, mesothelioma	Ber-EP4; MOC31; Claudin-4 +; CK7 +, CK20 +/–; WT-1 -; Calretinin -; CDX2 +/– (60%); HER2 (20%)	ERBB2 (16%); NTRK (2%); EGFR (6%); MET (3%)	ESCAT I; ESCAT II
	Pancreatic ductal Adenocarcinoma	PE: 3% PerE: 11%	• Architecture: single cells or rounded clusters or cells in sheets (drunken honeycomb) • Cellular features: atypical ductal cells, cytoplasmic mucin vacuoles • Nuclear overlap and molding, marked loss of nuclear polarity, anisonucleosis > 4:1	Lung, breast, stomach, colon, ovarian	Ber-EP4; MOC31; Claudin-4 +; CK7 +, CK20 +/–; WT-1 -; Calretinin -; IMP3 + (>90%); Placental S100 + (>90%); SMAD4 loss (54%); Pvhl -/loss (>90%); MUC 4 +	BRCA1/2 germline (4-7%); NTRK (<1%); KRAS (90%-92%); PALB2 germline (3-4%); NRG1 (7%); CDKN2A (90%); TP53 (75%); SMAD4 (55%)	ESCAT I; ESCAT II; Pathogenic
	Colorectal Adenocarcinoma	PE: 1% PerE: 10%	• Variably macronucleoli • Architecture: clusters, syncytial fragments • Cellular features: columnar-shaped • Nuclear pleomorphic, enlarged ovoid nuclei, high N/C ratio • Variably prominent nucleoli	Lung, breast, ovarian, stomach, pancreas	Ber-EP4; MOC31; Claudin-4 +; CK7 -, CK20 +; WT-1 -; Calretinin -; CDX2 + (86%–100%); SATB2 +	BRAF^V600E (8.5%); KRAS p.G12C (4%); NTRK1 (0.5%); ERBB2 (2%); KRAS (44%); NRAS (4%)	ESCAT I; ESCAT II; Pathogenic
	NUT Carcinoma	PE: rare PerE: rare	• Architecture: cohesive clusters • Cellular features: small to medium size, minimal indistinct to clear cytoplasm, dense eosinophilic cytoplasm (squamous differentiations) • Monotonous round to oval nuclei, high mitotic rate • Variably prominent nucleoli	Poorly differentiated adenocarcinoma, small cell carcinoma, mesothelioma, lymphoma	Ber-EP4; MOC31; Claudin-4 -; Pancytokeratin +; WT-1 -; Calretinin -; NUT 1 + (speckled) (87%); P40/p63 + (67%); EMA +; TFF1 -; CD 99 -; Synaptophysin -	NUT gene 15q14 translocation; BRD4-NUT (15p13) fusion (67%); BRD3-NUT or NSD3-NUT fusions	Pathogenic

						Pathogenic
Non-Epithelial: Non-cohesive, individual, solitary neoplastic cells, scattered across smears or forming loose, indistinct clusters	Mesothelioma	PE: 1%–6% PerE: 1%–3%	• Architecture: single cells or rounded clusters (papillary, morules, spheres) • Cellular features: cells with dense cytoplasm, pale rim/ectoplasm (skirts), displaying a narrow space in between cells when grouped (window) • Nuclear size variation, pleomorphism, irregular nuclear contours, frequent binucleation or multinucleation, macronucleoli • Overlap reactive mesothelial cells • Softer signs: metachromatic/2 tone cytoplasm, large variation in size (from normal to gigantic), pseudokeratotic cells (pyknotic, eosinophilic, or orangeophilic cells)	Adenocarcinoma	Ber-EP4; MOC31; Claudin-4 - CK7 +, CK20 - WT-1 +; Calretinin + (91%–96%) BAP 1 loss (55%–80%) D2-40 +; Mesothelin +; EMA + (87%–90%); CEA –	CDKN2A (60%) NF2 (50%–60%) BAP1 (60%–80%)
	Melanoma	PE: 5%–6% PerE: 2%	• Architecture: single cells pattern • Cellular features: pigmented cells (sparse, blue-black quality on Romanowsky- based stains and brown-black on Papanicolaou stain) • Nuclear pleomorphism, nuclear membrane irregularities, coarse chromatin, binucleation, multinucleation, intranuclear pseudoinclusions • Prominent nucleoli and mitotic activity • Numerous pigmented histiocytes	Mesothelioma, adenocarcinoma	Ber-EP4; MOC31 - WT-1 +; Calretinin - HMB45 + Melan-A (MART1) + S100 + SOX10 + Tyrosinase + MITF + PRAME +	ESCAT I BRAF^V600E 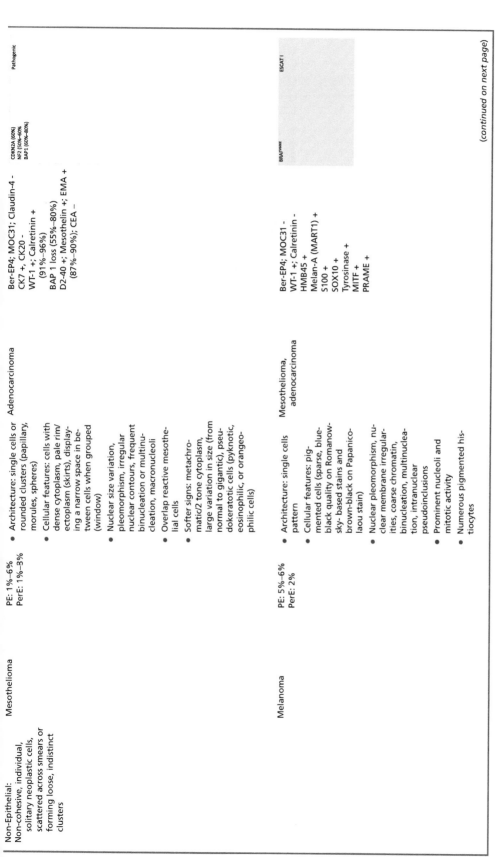

(continued on next page)

Table 1
(continued)

Malignant Effusion[29]	Diagnosis	Prevalence[30-32]	Cytomorphology[17,30,33-36]	Differential Diagnosis	IHC Profile[17,37-43]	Actionable Genomic Alterations or Pathogenic Alterations Related (Prevalence)[34,35,44,45]		
	Lymphoma	PE: 3%–16% PerE: 5%–12%	• Architecture: single cells pattern • Cellular features: small cells (<2 × of resting lymphocyte or <1 × histiocyte nuclei); large cells (≥2 × of resting lymphocyte or >1 × histiocyte nuclei) • High N/C ratio, clumped chromatin • Variable nucleoli (depends on subtype) • Lymphoglandular bodies in background	Small cell carcinoma, melanoma, poorly differentiated non-small cell carcinoma	• Small cell: flow cytometry (kappa light chain, lambda light chain); • Large cell: IHC CD20, CD79a, PAX5 (B cell marker) CD3 (T cell marker) CD138 (plasma cell marker) HHV8 (primary effusion lymphoma)	Follicular lymphoma: t(14;18) BCL2-IgH fusion Mantle cell lymphoma: t(11;14) (q13;q32); BCL1-IgH fusion Burkitt lymphoma: t(8;14) (q24;q32); cMYC-IgH fusion		Pathogenic
	Sarcoma	3%–6% in ME	• Architecture: single cells pattern • Cellular features: spindle cells • Nuclei: round to oval, fusiform or spindle-shaped; chromatin clumping • Prominent nucleoli	Melanoma, lymphoma, small cell carcinoma	Depend on subtype Leiomyosarcoma caldesmon+, Desmin+, SMA+ GIST c-kit + DOG1+ Endometrial stromal sarcoma: CD10+ Synovial sarcoma Keratin+, EMA+, TLE1+, CD99+ Alveolar soft part sarcoma TFE3+, EMA−, S100+/−, desmin+/−, keratin−, HMB45− Ewing sarcoma CD99+, NKX2.2+, FLI1+	cKit mutations ALK mutations CD4 amplification GIST: KIT mutations PDGFRA mutations Endometrial stromal sarcoma : JAZF1-SUZ1 Synovial sarcoma SS18-SSX1, SS18-SSX2 Alveolar soft part sarcoma ASPCR1-TFE3 Ewing sarcoma EWSR1-FLI1, EWSR1-ERG	ESCAT I ESCAT II	Pathogenic

Abbreviations: ESCAT, ESMO scale for clinical actionability of molecular targets; GIST, gastrointestinal stromal tumor; IHC, immunohistochemistry; ME, malignant effusion; N/C, nucleus/cytoplasm; PCE, pericardial effusion; PE, pleural effusion; PerE, peritoneal effusion.

Table 2
Features of the types of cytologic preparations for molecular assays[11,55,56]

	Smears	Liquid-Based Cytology	Cell Block
Advantages	• High-quality nucleic acids • Immediate adequacy assessment	• Efficiency in rapidly collecting and aspirating effusion samples	• It does not need additional validation for molecular tests • Efficiently preserves diagnostic material
Limitations	• Require validation • Need to remove the lamella/scrapping • Slide sacrificing	• Quality of nucleic acids may vary depending on the fixative used	• Lower quality DNA • Limited number of cells
Fixation	• Alcohol-fixed or air-dried • Nucleic acids are better preserved in alcohol than in formalin • Air-dried has impact on RNA	• DNA yield from the CytoLyt™ fixed cells (Hologic corporation, Marlborough, MA, United States) was 5-fold that retrieved from CytoRich Red™ fluid (BD TriPath™, Burlington, NC, United States)	• Formalin fixation has a negative effect on the extracted DNA, which is usually suboptimal in quality • Formalin has a particularly harmful impact on RNA
Staining	• Papanicolaou or Diff Quik staining methods • Better results were observed with spray or ethanol-fixed slides in comparison to air-dried slides stained with Romanowsky method • For RNA molecular test: staining Papanicolaou	• Papanicolaou staining	• Hematoxylin and eosin
Removal and Extraction	• To remove coverslips—xylene for crystal coverslips; acetone for plastic coverslips. • To remove a glass coverslip: immersing the slide in xylene overnight. • Freezing Technique: The slide is positioned horizontally inside a deep freezer set at a temperature of −20°C for a duration of 1–3 min, allowing for the prompt removal of the coverslip. • Destaining the slides is not need. • Scraping or cell lifting with Pinpoint solution to extract the cells.		
Archival Slides	• Archived smears can be successfully isolated for various molecular tests. • Direct scraping of archival slides has a higher nucleic acid yield than cell lifting. • Stained slides archived in room temperature longer than 6 months may also not give satisfactory results.		

A malignant cell fraction exceeding 10% to 20% is deemed the lower acceptable threshold for molecular methods; at least 1 to 10 ng from 100 to 200 tumor cells is needed to obtain enough DNA for next-generation sequencing (NGS). It has been noted that 20% tumor cells are the minimum threshold to avoid the false-negative molecular test.[7] For isolating 10 ng of nucleic acids necessitates approximately 3 to 4 times more cells from an FFPE sample compared to ethanol-fixed material.[58] In cytology material samples, 100 to 2000 cells are categorized as low levels, 2000 to 5000 as intermediary levels, and those surpassing 5000 cells are deemed suitable for any NGS, including large panels.[59]

TECHNIQUES

Common molecular techniques in clinical cytopathology include fluorescence in situ hybridization (FISH), polymerase chain reaction (PCR), and NGS. Most molecular techniques show similar efficacy in serous effusions.[6] PCR, highly sensitive and specific, requires specific target DNA, while FISH uses DNA probes for target detection, necessitating well-preserved tumor cells. NGS, allowing rapid, whole-genome sequencing, is not target-specific, offering advantages in studying large numbers of target DNAs but may have limitations in terms of cost and data analysis complexity.[7]

KEY MOLECULAR THERAPEUTIC AND PROGNOSTIC TARGETS IN EFFUSIONS

The cytologist's role in molecular testing for effusion samples starts with an initial assessment and provisional diagnosis moving on to cellular area evaluation and viable cell labeling. Subsequently, the focus is on determining of tumor typing through immunostaining or targeted diagnostic molecular testing. The next stage is to use cell preparations specific to each case, which include cell blocks and stained slides for FISH, cell blocks and cell pellets for PCR, and cell blocks, cell pellets, and stained slides for NGS. For optimal molecular testing in cytology samples, Pinto and Schmitt[6] propose ordering a routine cell block with immediate evaluation for adequacy. If adequate, conduct testing; if not, perform molecular testing on smears or slides, considering digitalization for archival purposes. The final interpretation of results is carried out by the cytopathologist.[9]

PLEURAL AND PERICARDIAL EFFUSION

Most malignant pleural effusions are secondary to metastases to the pleura, most often from lung or breast cancer. Cytology of pleural fluid has a mean sensitivity of approximately 60% in diagnosing metastatic malignancy and is even lower for mesothelioma.

Mesothelioma

Mesothelioma stands out as the predominant primary pleural tumor, with over 90% of cases manifesting as malignant effusion.[60] The integration of novel molecular biomarkers in routine diagnostic panels, including BAP1, MTAP, and CDKN2A/p16 homozygous deletion, is increasingly pivotal for achieving a precise diagnosis of malignant mesothelioma.[61,62]

Cytology effusions are often the only material available for diagnosing malignant pleural mesothelioma. The detection of these molecular alterations from cytologic samples is becoming more common and reliable in cell block preparations.[63] In a comprehensive literature review encompassing 71 studies, Girolami and colleagues revealed that the BAP1 gene remains intact in reactive mesothelial cells but is frequently lost in mesothelioma cases. The specificity was high, reaching 0.99 for BAP1 loss and 100% for MTAP loss and p16. Moreover, the sensitivity can be significantly enhanced by employing a combination of 2 biomarkers, such as BAP1 and CDKN2A with fluorescence in situ hybridization, or a combination of BAP1 and MTAP with immunohistochemistry.[64]

Chevrier and colleagues suggest improving cytology diagnostic accuracy by incorporating routine BAP1 immunohistochemistry and p16 fluorescence in situ hybridization as adjunctive tests. This approach shows promise in enabling earlier detection of malignant mesothelioma.[65] Along these lines, an interesting study detected abnormalities in BAP1 and CDKN2A before cytomorphologic features diagnostic of pleural mesothelioma, thereby highlighting a possible cytologic equivalent for mesothelioma in situ.[66]

Lung

Malignant pleural and pericardial effusions are common occurrences in the progression of lung adenocarcinoma, affecting a significant proportion of patients, typically 30% to 50%. Once these effusions are histologically confirmed to be malignant, it indicates advanced disease; in lung cancer, the presence of stage IV disease, for which molecular testing becomes clinically necessary.[67]

The presence of genetic alterations in tumor cells, such as EGFR and BRAF gene mutations, as well as ALK and ROS1 gene rearrangements, are indications for targeted therapies. There are several first-line systemic therapy options for patients with newly diagnosed stage IV NSCLC.[68]

Nonetheless, there is growing evidence that certain patient groups with oligometastatic disease, which may have a more indolent biological nature than widespread metastatic diseases, may survive longer if definitive local treatment is administered to all metastatic sites. As a result of rapidly emerging systemic therapies, such as immune checkpoint inhibitors and a growing number of targeted therapies, more patients with this uncommon clinical opportunity have been identified and have received greater clinical attention.[69]

Using pleural effusion samples, various groups have effectively established canonical driver oncogenes using NGS techniques, whether in small or large panels. A comprehensive meta-analysis,[70] encompassing 15 studies with a total of 1266 cases, has indicated that the detection of EGFR mutations in pleural effusion samples holds promise as a viable alternative to tumor tissue for EGFR mutation testing in NSCLC patients. The analysis revealed an impressive sensitivity of 87% and a commendable specificity of 93%.

In a recent study conducted by Man Ng and colleagues,[71] EGFR testing was carried out in a total of 1855 cases, with 913 of them involving effusion fluid samples. The results revealed a notably higher EGFR detection (positive) rate in cell block pleural fluid when compared to biopsy specimens. Additionally, among all cytology materials, fluid specimens consistently displayed the highest detection rate.

Dalvi and colleagues[72] related specific criteria for pleural effusion samples from pulmonary or non-pulmonary sources. They found that a minimum volume of 20 mL, a cell count of 1000, and a tumor-to-non-tumor (T:NT) proportion between 20% and 50% were necessary for successful molecular analysis. In cases with a T:NT proportion below 20%, a minimum of 300 tumor cells was required for effective analysis. These criteria were based on the use of a comprehensive NGS panel detecting 324 genetic alterations.

Utilizing cell block preparations, a study explored the feasibility and clinical value of targeted NGS obtained from malignant effusions of metastatic lung adenocarcinoma patients. The custom target panel encompassed over 100 genes recurrently mutated in solid tumors, including key driver oncogenes specific to lung adenocarcinoma (such as KRAS, EGFR, BRAF, ROS1, ALK, RET, MET, ERBB2, PIK3CA, NRAS, AKT1, and MAP2K1), along with other frequently altered genes in lung cancer (eg, TP53, STK11, KEAP1, CDKN2A, and RB1). The sequencing reads exhibited robust quality control parameters, and variant allele frequencies were positively associated with tumor cellularity. Notably, a

substantial 88% of cell block samples provided adequate DNA for sequencing (1 ng/mL), with a median genomic concentration of 13.2 ng/mL and a quantity of 0.66 ng. These results compare favorably with success rates achieved in other NGS studies utilizing core-needle biopsy and fine-needle aspirate specimens, which typically range from 50% to 90%.[4]

Breast

Breast carcinoma cells in primary carcinomas and metastatic breast cancer (MBC) in effusions have different gene expression signatures.[73,74] Biomarker conversion at metastatic sites from the primary breast carcinoma is reported rates ranging from 14% to 24% for ER and 5% to 12% HER-2, which necessitates the revision of therapeutic intervention.[59] The prognosis and treatment planning for patients with metastatic disease localized to the serosal cavities may be significantly impacted by these variations.

ERBB2, PIK3CA, and germline BRCA1/2 alterations are biomarkers prospectively validated in breast cancer, driving the selection of targeted therapies. Agnostic biomarkers, namely microsatellite instability, NTRK fusions, and high tumor mutational burden, demonstrated similar activity across different tumor types. Additionally, emerging molecular biomarkers include somatic BRCA1/2 mutations, germline PALB2 mutations, HER2-low expression, ERBB2 mutations, PTEN deletions, AKT1 mutations, and ESR1 resistance mutations.[45]

ERBB2 amplifications are typically evaluated through immunochemistry or in situ hybridization. BRCA1/2 mutations are assessed via germline testing, while PIK3CA status can be determined by PCR targeting the 3 hotspots.[44] For workflow effusion samples, opting for a multigene NGS panel appears to be a more suitable approach.

Studies demonstrated the detection of ERBB2 gene amplification in effusion samples using FISH techniques, including cytospin preparations and archival smears May-Grünwald-Giemsa stained, even in cases with minimal cellular content.[75,76] In the context of hormone receptor-positive/HER2-negative MBC, TP53, ESR1, ERBB2, ARID1A, NF1, and KMT2D exhibit a higher frequency of mutations in the metastatic setting compared to early tumors.[77]

PERITONEAL EFFUSION

Fluid accumulation in the peritoneal cavity is prevalent in ovarian, colorectal, pancreatic, gastric, and primary peritoneal cancers. Molecular profiling studies on malignant ascites contents

Table 3
Applications and findings of molecular tests in supernatant and cell-free effusion samples

Publication	Number of Cases	Effusion Type	Diagnosis	Extraction Source	Volume	Mean DNA/RNA Yield (ng/μL)	Molecular Assay	Genomic Markers	Conclusions
Liu et al,[86] 2013	27	PE	NSCLC	Supernatant	NI	NI	ARMS	EGFR	• EGFR mutation rate in Supernatant MPE: 48.1% • Supernatant Sensitivity (compared with tissue samples): 63.6% • Supernatant Specificity (compared with tissue samples): 100%
Liu et al,[87] 2014	41	PE	Lung adenocarcinoma	Supernatant	10 mL	NI	ARMS	EGFR	• EGFR mutation rate in MPE: 56.3% • Supernatant Sensitivity (compared with tissue samples): 84.2% • Supernatant Specificity (compared with tissue samples): 90.9%

Study	N			Source	Volume		Method	Gene	Findings
Husain et al,[88] 2017	6	PE PerE	MST	cfDNA from supernatant	30 mL	DNA: 3.9–38.4	NGS	BRAF, EGFR, IDH1, IDH2, KRAS, NRAS, PIK3CA, PTEN, TP53	• cfDNA from Asc and PE may provide additional information not detected with tumor and plasma cell-free DNA
Asaka et al,[89] 2018	9	PE	NSCLC	cfDNA from supernatant	1.5 mL	DNA: 7.4	dd-PCR	EGFR	• Concordance rates between cfDNA supernatant and cell-pellet: 96.7% • EGFR mutations detected in cfDNA supernatants for which the cytologic diagnoses of the corresponding cell pellets were 'suspicious for malignancy', 'atypical' or 'negative for malignancy' • Sensitivity: MPE supernatant vs tissue: 100%
Han et al,[90] 2018	58	PE	Lung adenocarcinoma	cfDNA from supernatant	0.5 mL	NI	PCR	EGFR	• cfDNA Supernatant > Accuracy: 96% vs 46%–65% in Plasma • cfDNA Supernatant > Sensitivity: 97% vs 55%–71% in Plasma

(continued on next page)

Table 3
(continued)

Publication	Number of Cases	Effusion Type	Diagnosis	Extraction Source	Volume	Mean DNA/RNA Yield (ng/μL)	Molecular Assay	Genomic Markers	Conclusions
Tong et al,[91] 2019	63	PE	Lung cancer	cfDNA from supernatant	3–6 mL	DNA: 278.1	NGS	416 cancer-related genes	• cfDNA Supernatant contain more abundant tumor DNA than PE Sediments and Plasma samples • cfDNA Supernatant > mutation detection rate: 98.4% vs 90.5% in PE Sediments vs 87% in Plasma • cfDNA Supernatant > detection rate of EGFR driver mutations: 71% vs 68% in PE sDNA vs 59% in plasma cfDNA • cfDNA Supernatant > Tumor mutational burden (TMB): 6.4 vs 3.4 in Plasma vs 3.3 PE Sediments • cfDNA Supernatant = Tumor mutational burden (TMB): median 6.4 vs median 5.6 in Tissue

et al,[92] 2019	MST			supernatant					effusion can be used to detect driver mutations as well as resistance mechanisms like EGFR T790 M in pleural effusion with high accuracy
Xiang et al,[93] 2020	47	PE	NSCLC	cfTNA from supernatant	1 mL	DNA: 65.8	NGS	ALK, BRAF, EGFR, ERBB2, KRAS, MAP2K1, MET, NRAS, PIK3CA, RET, ROS1	• cfTNA isolated from pleural fluids can be effectively used in clinical practice for molecular analysis by NGS, even in cases where corresponding cell pellets or tumor tissues yield insufficient material • cfDNA Supernatant > somatic mutation detection rate: 89.1% vs 54.3% in Cell Pellets • cfDNA Supernatant + Cell Pellets showed a high concordance (88.3%) of variant detection with their respective tumor tissue specimens

(continued on next page)

Table 3
(continued)

Publication	Number of Cases	Effusion Type	Diagnosis	Extraction Source	Volume	Mean DNA/RNA Yield (ng/µL)	Molecular Assay	Genomic Markers	Conclusions
Yang et al,[94] 2020	21	PE PerE PericE	MST	cfDNA from supernatant	5 mL	DNA: 10.3	NGS	Panel of 130 cancer-relevant genes	• Supernatant samples show similar preanalytical and sequencing quality control metrics when compared with FFPE testing • All effusions were successfully sequenced to a median depth of >1000, revealing a wide spectrum of genomic changes such as single nucleotide variations, minor insertions and deletions, amplifications, and fusions

Mayo-de-Las-Casas et al,[95] 2020	50	PerE	Endometrial cancer	cfDNA from supernatant	2–4 mL	DNA: 4–20	PCR	KRAS, PIK3CA	• cfDNA mutational analysis in peritoneal lavages and blood from early stage endometrial cancer is feasible • The mutations found from cfDNA peritoneal lavages were coincident with those detected in tumor tissue by NGS
Leick et al,[96] 2020	37	PerE	Gastrointestinal cancer with peritoneal carcinomatosis	cfDNA	NI	NI	dd-PCR	KRAS	• cfDNA PerE may enable prediction of disease burden • cfDNA with mean allele frequency > 1% had significantly higher surgical peritoneal cancer index scores: 27 vs 13 • cfDNA with mean allele frequency > 1% tended to have higher radiological peritoneal cancer index

(continued on next page)

Table 3
(continued)

Publication	Number of Cases	Effusion Type	Diagnosis	Extraction Source	Volume	Mean DNA/RNA Yield (ng/μL)	Molecular Assay	Genomic Markers	Conclusions
Chen et al,[97] 2021	77	PE	NSCLC	cfDNA and cfRNA from supernatant	NI	DNA: > 2 RNA 10–500	rt-PCR	EGFR, KRAS, BRAF, NRAS, HER2, PIK3CA, ALK, ROS1, RET	• Supernatant Specificity for driver gene alteration: 100% • Supernatant > Sensitivity: 81.5% for SNV/Indels by cfDNA and 80% for fusions by cfRNA vs 71% by cell blocks vs 66.7% by cell sediments • cfRNA Supernatant Concordance for fusions with paired tissue samples: 97.9% • Supernatant TAT workflow for molecular testing: 4 h against 3 d of traditional workflow using cell blocks for molecular detection

Study	N	Effusion	Cancer	Analyte	Volume	DNA concentration	Method	Genes	Findings
Mokánszki et al,[98] 2021	65	PE	Lung cancer	cfDNA	5 mL	DNA: 0.21–46.8	Reverse-Hybridization Assay	EGFR, KRAS, BRAF	• Gene mutations could be safely demonstrated from the PE cfDNA • cfDNA PE > Concentration: 23.2 vs 4.8 ng/μL in Plasma samples
Kock et al,[99] 2021	5	PE	Lung cancer	cfDNA from supernatant	8 mL	NI	ddPCR	EGFR, KRAS, BRAF	• cfDNA Supernatant > Concentration and Fractional Abundance than Plasma samples • Longitudinal ctDNA PE Supernatant better reflects the course of the disease and therapy response compared to plasma
Suenaga et al,[100] 2021	89	PerE	Pancreatic ductal adenocarcinoma	cfDNA	100 mL (peritoneal washing)	DNA: 5.5–81.5	dd-PCR	KRAS	• cfDNA PerE was found not only in all the patients with peritoneal lavage cytology positive but also in patients with peritoneal

(continued on next page)

Table 3
(continued)

Publication	Number of Cases	Effusion Type	Diagnosis	Extraction Source	Volume	Mean DNA/RNA Yield (ng/μL)	Molecular Assay	Genomic Markers	Conclusions
									lavage cytology negative. • The cfDNA biomarker had a much higher sensitivity for peritoneal recurrence than cytology, whereas cytology had higher specificity • cfDNA PerE may predict poor prognosis and peritoneal recurrence in pancreatic ductal adenocarcinoma
Van't Erve et al,[101] 2021	20	PerE	Colorectal cancer	cfDNA	5 mL (ascites); 50 mL (peritoneal washing)	DNA: 0.12–36.6	dd-PCR	KRAS, BRAF	• In patients with CRC-peritoneal metastases, PerE (high detectability of cfDNA) may serve as a more useful source of cfDNA than plasma • In patients with CRC-peritoneal

No.	Author, Year	Cancer	Source	Analyte	Volume		Method	Panel	Findings
									metastases, cfDNA PerE > Mutant Allele Fraction: 16.4% X vs 0.28% in Plasma • In patients with CRC-peritoneal metastases, cfDNA analysis of peritoneal washes may offer an alternative to detect and monitor peritoneal spread
4	Ju et al,[102] 2022	Endometrial cancer	PerE	cfDNA	10 mL	NI	Whole-exome Sequencing	Panel of 666 cancer-relevant genes	• ctDNA from PerE might be a suitable biomarker for identifying the mutational landscape of EC and could complement tumor heterogeneity • cfDNA PerE > Coverage of Sequencing Depth: 199.0X vs 171.2X in Plasma • ctDNA of Negative PerE > total mutation numbers than Positive PerE and Tissue samples

(continued on next page)

Table 3
(continued)

Publication	Number of Cases	Effusion Type	Diagnosis	Extraction Source	Volume	Mean DNA/RNA Yield (ng/μL)	Molecular Assay	Genomic Markers	Conclusions
Wu et al,[103] 2022	491	PE PerE	Lung cancer, gastrointestinal cancer	cfDNA from supernatant	NI	NI	NGS	Panel of 59 or 1021 cancer-relevant genes	• cfDNA Asc Supernatant > Maximum somatic allele frequency: 50% vs 3% in Plasma samples • cfDNA PE Supernatant > Maximum somatic allele frequency: 28.5% vs 1.30% in Plasma samples • cfDNA PE Supernatant > Actionable Mutation rate: 80.3% vs 48.4%,in Plasma samples • cfDNA PE Supernatant > frequency of uncommon variations than the Plasma regardless of distant organ metastasis

Abbreviations: ARMS, amplification refractory mutation system; Asc, ascites; cfDNA, cell-free DNA; cfRNA, cell-free RNA; cfTNA, cell-free total nucleic acid; ddPCR, droplet digital PCR; EC, effusion cytology; MPE, malignant pleural effusion; MST, metastatic solid tumor including of the lung cancer, breast cancer, pancreas cancer, colon cancer, rectal cancer, appendiceal carcinoma, renal cell carcinoma, and adenocarcinoma of unknown primary; NI, not informed; NGS, next generation sequencing; NSCLC, non-small cell lung cancer; PCR, polymerase chain reaction; PE, pleural effusion; PerE, peritoneal effusion; PericE, pericardial effusion; rt-PCR, real time PCR; TAT, turnaround time.

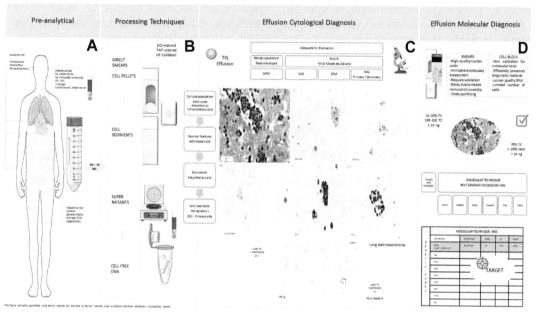

Fig. 1. Schematic of the workflow and molecular approach to effusion cytopathology. (*A*) Pre-analytical step: main standardizations for the acquisition and preservation of effusion samples; (*B*) Effusion fluids processing techniques; (*C*) Cytological examination of the effusion—exemplification of a cytological diagnosis in a patient with pleural effusion and cytological diagnosis of lung adenocarcinoma: classification of the sample in the TIS categories, main criteria, and cytomorphological findings (HE, 40 ×), immunocytochemical (40 ×) study with positivity for Ber-EP4, MOC-31, CK-7, TTF-1 and Calretinin negativity, PD-L1 expression (clone 22C3) in neoplastic cells less than 1%; (*D*) Effusion molecular diagnosis—steps of molecular profiling for a cytological effusion sample with a confirmed diagnosis of lung adenocarcinoma: advantages and disadvantages of the cytological preparations used; assessment of tumor cellularity; application of a high-sensitivity molecular technique and gene multipanel; molecular result with detection of actionable genetic alteration with target therapy.

(soluble molecules, extracellular vesicles, and cells) offer insights for new biomarkers and therapies.[78] Approximately 10% to 40% of patients with gastric cancer and colorectal cancer have peritoneal metastases.[79] Examination of ascites and peritoneal washing fluids from patients with gastrointestinal (GI) cancers can help in the tumor staging and prognosis.[80]

A study by Nokavi and colleagues showed that archival cytologic specimens for ascitic fluid samples could be used for genomic analysis and can identify alterations for large panels without interventional surgery or biopsy. In this series, molecular cytology of ascitic fluid may yield a more comprehensive picture of the entire abdominal cavity, detecting changes not identified by FFPE samples, even with a smaller quantity of extracted DNA, but of better quality.[81]

Current guidelines recommend that all women diagnosed with epithelial ovarian, fallopian tube, and/or peritoneal cancers should be offered genetic screening for BRCA mutations. BRCA mutations (germline or somatic) are eligible for treatment with poly (ADP-ribose) polymerase inhibitors (PARPi).[82] Gornjec and colleagues demonstrated 100%

concordance in BRCA mutation testing between effusion cytologic samples (at least 30 mL of ascites or pleural effusion) from ovarian cancer patients and histologic samples. Cytologic samples with adequate percentage of tumor cells (average per sample: 53.1%) was equivalent to FFPE samples in determining BRCA mutations by NGS.[83]

With parallel findings, Lou and colleagues determined that effusion cytologic samples from high-grade serous carcinoma (HGSC) serve as excellent resources for NGS testing of BRCA1/2 genetic alterations, particularly when a substantial tumor cellularity (averaging 58%) is available. Moreover, there was an equivalency observed among fresh, alcohol-fixed, and FFPE cytologic specimens for NGS assessment of BRCA1/2. NGS testing on HGSC cytologic samples also exhibits strong concordance with the BRCA1/2 status found in surgical specimens.[84]

Bae and colleagues analyzed NGS targets tumor-derived DNA of ascites and peritoneal washing fluids from patients with GI cancers, compared with tissue samples, and correlates with cytopathologic findings. Fluid and tissue genotyping showed a 25% correlation and 21.43%

sensitivity. Detecting somatic mutations increased to 69.2% in samples with greater than 2% tumor volume. In ascitic fluid analysis, mutations were identified in patients with gastric cancer, which included KRAS, TP53, and APC mutations. In pancreatic cancer, KRAS, TP53, and CDH1 mutations.[85]

FUTURE TRENDS

SUPERNATANT AND CELL-FREE DNA

Supernatant fluid is obtained after cell pelleting and centrifugation during cytology specimen preparation. In the past, supernatants from effusion samples centrifugation were discarded. However, effusion supernatants are also informative, as they contain DNA, RNA, microRNA, and proteins. Nucleic acid residues in these supernatant solutions can be extracted for potential utilization in various molecular tests such as PCR and NGS.

A small proportion of cell-free DNA (cfDNA) originates from primary sites, metastatic sites, or circulating tumor cells. Serous effusions are routinely collected in clinical practice and can be easily processed for cfDNA extraction. This material from peritoneal fluid can provide additional genomic information that cannot be obtained from tumor and plasma of various cancers.

Effusion supernatants and cfDNA are therefore drawing increasing attention to their potential as part of the rapidly expanding area of liquid biopsies. Furthermore, compared to traditional workflows, the use of this sample standard improved cost and turnaround time, facilitating faster mutation detection in clinical practice and making them a convenient and cost-effective alternative to tissue or plasma samples. Table 3 displays the studies applying this approach along with the principal technical standards and the corresponding revealed results.

NEGATIVE CYTOLOGY AND ARTIFICIAL INTELLIGENCE

Insufficient specimen volume and low tumor cellularity pose inherent limitations in both conventional and innovative cytopathological analyses of patient effusion samples. These constraints not only restrict the diagnostic capacity but also impede subsequent molecular investigates aimed at identifying actionable therapeutic targets.[104]

Recent studies have offered insights into mitigating or overcoming limitations associated with effusion samples. On the one hand, revealing the feasibility of detecting actionable genetic changes in cytological-negative, although these findings

are based on small number of cases.[5,105] For instance, Song and colleagues demonstrated a high mutation detection rate, reaching 99.2% in malignant pleural effusions and 100% in 40 cytologically-negative pleural effusion supernatant samples. Their results indicated superior performance compared to tumor tissues in identifying EGFR mutations.[106] Another study emphasized that EGFR mutations can be identified in cytologically-negative effusions when utilizing a sensitive method, with a detection rate of 45.7% in sediment samples from such effusions.[107]

On another note, an interesting study, utilizing supervised deep learning, developed an AI-driven technology platform for identifying, classifying, and isolating carcinoma cells in a background of benign cells typically found in effusions and from diverse cancer ascites and pleural effusion specimens.[108]

CLINICS CARE POINTS

- Advancements in "innovate-cytology sample" introduce as a cancer-specific biomarker, offering the potential to act as a surrogate for detecting early disease metastases, therapies response, tumor heterogeneity, and disease progression.

- Effusion cytology improves cost and turn-around in molecular analysis, aligning with the concept that less can be more, and the process can also be faster and cheaper.

- Pathologists play a pivotal role in navigating the intricate landscape of diagnostic and molecular testing procedures.

- The precision medicine translates into minimal invasive diagnosis associated with molecular assay.

- The approaches to effusion cytopathology (Fig. 1) discussed in this article represent a mirror of the current state-of-the-art practices and the established standards in contemporary medical care.

DISCLOSURE

The authors have nothing to disclose.

REFERENCES

1. Bibby AC, Dorn P, Psallidas I, et al. ERS/EACTS statement on the management of malignant pleural effusions. Eur Respir J 2018;52(1):1800349.

2. Michael CW. Serous fluid cytopathology: Past, present, and future. Diagn Cytopathol 2021;49(5):577–81.

3. Davidson B. Molecular testing on serous effusions. Diagn Cytopathol 2021;49(5):640–6.

4. Yang SR, Lin CY, Stehr H, et al. Comprehensive genomic profiling of malignant effusions in patients with metastatic lung adenocarcinoma. J Mol Diagn 2018;20(2):184–94.

5. Steinfort DP, Kranz S, Dowers A, et al. Sensitive molecular testing methods can demonstrate NSCLC driver mutations in malignant pleural effusion despite non-malignant cytology. Transl Lung Cancer Res 2019;8(4):513–8.

6. Pinto D, Schmitt F. Current applications of molecular testing on body cavity fluids. Diagn Cytopathol 2020;48(9):840–51.

7. Sahu S, Gupta P, Dey P. Molecular testing on serous effusion: An update. CytoJournal 2021;18:35.

8. Medenica M, Medenica M, Cosovic D. Pleural effusions in lung cancer: detection and treatment. In: Torres AFC, editor. Lung cancer - strategies for diagnosis and treatment. InTech; 2018.

9. Dermawan JKT, Policarpio-Nicolas ML. Malignancies in pleural, peritoneal, and pericardial effusions. Arch Pathol Lab Med 2020;144(9):1086–91.

10. Allan Z, Witts S, Tie J, et al. The prognostic impact of peritoneal tumour DNA in gastrointestinal and gynaecological malignancies: a systematic review. Br J Cancer 2023. https://doi.org/10.1038/s41416-023-02424-6.

11. Turner SA, Abou Shaar R, Yang Z. The basics of commonly used molecular techniques for diagnosis, and application of molecular testing in cytology. Diagn Cytopathol 2023;51(1):83–94.

12. Engels M, Michael C, Dobra K, et al. Management of cytological material, pre-analytical procedures and bio-banking in effusion cytopathology. Cytopathology 2019;30(1):31–8.

13. Michael CW, Davidson B. Pre-analytical issues in effusion cytology. Pleura Peritoneum 2016;1(1):45–56.

14. Guzman J, Arbogast S, Bross KJ, et al. Effect of storage time of pleural effusions on immunocytochemical cell surface analysis of tumor cells. Anal Quant Cytol Histol 1992;14(3):203–9.

15. Guzman J, Arbogast S, Bross KJ, et al. Effect of storage time on the analysis of lymphocyte subpopulations in pleural effusions. Acta Cytol 1993;37(3):267–71.

16. Manosca F, Schinstine M, Fetsch PA, et al. Diagnostic effects of prolonged storage on fresh effusion samples. Diagn Cytopathol 2007;35(1):6–11.

17. Chandra A, Crothers B, Kurtycz D, et al, editors. The international system for serous fluid cytopathology. Cham: Springer Nature Switzerland AG; 2020. https://doi.org/10.1007/978-3-030-53908-5.

18. Coconubo DM, Baskota SU, Li R, et al. Reassessing the optimal volume for malignancy detection in serous fluid cytology. Cancer Cytopathol 2022;130(7):551–7.

19. Rooper LM, Ali SZ, Olson MT. A specimen volume of ≥80 mL improves cytologic sensitivity for malignant ascites: a retrospective analysis of 2665 cases. J Am Soc Cytopathol 2016;5(5):301–5.

20. Rooper LM, Ali SZ, Olson MT. A minimum volume of more than 60 mL is necessary for adequate cytologic diagnosis of malignant pericardial effusions. Am J Clin Pathol 2016;145(1):101–6.

21. Shidham VB, Layfield LJ. Approach to diagnostic cytopathology of serous effusions. CytoJournal 2021;18:32.

22. Garcia LW, Ducatman BS, Wang HH. The value of multiple fluid specimens in the cytological diagnosis of malignancy. Mod Pathol 1994;7(6):665–8.

23. VandenBussche CJ, Crothers B, Chandra A, et al. The International system for reporting serous fluid cytopathology: The initial project survey. Cytopathology 2023;34(3):191–7.

24. Mikou P, Pergaris A, Engels M, et al. Review of the impact of the International System for Serous Fluid Cytopathology. Cytopathology 2023. https://doi.org/10.1111/cyt.13313.

25. Pinto D, Cruz E, Branco D, et al. Cytohistological Correlation in Pleural Effusions Based on the International System for Reporting Serous Fluid Cytopathology. Diagnostics 2021;11(6):1126.

26. Lobo C, Costa J, Petronilho S, et al. Cytohistological correlation in serous effusions using the newly proposed International System for Reporting Serous Fluid Cytopathology: Experience of an oncological center. Diagn Cytopathol 2021;49(5):596–605.

27. Zuna RE. Diagnostic cytopathology of peritoneal washings. CytoJournal 2022;19:9.

28. Gokozan HN, Harbhajanka A, Lyden S, et al. Root cause analysis of indeterminate diagnoses in serous fluids cytopathology. Diagn Cytopathol 2021;49(5):633–9.

29. Russell DK, Jain D. Cytopreparatory techniques. In: Chandra A, Crothers B, Kurtycz D, et al, editors. The international system for serous fluid cytopathology. Cham: Springer Nature Switzerland AG; 2020. p. 239–65. https://doi.org/10.1007/978-3-030-53908-5_10.

30. Lepus CM, Vivero M. Updates in effusion cytology. Surg Pathol Clin 2018;11(3):523–44.

31. Pantanowitz L, Chivukula M. Serous fluid: Metastatic sarcomas, melanoma, and other non-epithelial neoplasms. CytoJournal 2022;19:15.

32. Vemireddy LP, Jain N, Aqeel A, et al. Lung Adenocarcinoma Presenting as Malignant Pericardial Effusion/Tamponade. Cureus 2021;13(3):e13762.

33. Jhala N, Arriola A, Pantanowitz L. Serous cavity metastasis: Evaluation of unknown primary. CytoJournal 2022;19:16.

34. Gabali A. Serous fluids and hematolymphoid disorders. CytoJournal 2022;19:17.

35. Gabali A. Flow cytometry, molecular analysis, and other special techniques (in Serous Fluid Cytopathology). CytoJournal 2022;19:18.

36. Dutta R, Nambirajan A, Mittal S, et al. Cytomorphology of primary pulmonary NUT carcinoma in different cytology preparations. Cancer Cytopathology 2021;129(1):53–61.

37. Sundling KE, Cibas ES. Ancillary studies in pleural, pericardial, and peritoneal effusion cytology. Cancer Cytopathol 2018;126(Suppl 8):590–8.

38. Shen Y, Pang C, Shen K, et al. Diagnostic value of thyroid transcription factor-1 for pleural or other serous metastases of pulmonary adenocarcinoma: a meta-analysis. Sci Rep 2016;6:19785.

39. Baskota SU, Qazi D, Chandra A, et al. Comprehensive review of metastatic breast carcinoma in cytology specimens. J Mol Pathol 2022;3(4):293–306.

40. Bradt A, Jing X, Smola BS, et al. Comparative expression of TRPS1, GATA3, SOX10, mammaglobin, and GCDFP-15 in effusion specimens with breast carcinoma. Diagn Cytopathol 2023;51(11):665–73.

41. Li D, Wang D, Long H, et al. Diagnostic accuracy of calretinin for malignant mesothelioma in serous effusions: a meta-analysis. Sci Rep 2015;5:9507.

42. Lin W, Liu X, Cen Y. Diagnostic accuracy of epithelial membrane antigen for malignant effusions: a meta-analysis. Int J Biol Markers 2016;31(1):e11–6.

43. Kanber Y, Pusztaszeri M, Auger M. Immunocytochemistry for diagnostic cytopathology-A practical guide. Cytopathology 2021;32(5):562–87.

44. Mosele MF, Westphalen CB, Stenzinger A, et al. Recommendations for the use of next-generation sequencing (NGS) for patients with advanced cancer in 2024: a report from the ESMO Precision Medicine Working Group. Annals of Oncology 2024;0(0). https://doi.org/10.1016/j.annonc.2024.04.005.

45. Crimini E, Repetto M, Aftimos P, et al. Precision medicine in breast cancer: From clinical trials to clinical practice. Cancer Treat Rev 2021;98:102223.

46. Tan AC, Bagley SJ, Wen PY, et al. Systematic review of combinations of targeted or immunotherapy in advanced solid tumors. J Immunother Cancer 2021;9(7):e002459.

47. Layfield LJ, Zhang T, Esebua M. PD-L1 immunohistochemical testing: A review with reference to cytology specimens. Diagn Cytopathol 2023;51(1):51–8.

48. Satturwar S, Girolami I, Munari E, et al. Program death ligand-1 immunocytochemistry in lung cancer cytological samples: A systematic review. Diagn Cytopathol 2022;50(6):313–23.

49. Song Z, Cheng G, Zhang Y. PD-L1 expression in malignant pleural effusion samples and its correlation with oncogene mutations in non-small cell lung cancer. J Thorac Dis 2020;12(4):1385–92.

50. Hagmeyer L, Schäfer S, Engels M, et al. High sensitivity of PD-L1 analysis from pleural effusion in nonsmall cell lung cancer. ERJ Open Res 2021;7(1):00787–2020.

51. Mansour MSI, Seidal T, Mager U, et al. Higher concordance of PD-L1 expression between biopsies and effusions in epithelioid than in nonepithelioid pleural mesothelioma. Cancer Cytopathol 2021;129(6):468–78.

52. Mansour MSI, Huseinzade A, Seidal T, et al. Comparison of immunohistochemical mesothelial biomarkers in paired biopsies and effusion cytology cell blocks from pleural mesothelioma. Cytopathology 2023. https://doi.org/10.1111/cyt.13265.

53. Lindeman NI, Cagle PT, Aisner DL, et al. Updated Molecular Testing Guideline for the Selection of Lung Cancer Patients for Treatment With Targeted Tyrosine Kinase Inhibitors: Guideline From the College of American Pathologists, the International Association for the Study of Lung Cancer, and the Association for Molecular Pathology. J Thorac Oncol 2018;13(3):323–58.

54. Roy-Chowdhuri S, Dacic S, Ghofrani M, et al. Collection and Handling of Thoracic Small Biopsy and Cytology Specimens for Ancillary Studies: Guideline From the College of American Pathologists in Collaboration With the American College of Chest Physicians, Association for Molecular Pathology, American Society of Cytopathology, American Thoracic Society, Pulmonary Pathology Society, Papanicolaou Society of Cytopathology, Society of Interventional Radiology, and Society of Thoracic Radiology. Arch Pathol Lab Med 2020. https://doi.org/10.5858/arpa.2020-0119-CP.

55. Huang M, Wei S. Overview of molecular testing of cytology specimens. Acta Cytol 2020;64(1–2):136–46.

56. Zhou W, Geiersbach K, Chadwick B. Rapid removal of cytology slide coverslips for DNA and

RNA isolation. J Am Soc Cytopathol 2017;6(1):24–7.

57. Pisapia P, Pepe F, Sgariglia R, et al. Next generation sequencing in cytology. Cytopathology 2021;32(5):588–95.

58. Penault-Llorca F, Kerr KM, Garrido P, et al. Expert opinion on NSCLC small specimen biomarker testing — Part 1: Tissue collection and management. Virchows Arch 2022. https://doi.org/10.1007/s00428-022-03343-2.

59. Souza Da Silva R, Schmitt F. Optimal assessment of metastatic breast carcinoma: the value of cytopathology combined with molecular analysis. JMP 2022;3(4):329–38.

60. Brims F. Epidemiology and clinical aspects of malignant pleural mesothelioma. Cancers 2021;13(16).

61. Churg A, Nabeshima K, Ali G, et al. Highlights of the 14th international mesothelioma interest group meeting: Pathologic separation of benign from malignant mesothelial proliferations and histologic/molecular analysis of malignant mesothelioma subtypes. Lung Cancer 2018;124:95–101.

62. Cw M. The cytologic diagnosis of mesothelioma: are we there yet? J Am Soc Cytopathol 2023;12(2).

63. Eccher A, Girolami I, Lucenteforte E, et al. Diagnostic mesothelioma biomarkers in effusion cytology. Cancer Cytopathol 2021;129(7):506–16.

64. Girolami I, Lucenteforte E, Eccher A, et al. Evidence-based diagnostic performance of novel biomarkers for the diagnosis of malignant mesothelioma in effusion cytology. Cancer Cytopathol 2022;130(2):96–109.

65. Chevrier M, Monaco SE, Jerome JA, et al. Testing for BAP1 loss and CDKN2A/p16 homozygous deletion improves the accurate diagnosis of mesothelial proliferations in effusion cytology. Cancer Cytopathol 2020;128(12):939–47.

66. Louw A, van Vliet C, Peverall J, et al. Analysis of early pleural fluid samples in patients with mesothelioma: A case series exploration of morphology, BAP1, and CDKN2A status with implications for the concept of mesothelioma in situ in cytology. Cancer Cytopathol 2022;130(5):352–62.

67. Gayen S. Malignant pleural effusion: presentation, diagnosis, and management. Am J Med 2022;135(10):1188–92.

68. Pacheco JM. Approach to stage IV non-small-cell lung cancer: how to select among first-line therapy options? Curr Opin Pulm Med 2020;26(4):311–20.

69. Na KJ, Kim YT. The "new" oligometastatic disease state and associated therapies in non-small cell lung cancer: A narrative review. J Surg Oncol 2023;127(2):282–7.

70. Pang C, Ma H, Qin J, et al. Pleural effusion as a substitute for tumor tissue in detecting EGFR/ALK mutations in non-small cell lung cancer: A systematic review and meta-analysis. Medicine (Baltim) 2019;98(18):e15450.

71. Man Ng JK, Chow C, Kin Chan RC, et al. EGFR testing in paraffin-embedded cell block cytology material is reliable with increased detection for effusion fluid. Lung Cancer 2022;174:97–103.

72. Dalvi SD, Chau K, Sajjan S, et al. Adequacy of pleural fluid cytology for comprehensive molecular analysis of lung adenocarcinoma: Experience of a large health-care system. CytoJournal 2022;19:7.

73. Konstantinovsky S, Smith Y, Zilber S, et al. Breast carcinoma cells in primary tumors and effusions have different gene array profiles. JAMA Oncol 2010;2010:969084.

74. Whitfield HJ, Berthelet J, Mangiola S, et al. Single-cell RNA sequencing captures patient-level heterogeneity and associated molecular phenotypes in breast cancer pleural effusions. Clin Transl Med 2023;13(9):e1356.

75. B S, R G, D S, et al. Combined detection of Her2/neu gene amplification and protein overexpression in effusions from patients with breast and ovarian cancer. J Cancer Res Clin Oncol 2010;136(9). https://doi.org/10.1007/s00432-010-0790-2.

76. K A, M O, K O, et al. Discordant HER2 status between primary breast carcinoma and recurrent/metastatic tumors using fluorescence in situ hybridization on cytological samples. Jpn J Clin Oncol 2013;43(1). https://doi.org/10.1093/jjco/hys187.

77. Razavi P, Chang MT, Xu G, et al. The genomic landscape of endocrine-resistant advanced breast cancers. Cancer Cell 2018;34(3):427–38.e6.

78. Han MY, Borazanci EH. Malignant ascites in pancreatic cancer: Pathophysiology, diagnosis, molecular characterization, and therapeutic strategies. Front Oncol 2023;13:1138759.

79. Sánchez-Hidalgo JM, Rodríguez-Ortiz L, Arjona-Sánchez Á, et al. Colorectal peritoneal metastases: Optimal management review. World J Gastroenterol 2019;25(27):3484–502.

80. Taffon C, Giovannoni I, Mozetic P, et al. Seriate cytology vs molecular analysis of peritoneal washing to improve gastric cancer cells detection. Diagn Cytopathol 2019;47(7):670–4.

81. Nozaki T, Sakamoto I, Kagami K, et al. Molecular analysis of ascitic fluid cytology reflects genetic changes of malignancies of the ovary equivalent to surgically resected specimens. Cancer Cytopathol 2022;130(8):640–9.

82. Tew WP, Lacchetti C, Ellis A, et al. PARP inhibitors in the management of ovarian cancer:

ASCO Guideline. J Clin Oncol 2020;38(30): 3468–93.

83. Gornjec A, Novakovic S, Stegel V, et al. Cytology material is equivalent to tumor tissue in determining mutations of BRCA 1/2 genes in patients with tubo-ovarian high grade serous carcinoma. BMC Cancer 2019;19(1):296.

84. Lou SK, Grenier S, Care M, et al. Validation of BRCA testing on cytologic samples of high-grade serous carcinoma. Cancer Cytopathol 2021; 129(11):907–13.

85. Bae GE, Kim SH, Choi MK, et al. Targeted sequencing of ascites and peritoneal washing fluid of patients with gastrointestinal cancers and their clinical applications and limitations. Front Oncol 2021;11:712754.

86. Liu X, Lu Y, Zhu G, et al. The diagnostic accuracy of pleural effusion and plasma samples versus tumour tissue for detection of EGFR mutation in patients with advanced non-small cell lung cancer: comparison of methodologies. J Clin Pathol 2013; 66(12):1065–9.

87. Liu D, Lu Y, Hu Z, et al. Malignant pleural effusion supernatants are substitutes for metastatic pleural tumor tissues in EGFR mutation test in patients with advanced lung adenocarcinoma. PLoS One 2014;9(2):e89946.

88. Husain H, Nykin D, Bui N, et al. Cell-Free DNA from ascites and pleural effusions: molecular insights into genomic aberrations and disease biology. Mol Cancer Therapeut 2017;16(5): 948–55.

89. Asaka S, Yoshizawa A, Saito K, et al. Rapid point-of-care testing for epidermal growth factor receptor gene mutations in patients with lung cancer using cell-free DNA from cytology specimen supernatants. Int J Oncol 2018;52(6): 2110–8.

90. Han AL, Kim HR, Choi KH, et al. Comparison of cobas EGFR Mutation Test v2 and PANAMutyper-R-EGFR for Detection and Semi-Quantification of Epidermal Growth Factor Receptor Mutations in Plasma and Pleural Effusion Supernatant. Ann Lab Med 2019;39(5):478–87.

91. Tong L, Ding N, Tong X, et al. Tumor-derived DNA from pleural effusion supernatant as a promising alternative to tumor tissue in genomic profiling of advanced lung cancer. Theranostics 2019;9(19): 5532–41.

92. Hummelink K, Muller M, Linders TC, et al. Cell-free DNA in the supernatant of pleural effusion can be used to detect driver and resistance mutations, and can guide tyrosine kinase inhibitor treatment decisions. ERJ Open Res 2019;5(1): 00016–2019.

93. Xiang C, Huo M, Ma S, et al. Molecular profiling for supernatants and matched cell pellets of pleural effusions in non-small-cell lung cancer. J Mol Diagn 2020;22(4):513–22.

94. Yang SR, Mooney KL, Libiran P, et al. Targeted deep sequencing of cell-free DNA in serous body cavity fluids with malignant, suspicious, and benign cytology. Cancer Cytopathol 2020;128(1):43–56.

95. Mayo-de-Las-Casas C, Velasco A, Sanchez D, et al. Yang. Int J Cancer 2020;147(1):277–84.

96. Leick KM, Kazarian AG, Rajput M, et al. Peritoneal cell-free tumor DNA as biomarker for peritoneal surface malignancies. Ann Surg Oncol 2020; 27(13):5065–71.

97. Chen X, Li K, Liu Z, et al. Multigene PCR using both cfDNA and cfRNA in the supernatant of pleural effusion achieves accurate and rapid detection of mutations and fusions of driver genes in patients with advanced NSCLC. Cancer Med 2021;10(7): 2286–92.

98. Mokánszki A, Bádon ES, Mónus A, et al. Cell-free DNA From Pleural Effusion Samples: Is It Right for Molecular Testing in Lung Adenocarcinoma? Pathol Oncol Res 2021;27:613071.

99. de Kock R, Knoops C, Baselmans M, et al. Sensitive cell-free tumor DNA analysis in supernatant pleural effusions supports therapy selection and disease monitoring of lung cancer patients. Cancer Treat Res Commun 2021;29:100449.

100. Suenaga M, Fujii T, Yamada S, et al. Peritoneal lavage tumor DNA as a novel biomarker for predicting peritoneal recurrence in pancreatic ductal adenocarcinoma. Ann Surg Oncol 2021;28(4): 2277–86.

101. Van't Erve I, Rovers KP, Constantinides A, et al. Detection of tumor-derived cell-free DNA from colorectal cancer peritoneal metastases in plasma and peritoneal fluid. J Pathol Clin Res 2021;7(3):203–8.

102. Ju HY, Ho JY, Kang J, et al. Whole-exome sequencing reveals clinical potential of circulating tumor DNA from peritoneal fluid and plasma in endometrial cancer. Cancers 2022; 14(10):2506.

103. Wu H, Ji H, Yang W, et al. Liquid biopsy using ascitic fluid and pleural effusion supernatants for genomic profiling in gastrointestinal and lung cancers. BMC Cancer 2022;22(1):1020.

104. Sadik H, Pritchard D, Keeling DM, et al. Impact of clinical practice gaps on the implementation of personalized medicine in advanced non-small-cell lung cancer. JCO Precis Oncol 2022;6: e2200246.

105. Kawahara A, Fukumitsu C, Azuma K, et al. A Combined test using both cell sediment and supernatant cell-free DNA in pleural effusion shows increased sensitivity in detecting activating EGFR mutation in lung cancer patients. Cytopathology 2018;29(2):150–5.

106. Song Z, Wang W, Li M, et al. Cytological-negative pleural effusion can be an alternative liquid biopsy media for detection of EGFR mutation in NSCLC patients. Lung Cancer 2019;136: 23–9.

107. Chiang CL, Shen CI, Huang HC, et al. Cytology-Based Specimen Triage for Epidermal Growth Factor Receptor Mutation Testing of Malignant Pleural Effusions in Non-Small Cell Lung Cancer. Front Oncol 2022;12:810124.

108. Mavropoulos A, Johnson C, Lu V, et al. Artificial intelligence-driven morphology-based enrichment of malignant cells from body fluid. Mod Pathol 2023;36(8):100195.

Soft Tissue Fine-Needle Aspiration
Current and Future Impact on Patient Care

Sigfred Lajara, MD[a], Vickie Y. Jo, MD[b],*

KEYWORDS

- Sarcoma • Soft tissue • FNA • Immunohistochemistry • FISH • Fusion gene

Key points

- Soft tissue cytology is diagnostically challenging, and a pattern-based approach is practical for guiding differentials and selection of ancillary tests.

- Many soft tissue tumors have characteristic immunophenotypes and molecular alterations that can be targeted by ancillary testing.

- Immunohistochemistry allows efficient workup of small biopsies, and available markers include lineage-specific markers and surrogate molecular markers that detect protein products of specific gene alterations.

- In most scenarioes, molecular testing serves to support a provisional diagnosis after morphologic evaluation and immunohistochemical workup, although next-generation sequencing platforms are gaining favor and have many applications in soft tissue pathology.

- The recurrent molecular alterations in soft tissue neoplasms include many potential therapeutic targets, and applications of "precision medicine" for the treatment of sarcomas are expected to expand in the coming years.

ABSTRACT

Soft tissue neoplasms pose many diagnostic challenges on fine-needle aspiration (FNA), owing largely to their rarity, large number of entities, and histologic diversity. Advances in ancillary testing now allow detection of the characteristic immunophenotypes and molecular alterations for many neoplasms and include reliable surrogate immunohistochemical markers for underlying molecular events that are highly efficient in small biopsies. A morphology-based framework is recommended to guide appropriate differentials and judicious selection of ancillary tests for small biopsies. The accurate diagnosis of soft tissue tumors is crucial for patient management and prognostication, with many potential implications in this era of precision medicine.

OVERVIEW

There are numerous challenges in the cytologic diagnosis of soft tissue tumors, which are rare but histologically diverse, and are increasingly encountered in all practice settings with the rise of minimally invasive biopsy procedures. There are unique challenges and considerations for fine-needle aspiration (FNA) of soft tissue lesions, such as frequent overlap of morphologic features, limited ability to evaluate architectural clues, and the requirement of specimen triage for ancillary testing. However, definitive cytologic diagnosis is now

[a] Department of Pathology, UPMC Shadyside Hospital, Cancer Pavilion, Suite 201, 5150 Centre Avenue, Pittsburgh, PA 15232, USA; [b] Brigham and Women's Hospital, Harvard Medical School, 75 Francis Street, Boston, MA 02115, USA
* Corresponding author.
E-mail address: vjo@bwh.harvard.edu

Surgical Pathology 17 (2024) 483–507
https://doi.org/10.1016/j.path.2024.04.009
1875-9181/24/© 2024 Elsevier Inc. All rights reserved.

surgpath.theclinics.com

possible for many soft tissue neoplasms with our ability to detect their specific immunophenotypes and defining molecular alterations. A recent large meta-analysis has shown that FNA has high sensitivity and specificity for bone and soft tissue tumors, supporting it as a viable option for the initial workup of patients.[1] According to the National Comprehensive Cancer Network (NCCN) guidelines, biopsies of soft tissue lesions should provide information regarding malignancy, and if possible, a specific diagnosis and grade.[2] Accurate classification of soft tissue tumors on FNA is crucial for appropriate patient management, and even when definitive classification is not possible it is still informative to convey information regarding biologic behavior.

Molecular techniques have expanded since conventional karyotyping and include fluorescent in situ hybridization (FISH), reverse transcriptase–polymerase chain reaction (RT-PCR), and more recently next-generation sequencing (NGS; ie, massively parallel sequencing) platforms. Immunohistochemistry has also evolved and there are now many reliable biomarkers that act as surrogates for the detection of protein products of specific molecular alterations, in conjunction with traditional lineage-specific markers used to determine line of differentiation. Formalin-fixed, paraffin-embedded cell blocks are the favored substrate for immunohistochemistry and molecular testing, although cytologic preparations have proven to provide adequate material for NGS.[3]

Practically, FNAs of soft tissue lesions should be approached first by morphologic assessment (ideally both air-dried and alcohol-fixed smears) to generate a differential diagnosis, followed by immunohistochemical panels to refine the differential and selection of relevant molecular testing to support a provisional diagnosis based on the workup. In most scenarios, "rule in" methods of FISH (or RT-PCR) can be used to support the immunohistochemical workup. NGS platforms such as fusion panels are efficient in the workup sarcomas, however, currently routinely used primarily at tertiary referral centers.[4–7]

This review aims to provide a practical guide for the FNA diagnosis of common soft tissue tumors and differentials within a morphology-based framework, with emphases on clinical correlations and updates in ancillary testing. Most soft tissue lesions fall into one of the following 6 morphologic patterns: adipocytic, myxoid, spindle, round cell, epithelioid, and pleomorphic (though many entities can show overlapping patterns). We will also briefly discuss current and emerging precision medicine treatment paradigms, which underscore the clinical impact of accurate classification.

ADIPOCYTIC TUMORS

This group of lesions showing prominent fatty components, including mature white fat, lipoblasts, and brown fat; many have characteristic immunohistochemical and molecular features (Table 1).

Benign lipomas are common and most are easily recognized by their composition of mature white fat; most are superficial and small (<5 cm). Large tumors and tumors arising in unusual locations must be distinguished from atypical lipomatous tumor/well-differentiated liposarcoma (ALT/WDL). The recognition of ALT/WDL is especially important given its associated risks for recurrence and progression to dedifferentiated liposarcoma (DDLPS). Most cases of ALT/WDL arise in the retroperitoneum, but they also present in the deep tissues of the extremities, mediastinum, and other visceral sites. The diagnostic atypical stromal cells and variation in adipocyte size may not be well visualized or sampled, and cases may appear deceptively bland and mimic lipoma or fat necrosis. The enlarged hyperchromatic nuclei of tumor cells are seen in between adipocytes or within collagenous stroma[8–11] (Fig. 1A). ALT/WDL and DDLPS are characterized by amplification of chromosome 12q13-15. This region includes the MDM2 and CDK4 gene loci, and immunohistochemistry for MDM2 and CDK4 shows corresponding nuclear staining in ALT/WDL.[12] Inconclusive immunohistochemical results can be resolved by the more sensitive method of FISH to detect MDM2 amplification (Fig. 1B), which can be useful when there is prominent fat necrosis as histiocytes can show weak MDM2 staining. ALT/WDL should be considered for any adipocytic FNA from large tumors (>10.0 cm), deeply situated lesions, tumors in the retroperitoneum or viscera, or adipocytic tumors with atypical spindle cells. FNA of DDLPS may show associated ALT/WDL (and when present is a useful diagnostic clue); however, the component of malignant transformation typically shows nonlipogenic morphology and nearly any morphologic pattern (most often pleomorphic).

Hibernomas are rarer benign tumors that show brown fat differentiation; most arise in the subcutis of the extremities. Tumors show varying proportions of brown fat (adipocytes with small cytoplasmic vacuoles, sometimes appearing granular) and mature adipocytes, with rich capillaries.[13] While recognition of brown fat cells is usually straightforward, hibernomalike components can be seen in some liposarcomas. Testing for MDM2 amplification and DDIT3 rearrangement is

Table 1
Differential diagnosis: adipocytic and myxoid neoplasms and their diagnostic immunohistochemical and molecular features

Tumor Type	Immunohistochemistry	Molecular Features
Adipocytic Tumors		
Spindle cell/pleomorphic lipoma	CD34, Rb loss	13q deletions
Myxoid liposarcoma	DDIT3	*FUS::DDIT3* (majority) Rare *EWSR1::DDIT3*
ALT/WDL and DDLPS	MDM2, CDK4	*MDM2* amplification
ASCLT/APLT	CD34, variable desmin and S-100, Rb loss	13q deletions
Myxoid Tumors		
Intramuscular myxoma	CD34 variable, EMA rare	*GNAS* mutations
Soft tissue perineurioma	CD34, EMA, claudin-1	-
Low-grade fibromyxoid sarcoma	MUC4	*FUS::CREB3L2* (90%)
Myoepithelial neoplasms of soft tissue	Keratin, EMA, S-100, SOX10, p63 (50%)	*EWSR1* rearrangements
Extraskeletal myxoid chondrosarcoma	INSM1, S-100 (50%)	*EWSR1::NR4A3* *TAF15::NR4A3*
Ossifying fibromyxoid tumor	Variable S-100 desmin	*PHF1* fusions
DDLPS	MDM2, CDK4	*MDM2* amplification

Abbreviations: ALT, atypical lipomatous tumor; APLT, atypical pleomorphic lipomatous tumor; ASCLT, atypical spindle cell lipomatous tumor; DDLPS, dedifferentiated liposarcoma; WDL, well-differentiated liposarcoma.

useful in excluding ALT/WDL/DDLPS and myxoid liposarcoma, respectively.

Pleomorphic liposarcoma is the rarest liposarcoma subtype; most cases arise as deep-seated masses in the limbs. The presence of pleomorphic lipoblasts, often enlarged, is the sole diagnostic feature; however, recognition can be challenging depending on sampling as the high-grade spindle and pleomorphic component may predominate and myxoid stroma may be present.[14,15] These tumors lack specific immunohistochemical and molecular features; they should be tested for *MDM2* amplification to exclude examples of DDLPS with "homologous" lipoblastic differentiation.[16]

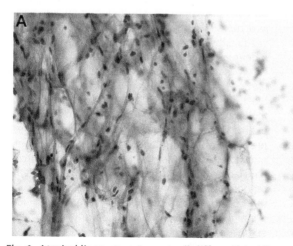
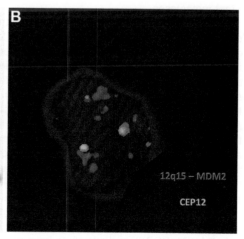

Fig. 1. Atypical lipomatous tumor/well-differentiated liposarcoma. (*A*) Tissue fragments show variation in adipocyte size and atypical tumor cells with enlarged hyperchromatic nuclei (Papanicolaou stain). (*B*) FISH analysis shows high-level amplification of *MDM2*.

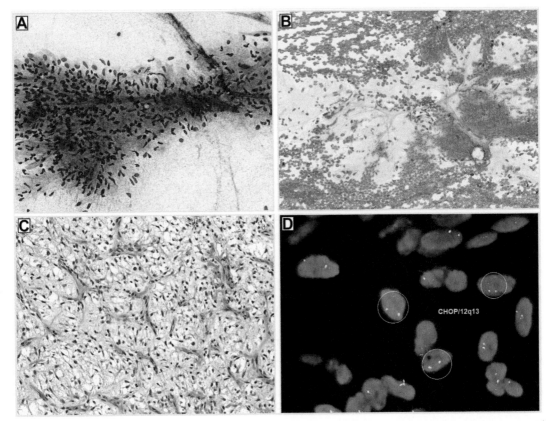

Fig. 2. Myxoid liposarcoma. (*A*) Uniform ovoid and spindle cells embedded in myxoid stromal fragments, with scattered "signet-ring"-like lipoblasts (Romanowsky stain). (*B*) Myxoid stroma with the characteristic delicate branching vessel pattern (Papanicolaou stain). (*C*) The core needle biopsy demonstrates the rich capillary network, monotonous tumors cells, and lipoblasts within an abundant myxoid stroma. (*D*) *DDIT3* (*CHOP*) rearrangement is confirmed on FISH (*nuclei circled*). (*Courtesy of* Dale W. Lewis.)

Pleomorphic liposarcoma is more aggressive, with local recurrence and metastatic rates up to 50%; in contrast, DDLPS shows local recurrence rates of approximately 40% and a 15% to 20% risk of distant metastases.

Myxoid liposarcoma commonly arises in the deep soft tissues of limbs of young and middle-aged adults. Aspirates show characteristic features of myxoid stroma, delicate branching capillaries; the presence of small univacuolated or bivacuolated lipoblasts is variable (**Fig. 2**).[17] The uniform spindle, ovoid, and round tumor cells are quite uniform. Tumors can appear hypocellular at the low-end of the spectrum with a predominance of myxoid stroma, while high-grade myxoid liposarcoma is cellular and often enters the differential of round cell sarcomas. Some examples may resemble spindle cell lipoma, while others may show overlapping features with DDLPS. Myxoid liposarcoma harbors *FUS::DDIT3* fusion (or rarely *EWSR1::DDIT3*), and surrogate immunohistochemistry for DDIT3 is highly sensitive and specific for the diagnosis.[18,19]

Spindle cell lipoma typically presented as superficial lesions in the posterior neck, back, and shoulder in adult men. These benign tumors show prominent myxoid stroma, with varying proportions of mature fat, short stubby spindle cells, and ropey collagen fibers; there is no significant vascularity.[20] Floret-like multinucleated cells are a feature of the variant pleomorphic lipoma.[21] CD34 is diffusely positive. Spindle cell lipomas harbor 13q14 deletions, which includes the retinoblastoma locus and corresponds with immunohistochemical loss of nuclear retinoblastoma (Rb) expression,[22] although this can be difficult to interpret in cell blocks. Spindle cell lipoma can mimic myxoid liposarcoma, but the latter has branching capillaries, frequent lipoblasts, and *DDIT3* rearrangement. The spindle cell component may raise the possibility of ALT/WDL; however, the clinical presentations of these 2 entities are distinct and spindle cell lipoma lacks atypia and is negative for MDM2/CDK4. Morphologically similar tumors located in the extremities and showing appreciable nuclear atypia represent atypical spindle cell lipomatous tumor/atypical pleomorphic lipo-matous tumor (ASCLT/APLT),[23] which are charac-terized by larger 13q alterations and Rb loss.[24–26] The distinction is not crucial on biopsy as ASCLT/APLT has only a low risk of local recur-rence (~ 12%) and does not metastasize or dedif-ferentiate; however, most cases should be tested for MDM2 and CDK4 to exclude ALT/WDL.

MYXOID TUMORS

A wide spectrum of tumor types show prominent extracellular myxoid matrix on cytologic prepara-tions, on which assessment of their characteristic histologic features is not possible. Assessment of cellularity and degree of atypia and pleomorphism is a useful first step in generating differentials, as most myxoid FNAs fall into 3 morphologic groups: hypocellular and bland; morphologically malignant (overlapping with the differential of pleomorphic sarcomas); and cellular, cytomorphologically monotonous. Myxoid lesions with prominent adi-pocytic components (spindle cell lipoma and myx-oid liposarcoma) were previously discussed. Ancillary testing is helpful for in many cases (see **Table 1**).

Myxoid smears that are hypocellular with bland or minimally atypical lesional cells are frequently benign. Definitive classification may not be possible on FNA and the primary goal is to exclude low-grade sarcomas, after which a descriptive diagnosis of "benign myxoid spindle cell neoplasm" is appropriate. The most common diagnostic considerations in the limbs are intra-muscular myxoma, soft tissue perineurioma, and low-grade fibromyxoid sarcoma (LGFMS; **Fig. 3**). Smears from these entities show significant morphologic overlap, with abundant myxoid stroma and scattered bland spindle and stellate cells having scant to moderate cytoplasm, some with bipolar processes.[27–30] Entrapped normal multinucleated skeletal muscle fibers may be sampled in intramuscular myxoma, and some ex-amples of are cellular with increased stromal collagen (see **Fig. 3A**). Immunohistochemistry is often not helpful as cell blocks tend to be paucicel-lular and all three can show EMA positivity; CD34 and claudin-1 are variably positive in perineurioma and also challenging on cell blocks.[29] Intramus-cular myxoma harbors GNAS1 mutations, although molecular testing is not practical or necessary on biopsies.

The hypocellular smears of LGFMS appear deceptively bland, as the uniform plump ovoid and spindle tumor cells show at most mild nuclear atypia and pleomorphism[28,30] (see **Fig. 3B**). Some cases have more collagenous stroma and more

rarely nuclear palisading around acellular collagen. Gene expression profiling studies led to the identi-fication of MUC4 as a highly sensitive and specific immunohistochemical marker for LGFMS.[31] Inclu-sion of MUC4 is recommended in nearly all in-stances of a bland, hypocellular myxoid lesion; benign entities in the differential are consistently negative.[29] LGFMS harbors FUS::CREB3L2 (or rarely FUS::CREB3L1 or EWSR1::CREB3L1), although molecular testing (typically FUS FISH) is usually not needed given the reliability of MUC4.

For myxoid lesions with appreciable atypia and pleomorphism, the diagnosis of myxofibrosar-coma must be considered. Myxofibrosarcoma is one of the most common sarcomas, typically pre-senting in the superficial tissues of the limbs of older adults. Tumors have no specific immuno-phenotype or molecular features. Its diagnosis is based on the characteristic features of myxoid stroma and curvilinear collagenized vessels, and in many scenarios deferred to surgical resection. Myxofibrosarcoma shows a wide range of histo-logic grades based on cellularity, and the amount of myxoid stroma is often inversely related to grade.[32,33] Low-grade myxofibrosarcoma is hypo-cellular but is rarely mistaken as benign due to the presence of pleomorphic spindled and stellate tu-mor cells with atypical hyperchromatic nuclei. High-grade myxofibrosarcoma shows high cellu-larity and larger cohesive clusters, and the charac-teristic myxoid stroma and curvilinear vessels are less prominent. Histiocytes with cytoplasmic mucin may be present in myxofibrosarcoma and may mimic lipoblasts. The role of ancillary testing is primarily to exclude sarcomatoid carcinoma (with wide spectrum keratins) and other pleomor-phic sarcomas. MDM2 and CDK4 are also helpful since some examples of DDLPS can closely resemble myxofibrosarcoma. High grade myxofi-brosarcoma is discussed later in the pleomorphic differential.

Cellular myxoid aspirates with cytomorphologi-cally uniform tumor cell populations are commonly translocation-associated entities; these include myxoid liposarcoma (discussed previously), soft tissue myoepithelial neoplasms, extraskeletal myxoid chondrosarcoma (EMC), and ossifying fibromyxoid tumor (OFMT). Ancillary studies are helpful in this differential, which also includes car-cinoma and melanoma.

The family of myoepithelial tumors of soft tissue includes benign entities (myoepithelioma and benign mixed tumor) and myoepithelioma carci-noma of soft tissue and can arise across a wide anatomic range in patients of all ages. Myoepithe-lial neoplasms are well-known for their character-istic architectural and cytologic heterogeneity,

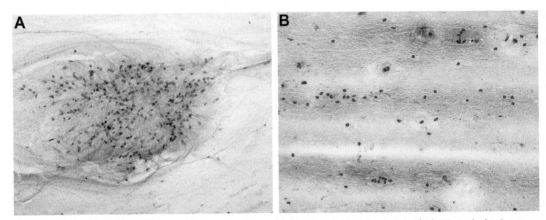

Fig. 3. The differential diagnosis of hypocellular myxoid lesions with bland cytomorphologic includes intramuscular (cellular) myxoma (*A;* Papanicolaou stain) and low-grade fibromyxoid sarcoma (LGFMS) (*B;* Romanowsky stain). Most scenarios require MUC4 immunohistochemistry, a highly sensitive and specific marker for LGFMS.

which accounts for the wide spectrum of cytomorphologic appearances. Chondromyxoid stroma is a consistent feature. The tumor cells appear variably epithelioid, spindled, and plasmacytoid and can also show clear cell and rhabdoid morphologies.[34–37] The tumor cells are singly dispersed and in clusters, often embedded in the stroma. Ductal structures are the diagnostic feature of benign mixed tumor, which are identical to pleomorphic adenoma of the salivary gland and similarly harbor *PLAG1* rearrangement.[38] Myoepithelial carcinoma is defined by cytologic atypia, and a predominant round cell morphology occurs in a subset (particularly pediatric tumors). Myoepithelial cells usually show positivity for a combination of keratins/EMA and S-100, SOX-10, and GFAP. Variable staining is seen for p63 and SMA. *EWSR1* arrangements occur in at least half of all myoepithelial neoplasms, involving a large spectrum of partner genes.[39] *EWSR1* FISH may be helpful, though rare cases have alternate *FUS* fusions or *SMARCB1* deletions,[40,41] the latter corresponding with immunohistochemical loss of SMARCB1.

Both EMC and OFMT show overlapping features with myoepithelial neoplasms. These rare entities typically arise in the limbs of adults. EMC is composed of epithelioid and spindle cells admixed with an abundant fibrillary metachromatic chondromyxoid stroma[42,43] (**Fig. 4**). Tumor cells frequently show nuclear grooves and wispy cytoplasmic extensions that may link to one another in a reticular fashion. While some tumor cells may appear situated in lacunae within stroma, it should be emphasized that EMC is a tumor of uncertain differentiation and shows no true cartilaginous differentiation. EMC is often positive for INSM1; S-100 staining is infrequent, and

keratins and EMA are negative. EMC harbors recurrent *NR4A3* fusions, and *NR4A3* FISH is recommended for confirming the diagnosis, which is more specific than *EWSR1* FISH. Smears of OFMT also show uniform epithelioid cells arranged singly or in clusters and cords in association with a fibromyxoid stroma.[44,45] The characteristic peripheral shell of bone is unlikely to be sampled by FNA. S-100 and Desmin are variably positive (70% and 50%, respectively) while keratins, EMA, SOX10, and S-100 are largely negative. OFMT is associated with frequent *PHF1* fusions[46]; rare cases harbor *BCOR* alterations and are positive for BCOR and pan-TRK.[47,48]

SPINDLE CELL TUMORS

A practical approach for spindle cell FNAs is to first determine whether the lesion appears morphologically low grade or high grade. In many scenarios, benign tumors and sarcomas can be easily separated. Some soft tissue neoplasms are understood to have intermediate biologic potential (either locally aggressive or rarely metastasizing) and can morphologically overlap with both benign and malignant tumors; these include gastrointestinal stromal tumor (GIST), desmoid fibromatosis, inflammatory myofibroblastic tumor (IMT), and solitary fibrous tumor (SFT). Thus, ancillary testing and clinical correlations are essential (**Table 2**). When definitive diagnosis is not possible, descriptive cytologic diagnoses conveying grade (ie, "low-grade spindle cell neoplasm," "atypical spindle cell neoplasm," or "malignant spindle cell neoplasm") are appropriate.

Low-grade spindle cell lesions show uniform spindle cells with mild or no atypia and lack necrosis and significant mitotic activity. Lesional cells are

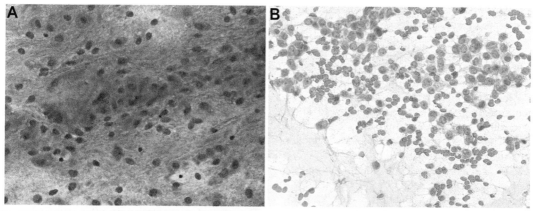

Fig. 4. Extraskeletal myxoid chondrosarcoma. Tumors show abundant fibrillary chondromyxoid stroma and monotonous ovoid and epithelioid cells with uniform nuclei and variable amounts of wispy cytoplasm (*A*, Romanowsky stain; *B*, Papanicolaou stain).

usually clustered in groups and sheets, often with clean backgrounds. Common benign tumors in this differential are schwannoma and leiomyoma. Schwannomas show jigsaw-puzzle-like fragments of syncytial spindle cells with oval and buckled tapering nuclei and wispy and fibrillary cytoplasm.[49,50] Diagnostic pitfalls include schwannomas with degenerative hyperchromatic (but smudgy) nuclear changes and the solidly cellular fascicles of cellular schwannoma. SOX-10 and S-100 are diffusely positive, a feature that distinguishes schwannoma from malignant peripheral

Table 2
Differential diagnosis: immunohistochemical and molecular features of spindle cell neoplasms

Tumor Type	Immunohistochemical Features	Molecular Features
Benign		
Schwannoma	S-100, SOX10	N/A
Leiomyoma	SMA, desmin, Caldesmon	N/A
Nodular fasciitis	SMA	*USP6::MYH9*
Intermediate Biologic Potential		
Gastrointestinal stromal tumor	KIT and DOG1	*KIT* mutations
Desmoid fibromatosis	β-catenin (80%), SMA variable	*CTNNB1* or *APC* mutations
Inflammatory myofibroblastic tumor	SMA, ALK (50%)	*ALK* rearrangements (50%)
Solitary fibrous tumor	STAT6, CD34	*NAB2::STAT6*
Dermatofibrosarcoma protuberans	CD34	*COL1A1::PDGFB*
Malignant		
Synovial sarcoma	SS18:SSX, SSX	*SS18::SSX*
MPNST	Rare S-100, SOX10, GFAP; H3K27me3 loss	*EED1* and *SUZ12* mutations
Spindle cell rhabdomyosarcoma	Desmin, MyoD1	*MyoD1* mutations
Leiomyosarcoma	SMA, desmin, caldesmon	N/A
DDLPS	MDM2, CDK4	*MDM2* amplification

Abbreviations: DDLPS, dedifferentiated liposarcoma; MPNST, malignant peripheral nerve sheath tumor.

nerve sheath tumor (MPNST), which is typically negative for these markers. Schwannomas can arise in any site and sometimes clinically mistaken as enlarged lymph nodes. In biopsies from the gastrointestinal tract, schwannoma must be distinguished from leiomyoma and GIST. Leiomyomas yield fascicular fragments of bland spindle cells often arranged parallel to one another.[51] Tumors are positive for SMA, desmin, and caldesmon; they are negative for β-catenin enabling distinction from desmoid fibromatosis.

GISTs are associated with variable behavior; over half arise in the stomach. Most GISTs are sporadic and arise in adulthood. Cytologic samples show uniform spindle cells arranged in clusters and singly dispersed, sometimes with stripped nuclei in the background; some cases show a mixed (or predominant) epithelioid morphology.[52,53] The uniform nuclei are ovoid or tapered, lacking atypia and pleomorphism, and the cytoplasm is often wispy with bipolar extensions. Most (95%) GISTs show diffuse and strong KIT immunoreactivity; however, KIT can be negative in cell blocks prepared from methanol-based fixative (such as CytoLyt). DOG1 is more sensitive and specific and identifies KIT-negative GISTs and is not affected by the cytology specimen processing method.[54,55] Most GISTs have activating KIT mutations; a small subset harbor PDGFRA mutations, and rarer alterations include NF1, BRAF, and KRAS mutations. KIT mutation status is an important prognostic and predictive factor (see later discussion). Among KIT-wild-type GISTS, it is important to recognize SDH-deficient GISTs (see Epithelioid Tumors).

Desmoid fibromatosis is a myofibroblastic neoplasm with a tendency for local recurrence but does not metastasize. Tumors are more common in women and can arise in the extremities, abdominopelvic cavity, and trunk, as well as the abdominal wall after pregnancy or cesarean section. Sporadic desmoids have CTNNB1 mutations, while tumors associated with familial adenomatous polyposis have APC mutations. Aspirates show long fascicular tissue fragments having collagenous stroma in which are embedded bland bipolar spindle cells.[56–58] Tumors are notoriously infiltrative and entrapped normal multinucleated skeletal muscle fibers can be sampled. SMA is frequently positive, and most (70%) show nuclear β-catenin expression.

Nodular fasciitis is a benign, self-limiting neoplasm, although smears can appear more cellular and heterogeneous (**Fig. 5**A–C). Tumors harbor USP6 rearrangements (most frequently partnered with MYH9).[59] Nodular fasciitis typically presents as a rapidly enlarging mass in subcutaneous soft tissues followed by spontaneous resolution. Most tumors are small (<2 cm), although the rapid growth may be concerning. Tumors sampled in the early proliferative phase show myxoid stromal fragments and appear increasingly collagenized with regression. There are numerous spindle, stellate, and polygonal myofibroblastic cells that are loosely clustered and singly dispersed, with bland ovoid nuclei and frequently wispy and tapering cytoplasmic ends.[60] A prominent chronic inflammatory infiltrate is seen. There may be mitotic activity; however, atypia and pleomorphism as absent, distinguishing lesions from IMT. The myofibroblasts are positive for SMA. The clinical presentation is often suggestive of the diagnosis, and the main goal is to exclude sarcoma to avoid mismanagement. Challenging cases can be resolved with USP6 FISH (**Fig. 5D**).

IMT is a myofibroblastic neoplasm that shows frequent local recurrence and a low risk of distant metastases. Tumors are most in children and young adults, frequently arising in the abdominal soft tissues. The cellular smears are composed of plump spindle cells that are singly dispersed and in loose clusters and aggregates.[61,62] There is a prominent infiltrate of lymphocytes and plasma cells, and myxoid matrix is common. Tumor cells have mild but appreciably atypical ovoid nuclei, small nucleoli, and tapering cytoplasm. IMT is frequently positive for SMA and occasionally positive for desmin and keratins. Half of all cases have ALK fusions involving a heterogeneous group of fusion partners and show resultant cytoplasmic ALK immunoreactivity.[63] Rare alternate fusions involve ROS1 and NTRK3. One pitfall is that the cytomorphologic mimic angiomatoid fibrous histiocytoma can show ALK positivity but lacks ALK rearrangement[64]; these tumors more likely arise in the limbs of young adults, are frequently positive for EMA, desmin, and CD99, and harbor EWSR1::-CREB1 fusions.

SFT arises in adults in a broad anatomic distribution and its biologic behavior is variable. The cellular smears are composed of cytologically uniform tumor cells having tapered and stubby nuclei with evenly distributed chromatin, smooth contours, and indistinct nucleoli.[65] The tumor cells are arranged in clusters and irregular fascicles, often in an anastomosing meshwork. Naked nuclei can be seen in the background, and distinction from low-grade spindle cell sarcomas can be difficult. SFT is positive for CD34 and STAT6.[66] Nuclear STAT6 is highly sensitive and specific for SFT, a surrogate for underlying NAB2::STAT6 fusion.[67,68] STAT6 is especially helpful in distinguishing SFT from dermatofibrosarcoma protuberans, which arise in the dermis of the trunk or

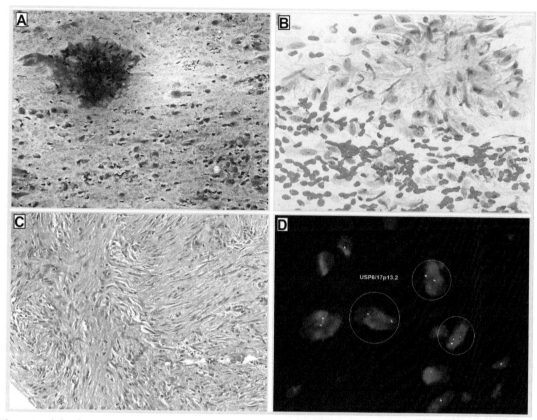

Fig. 5. Nodular fasciitis. (*A*) Dispersed spindle, stellate, and polygonal myofibroblastic cells and myxoid stromal fragments (Romanowsky stain). (*B*) The tumor cells have uniform round and ovoid nuclei with small or inconspicuous nucleoli and are loosely clustered within stroma (Papanicolaou stain). (*C*) Core needle biopsy shows tumor cells arranged in loose fascicular to vaguely storiform patterns within variably myxoid and collagenous stroma (H&E). (*D*) FISH confirms *USP6* rearrangement (*nuclei circled*). (*Courtesy of* Dale W. Lewis.)

limbs and may also show high-grade transformation. Tumors are also CD34 positive and carry *COL1A1::PDGFB*.

Most FNAs of spindle cell sarcomas can be recognized as malignant, although ancillary testing is often needed for classification. Aspirates are cellular with large cellular clusters and singly dispersed cells and nuclei, with malignant cells showing cytologic atypia, pleomorphism, and mitotic activity; necrosis is common. The workup should include MDM2/CDK4 for DDLPS (which can appear as a spindle cell sarcoma), melanocytic markers (Mart-1 and HMB-45) for spindle cell melanoma, and keratin for sarcomatoid carcinoma.

Synovial sarcoma is notable for its cytologic uniformity compared to other spindle cell sarcomas. Tumors most commonly arise in the limbs of young adults but are seen in almost any anatomic site. At low power, the smears have a distinctive appearance of alternating cellular clusters and dispersed single cells; transgressing vessels are common.[69–71]

The fusiform cells have uniform ovoid and round nuclei, with small or inconspicuous nuclei, and scant tapering cytoplasm (**Fig. 6**A). The tumor cell nuclei often spill off the edges of the cell clusters. Both monophasic (purely spindle cell) and biphasic synovial sarcomas show a predominant spindle cell appearance in cytologic samples; epithelial differentiation in biphasic synovial sarcoma is only infrequently evident by the presence of epithelial clusters and mucin. Synovial sarcoma harbors *SS18* rearrangements partnered with one of several *SSX* genes (*SSX1, SSX2,* or *SSX4*). Immunohistochemical surrogates for *SS18-SSX* fusion are available, and antibodies for *SS18-SSX* fusion protein and *SSX* C-terminus are highly sensitive, though the latter is slightly less specific[72,73] (**Fig. 6**B). These have largely replaced the conventional marker TLE1 which had low specificity and obviate the need for *SS18* FISH in many cases.

MPNST can arise sporadically or in the setting of neurofibromatosis type 1; tumors present in any site and some arise in association with

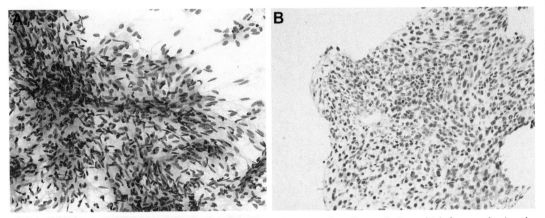

Fig. 6. (A) Synovial sarcoma is composed of a strikingly uniform spindle cell population which forms cohesive clusters, with tumor cells often spill off the edges to merge with singly dispersed in the background; delicate capillaries within clusters are common (Romanowsky stain). (B) Immunohistochemistry using an antibody targeting the SS18-SSX fusion protein shows strong nuclear staining.

neurofibroma or a peripheral nerve. The spindle cells have wavy, tapered, or hooked hyperchromatic nuclei and scant fibrillary stroma.[74,75] Low-grade tumors can appear cytologically uniform with mild atypia and resemble synovial sarcoma, but high-grade tumors show increased pleomorphism and necrosis. Immunohistochemistry can be challenging, as MPNST is frequently negative for S-100, SOX10, and GFAP, and positivity is only at most focal. Immunohistochemistry can detect loss of the trimethylation mark of histone H3 at lysine 27 (H3K27me3); H3K27me3 nuclear loss of expression reflects inactivation of the PRC2 complex secondary to mutations in *SUZ12* or *EED1*.[76] H3K27me3 loss occurs most frequently in high-grade MPNST but is often retained in many low- and intermediate-grade tumors.[77–79] High-grade MPNST with heterologous rhabdomyoblastic differentiation is positive for desmin, MyoD1, and myogenin; the differential then includes spindle cell rhabdomyosarcoma, which shows retained H3K27me3 and diffuse nuclear MyoD1 staining, correlating with frequent *MyoD1* mutations.[80]

Leiomyosarcoma usually arises in the retroperitoneum and deep tissues of the extremities. Apart from uterine tumors, many are associated with a large vessel. These show densely cellular fascicles with smoothly contoured edges; tumor cell nuclei are ovoid and rounded with blunt ends and have bipolar cytoplasmic extensions.[81] Immunohistochemistry is positive for smooth muscle markers SMA, desmin, and caldesmon. MDM2/CDK4 should be included for retroperitoneal tumors to exclude DDLPS with myogenic differentiation. Keratin staining occurs in a subset, a pitfall for sarcomatoid carcinoma.

ROUND CELL TUMORS

This group of "small round blue cell" sarcomas includes entities associated with specific clinical presentations, histologic features, and fusion genes, and definitive classification requires ancillary testing (**Table 3**). Several tumor types have specific and effective treatment regimens. While NGS fusion panels have high efficacy in this context, most cases can be efficiently worked up by immunohistochemistry and confirmatory FISH or RT-PCR. A panel approach is recommended for immunohistochemistry, and the inclusion of LCA, keratin, and S-100 allows identification of non-mesenchymal mimics (eg, lymphoma, neuroendocrine neoplasms, carcinoma, and melanoma). While many entities have characteristic immunophenotypes, there are also much overlap and many pitfalls, and an inclusive panel ultimately provides an informative context for interpreting molecular results.

Ewing sarcoma is the archetypal round cell sarcoma and harbors fusion genes involving a member of the FET family and a member of ETS family of transcription factors, most commonly *EWSR1::FLI1*. Rare fusion variants include *EWSR1::ERG* and fusions involving *FUS* in lieu of *EWSR1*. Ewing sarcoma typically arises as osseous tumors in patients younger than 20 years but can arise in extraosseous sites (especially in older individuals). The round cells have scant cytoplasm, usually with smooth nuclear contours and small or indistinct nucleoli[82] (**Fig. 7A–C**). A second population of smaller cells with hyperchromatic and angulated nuclei (considered to be degenerative features) is common. There may be glycogen-rich intracytoplasmic vacuoles or a tigroid

Table 3
Differential diagnosis: round cell sarcomas: immunohistochemical and molecular features

Tumor	Immunohistochemical Features	Molecular Features
Ewing sarcoma	CD99 (diffuse, membranous) NKX2.2	*EWSR1::FLI1* (majority) *EWSR1::ERG* (10%) *EWSR1::*ETS gene *FUS::*ETS gene
CIC-rearranged sarcoma	WT1, ETV4 CD99 variable	*CIC::DUX4* (majority) *CIC::NUTM1, CIC::FOXO4,* *CIC::LEUTX*
Sarcomas with *BCOR* alterations	BCOR SATB2, TLE1, Cyclin D1, Pan-TRK CD99 variable CCNB3 if *BCOR::CCNB3*	*BCOR::CCNB3* (majority) *BCOR* ITD
Alveolar rhabdomyosarcoma	FOXO1 Desmin, myogenin (diffuse), MyoD1	*PAX3::FOXO1A* (majority) *PAX7::FOXO1A*
Desmoplastic small round cell tumor	CD99 variable, keratin, desmin, NSE, WT1 (C-terminus antibody)	*EWSR1::WT1*
Poorly differentiated synovial sarcoma	SS18::SSX, SSX	*SS18::SSX*
High-grade myxoid liposarcoma	DDIT3	*FUS::DDIT3* Rare *EWSR1::DDIT3*
Myoepithelial carcinoma of soft tissue	Keratin, EMA, S-100, SOX10, p63 (50%)	*EWSR1* fusions (varied)

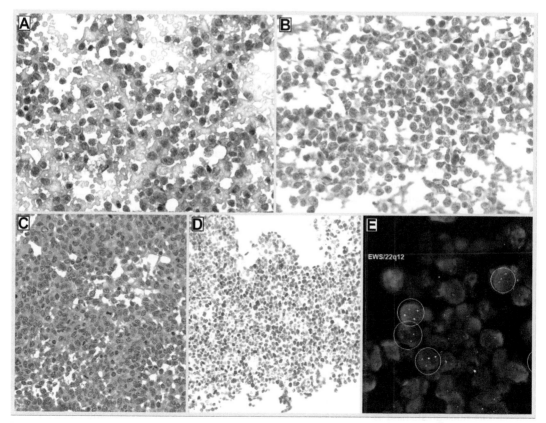

Fig. 7. Ewing sarcoma. Smears show a monotonous round cell population with clumped chromatin and occasional nucleoli; cytoplasm is sparse. Some tumor cells show degenerative changes with condensed chromatin (*A*, Romanowsky stain; *B*, Papanicolaou stain; *C*, H&E cell block). (*D*) Strong nuclear staining for NKX2.2 is a consistent feature. (*E*) *EWSR1* rearrangement is confirmed by FISH analysis (*nuclei circled*). (Photo courtesy of Dale W. Lewis.)

background of cytoplasmic fragments and naked nuclei. Immunohistochemistry for CD99 and NKX2.2 identifies most potential cases. Ewing sarcoma shows a characteristic diffuse membranous staining pattern for CD99; more variably staining patterns can be seen in many mimics, including CIC-rearranged sarcoma, sarcomas with BCOR alterations, and poorly differentiated synovial sarcoma. Nuclear NKX2.2 staining is highly sensitive for Ewing sarcoma, but specificity is more limited[83,84] (Fig. 7D). ERG is positive in rare cases with EWSR1::ERG. EWSR1 FISH is commonly used for confirmatory molecular testing (Fig. 7E); when available, fusion panels have the advantage of identifying the specific fusion partner, which is helpful in certain contexts since EWSR1 rearrangements are not unique to Ewing sarcoma.

CIC-rearranged sarcomas arise in deep soft tissue sites in patients of all ages. Before their recognition as a distinct entity, these tumors accounted for up to two-thirds of non-Ewing undifferentiated round cell sarcomas. While smears can largely resemble Ewing sarcoma, these tumors tend to show more cohesive groups, increased atypia and pleomorphism, prominent nucleoli, more cytoplasm, and spindled morphology[85,86] (Fig. 8A–C). Myxoid stroma and necrosis have been described, as well as rhabdoid and multinucleated forms. CD99 immunoreactivity ranges from negative to patchy (Fig. 8D). Most cases show dual positivity for WT1 and ETV4[87] and are negative for NKX2.2. DUX4 and NUTM1 immunohistochemistry are positive in cases with CIC::DUX4 and CIC::NUTM1, respectively. Approximately 95% of cases harbor CIC::DUX4 fusion which can be detected by FISH or sarcoma-specific NGS fusion panels.[88–90] CIC-rearranged sarcomas are aggressive, with significantly worse outcomes compared to Ewing sarcoma, and respond poorly to Ewing-specific regimens.[91]

Sarcomas with BCOR genetic alterations largely share the same cytomorphologic features with CIC-rearranged sarcoma but are rarer and often arise in bone. Two main groups are observed: sarcomas with BCOR-related fusions (most commonly BCOR::CCNB3) which arise in bones of young male individuals and tumors with BCOR internal tandem duplications (ITDs) of exon 15 which arise in the soft tissues of infants.[92–94] Spindle and rhabdoid cells, pseudopapillary structures, and vascular cores on smears have been described specifically in these tumors.[95] By immunohistochemistry, CD99 is positive in half of all cases. BCOR nuclear staining is consistent, but not specific. There is frequent positivity for cyclin B3, cyclin D1, TLE1, SATB2, Pan-Trk, which are also nonspecific but the constellation of positive

results helps identify potential cases.[48] Ultimately, molecular testing is necessary to detect BCOR fusion or ITD. Data indicate that BCOR::CCNB3 sarcomas behave similarly as Ewing sarcoma and show histologic responses to Ewing treatment regimens.[96]

Alveolar rhabdomyosarcoma harbors FOXO1 fusions, most commonly PAX3::FOXO1 and a smaller subset with PAX7::FOXO1, the latter associated with better prognosis. Tumor cells characteristically have enlarged, irregular and hyperchromatic nuclei with prominent nucleoli, and frequent binucleation, spindled cells, and rhabdomyoblasts.[97,98] Multinucleated giant cells with wreathlike arrangement of nuclei are helpful if present. Tumors show positivity for desmin and myoD1. Strong and diffuse nuclear staining for myogenin is characteristic and additionally helps distinguish alveolar rhabdomyosarcoma from embryonal rhabdomyosarcoma, which shows more heterogeneous staining.[99] This distinction is important because the prognosis of alveolar rhabdomyosarcoma is far worse. Immunohistochemistry for FOXO1 (using antibodies targeted at an epitope retained in the fusion oncoprotein) shows high sensitivity for alveolar rhabdomyosarcoma.[100] FOXO1 FISH can confirm the diagnosis of alveolar rhabdomyosarcoma.

Desmoplastic small round cell tumor (DSRCT) most commonly presents in teenage or young adult males as a large intra-abdominal mass. EWSR1::WT1 is the molecular hallmark. While DSRCT appears as a round cell neoplasm, the tumor cells are appreciably more cohesive, forming loosely sheets and tight clusters with angulated and molded nuclei; rosette-like structures may be present.[101,102] Desmoplastic stromal fragments, including fibroblastic foci, are seen. DSRCT shows a polyphenotypic immunophenotype, with positivity for keratin, EMA, NSE, and desmin; CD99 is often variable. Nuclear reactivity WT1 using antibodies targeting the carboxy terminus of WT1 is a surrogate for EWSR1::WT1; however, tumors are negative for the most widely used WT1 antibody against the amino terminus. EWSR1 FISH confirms the diagnosis, but should be interpreted in the context of clinical presentation, morphology, and immunohistochemical features; sequencing-based methods to identify EWSR1::ATF1 are most specific.

Cytopathologists should be aware of several entities that can show predominant round cell morphology and include relevant markers when necessary (see Table 3). As mentioned earlier, these include poorly differentiated synovial sarcoma (SS18-SSX and SSX immunohistochemistry or SS18 FISH), high-grade myxoid liposarcomas

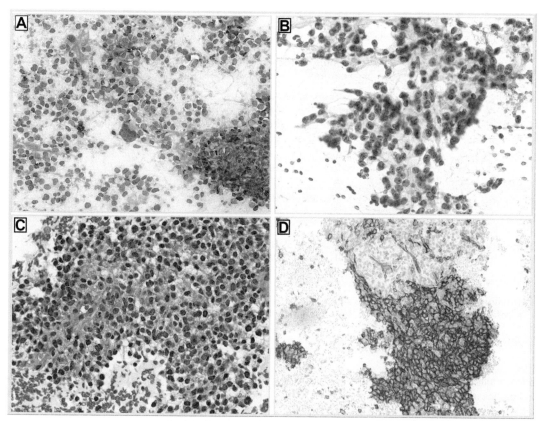

Fig. 8. *CIC*-rearranged sarcoma with *CIC::DUX4*. (*A*) The malignant round tumor cells show nuclear atypia and pleomorphism, with varying amounts of cytoplasm and fibrillary myxoid stroma (Romanowsky stain). (*B*) Tumor cell nuclei show nuclear contour irregularities prominent nucleoli (Papanicolaou stain). (*C*) The nuclear atypia and increased cytoplasm are evident on H&E cell blocks. (*D*) Heterogeneous CD99 immunoreactivity in tumor cells, ranging from negative to membranous.

(DDIT3 immunohistochemistry or *DDIT3* FISH), and myoepithelial carcinoma of soft tissue (keratins, EMA, SOX10, S-100, and GFAP; *EWSR1* FISH).

Last, many novel fusions are increasingly reported in small subsets of undifferentiated small round cell sarcomas. These include *EWSR1*-non-ETS fusions, such as *EWSR1/FUS::NFATC2* and *EWSR1::PATZ1*.[103] Current data are limited on the clinical significance of these molecularly defined but otherwise unclassified tumors. Practically, the workup of a round cell sarcoma should focus on identifying known entities with specific treatment and prognostic implications.

EPITHELIOID TUMORS

This morphologic pattern describes tumors having rounded cells with moderate-to-abundant cytoplasm, with centrally or eccentrically placed round nuclei. Most are sarcomas, but typically appear cytomorphologically uniform. In general, aspirates show an admixture of singly dispersed cells and cohesive sheets, appearing similar between entities despite their distinctive histologic appearances. Immunohistochemistry has a central role in the diagnostic workup (**Table 4**) and should also address the pitfalls of carcinoma and melanoma. Previously discussed cellular myxoid tumors may also enter this differential, particularly myoepithelial tumors of soft tissue.

Epithelioid sarcoma (ES) can show some variation in appearance depending on the subtype, but all cases have epithelioid tumor cells with large eccentric round nuclei and prominent nucleoli, with dense cytoplasm and distinct borders.[104,105] Cytoplasmic vacuoles and perinuclear pale zones are common. Proximal-type ES is composed of a uniform epithelioid tumor cell population, with occasional rhabdoid morphology; this variant arises in the proximal limbs of older adults. Admixed spindle cells, extracellular debris, and granulomatous-type structures are common in distal-type ES, which typically presents in the distal extremities of

Table 4
Differential diagnosis: epithelioid soft tissue tumors

Tumor	Immunohistochemical Features	Molecular Features
Epithelioid sarcoma	Keratin, EMA, CD34 (50%), SMARCB1 loss	SMARCB1 alterations
Epithelioid hemangioendothelioma	CD31, CD34, ERG, CAMTA1 TFE3 and loss of YAP1 if YAP1::TFE3	WWTR1::CAMTA1 Rare YAP1::TFE3
Clear cell sarcoma of soft tissue	S-100, SOX10, HMB-45, Melan-A	EWSR1::ATF1 (majority) EWSRR1::CREB1
PEComa	SMA, desmin, HMB-45, Melan-A	TSC mutations Subset with TFE3 fusions
Alveolar soft part sarcoma	TFE3	ASPSCR1::TFE3
SDH-deficient GIST	KIT, DOG1, SDHB loss SDHA loss if SDHA- mutant	SDHA, SDHB, SDHC, or SDHD mutations SDHC promoter hypermethylation
Epithelioid inflammatory myofibroblastic sarcoma	ALK Variable SMA, desmin, CD30	ALK::RANBP2

Abbreviation: GIST, gastrointestinal stromal tumor.

young adults and teenagers. Tumors are positive for keratins and EMA and show frequent CD34 staining. The loss of nuclear staining of SMARCB1 secondary to SMARCB1 alterations is diagnostic.[106] However, SMARCB1 loss can be seen in other tumor types, including malignant rhabdoid tumor, poorly differentiated chordoma, and a subset of soft tissue myoepithelial neoplasms, underscoring the importance of clinical correlations and inclusive immunohistochemical panels.

Epithelioid hemangioendothelioma (EHE) is a malignant vascular neoplasm that arises in both somatic and visceral soft tissue sites. On aspirate smears, EHE shows dispersed epithelioid cells with frequent nuclear pseudoinclusions and grooves; a helpful feature is the presence of prominent intracytoplasmic vacuoles.[107,108] Myxohyaline stroma is common. The endothelial markers CD34, CD31, and ERG are positive in EHE; 40% are positive for keratins which is a pitfall for carcinoma. Tumors harbor WWTR1::CAMTA1 fusion in most cases (90%), and CAMTA1 nuclear staining is diagnostic and discriminates EHE from other vascular tumors.[109,110] This is especially important for cases of epithelioid angiosarcoma, which are more aggressive than EHE. Epithelioid angiosarcoma also appears as epithelioid cells with cytoplasmic vacuoles, is positive for endothelial markers, and can show aberrant keratin staining; however, tumors tend to show more nuclear atypia and pleomorphism and are negative for CAMTA1. A small subset of EHE is characterized by

YAP1::TFE3 fusion which correlates with TFE3 nuclear staining and loss of YAP1[111,112]; this variant is more vasoformative with epithelioid cells having voluminous cytoplasm.

Both clear cell sarcoma (CCS) and PEComa show melanocytic differentiation but have distinctive clinical and molecular features. Melanoma must be excluded in affected patients. CCS mainly affects young adults, frequently arising in deep-seated tissues of the limbs, especially in the ankle or foot. On smears, tumor cell nuclei show prominent nucleoli and intranuclear inclusions and have vacuolated cytoplasm[113] (Fig. 9A–C). CCS is positive for S-100, SOX10, HMB-45 and Melan-A (Fig. 9D–E). CCS is characterized by EWSR1::ATF1 and molecular testing is required in most cases (Fig. 9F). PEComas are anatomically ubiquitous, arising over a wide age range with a female predominance; aspirates show epithelioid cells with abundant vacuolated cytoplasm, bare nuclei, and proliferating capillaries.[114] Tumors are positive for both smooth muscle (SMA, desmin, caldesmon) and melanocytic (HMB-45 and Melan-A) markers, but are negative for S-100 and SOX10. TSC2 alterations are common. A subset (15%) of PEComas have TFE3 fusions (with resultant nuclear TFE3 immunoreactivity); this variant tends to arise in younger patients and are negative for smooth muscle markers.[115]

Alveolar soft part sarcoma (ASPS) harbors ASPSCR1::TFE3. ASPS typically arises in the deep soft tissues of the limbs of young adults;

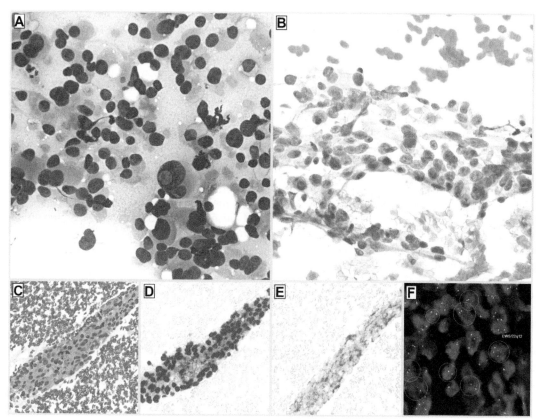

Fig. 9. Clear cell sarcoma. Dispersed epithelioid tumor cells have enlarged round nuclei and abundant cytoplasm. The nuclei have prominent nucleoli and nuclear pseudoinclusions (*A*, Romanowsky stain; *B*, Papanicolaou stain; *C*, cell block). Melanocytic differentiation is demonstrated by immunohistochemistry with nuclear positivity for SOX10 (*D*) and cytoplasmic staining for HMB-45 (*E*). (*F*) *EWSR1* rearrangement is confirmed by FISH (*nuclei circled*). (Photo courtesy of Dale W. Lewis.)

tumors in pediatric patients often involve the head and neck region. On cytologic preparations, epithelioid cells with fragile granular cytoplasm and naked nuclei are seen.[116,117] The immunophenotype is nonspecific apart from TFE3 nuclear staining; desmin and calretinin are positive in up to half of all cases. *TFE3* FISH can confirm the diagnosis. However, since *TFE3* fusions are also seen in subsets of PEComa and EHE, inclusion of melanocytic and vascular markers is necessary. One additional pitfall is that granular cell tumors show TFE3 expression while lacking *TFE3* rearrangements.[118] These benign tumors also show epithelioid morphology with abundant granular cytoplasm; however, the nuclear features are consistently bland and cases are positive for S-100, SOX10, inhibin, calretinin, and NKI-C3.

Epithelioid variants of certain tumor types are important to recognize. SDH-deficient GISTs show epithelioid morphology, arise exclusively in the stomach, and include the majority of pediatric cases (GISTs are otherwise rare in children).[119]

Tumors are still positive for KIT and DOG1. SDH-deficiency occurs secondary to inactivation in any of the 4 SDH-subunit genes and can be detected by SDHB immunohistochemistry, which is negative in tumor cells regardless of underlying mechanism.[120] Immunohistochemical loss of SDHA is specific for *SDHA*-mutant GISTs.[121] The behavior and prognosis of SDH-deficient GISTs differs from conventional GIST; tumors do not respond to imatinib but may still behave indolently even with liver metastases.[122] Patients are referred to genetic counseling given the syndromic associations, including the autosomal-dominant Carney–Stratakis syndrome (GIST–paraganglioma). Epithelioid inflammatory myofibroblastic sarcoma is an aggressive variant of IMT, and commonly arises as intra-abdominal masses in young male individuals.[123] Tumors show atypical epithelioid cells, frequent myxoid stroma, and infiltrating neutrophils[124]; tumors harbor *ALK::RNBP2* which corresponds with a nuclear membrane pattern staining for ALK.

PLEOMORPHIC TUMORS

The high-grade pleomorphic sarcomas of this group yield aspirates with enlarged, pleomorphic (often bizarre) tumor cells, mitotic activity frequently with atypical forms, and necrosis and can be challenging to distinguish from one another. For many tumors in this group, classification is possible by identifying a line of differentiation by immunohistochemistry, molecular testing, or defining morphologic features (Table 5), although this is not always feasible on cytologic samples. Several entities in this differential lack specific immunohistochemical and molecular profiles and often cannot be definitively diagnosed by FNA at initial presentation; such cases benefit from immunohistochemical workup to exclude other tumor types but ultimately are signed out descriptively. Since most patients are adults, sarcomatoid and undifferentiated carcinomas and melanoma should always be excluded in the workup.

DDLPS shows a broad morphologic range, and many appear as non-lipogenic pleomorphic sarcomas (Fig. 10A–D). Tumors harbor *MDM2* amplification and many are associated with precursor ALT/WDL. DDLPS is the prime consideration for tumors arising in the retroperitoneum, but testing for *MDM2* amplification is useful for almost any pleomorphic sarcoma encountered in practice. DDLPS has a lower risk of distant metastasis compared to other pleomorphic sarcomas. Most cases can be identified by nuclear staining for MDM2 and CDK4 immunohistochemistry; FISH may helpful (Fig. 10E) since weak nonspecific reactivity can be seen in other sarcoma types, such as myxofibrosarcoma and MPNST. DDLPS with heterologous differentiation should also be considered when a pleomorphic sarcoma shows myogenic or osteoblastic differentiation, and tumors with rhabdomyoblastic differentiation are associated with poorer prognosis.[125] Although infrequently sampled by FNA, intimal sarcoma also harbors *MDM2* amplification; clinical correlation is helpful as these are pleomorphic sarcomas that arise in large blood vessels (often in the thorax).

Immunohistochemistry has a role in identifying pleomorphic leiomyosarcoma and pleomorphic rhabdomyosarcoma, which are the most aggressive entities in this differential. Both are positive for desmin and are further distinguished by SMA and caldesmon positivity in leiomyosarcoma and myogenin and MyoD1 in rhabdomyosarcoma. Some cases of pleomorphic leiomyosarcoma show recognizable features of conventional leiomyosarcoma with fascicular fragments of spindle cells. Pleomorphic rhabdomyosarcoma shows large rhabdoid cells that are frequently bi- and multinucleated. Heterologous myogenic differentiation can occur in other tumor types, so exclusion of relevant entities may be necessary (eg,

Table 5
Differential diagnosis: pleomorphic sarcomas

Tumor Type	Helpful Features	Diagnostic Features
DDLPS	Most common in retroperitoneum or viscera ALT/WDL components (if present)	*MDM2* amplification (MDM2 and CDK4 IHC or *MDM2 FISH*)
Pleomorphic leiomyosarcoma	Conventional spindle cell morphology (if present)	IHC positive for SMA, desmin, Caldesmon
Pleomorphic rhabdomyosarcoma	Rhabdoid morphology	IHC positive for desmin (strong), myogenin, MyoD1
Extraskeletal osteosarcoma	IHC positive for SATB2	Osteoid matrix
Myxofibrosarcoma	Most common sarcoma in older patients; location in superficial tissues of limbs	Myxoid stroma and curvilinear collagenous vessels
Pleomorphic liposarcoma	Rare; location in deep soft tissues of limbs	Pleomorphic lipoblasts
Undifferentiated pleomorphic sarcoma	Location in deep soft tissues of limbs Diagnosis of exclusion	Diagnosis of exclusion

Abbreviations: ALT, atypical lipomatous tumor; DDLPS, dedifferentiated liposarcoma; FISH, fluorescent in situ hybridization; IHC, immunohistochemistry; WDL, well-differentiated liposarcoma.

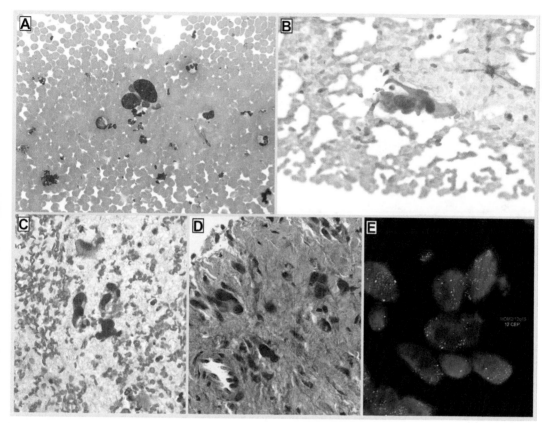

Fig. 10. Dedifferentiated liposarcoma. Smears show scattered intact large pleomorphic tumor cells and bare nuclei (many of which are bizarre) (*A*, Romanowsky stain; *B, C*, Papanicolaou stain). (*D*) The cell block shows pleomorphic cells set within a densely sclerotic stroma. (*E*) FISH analysis demonstrates *MDM2* amplification. (*Courtesy of* Dale W. Lewis.)

H3K27me3 for MPNST and MDM2/CDK4 for DDLPS).

Extraskeletal osteosarcoma arises in adults, most commonly in the extremities. Tumors show SATB2 positivity supporting osteoblastic differentiation, although many high-grade sarcomas can also show nonspecific SATB2 staining. The diagnosis requires the identification of extracellular osteoid matrix, which appears as metachromatic wiry and strandlike material intermingled with epithelioid and pleomorphic cells. Heterologous osteosarcomatous differentiation may occur in MPNST and DDLPS, and clinical correlation and immunohistochemistry are needed to exclude those possibilities.

High-grade myxofibrosarcoma and pleomorphic liposarcoma are in the differential of tumors arising in the limbs, and there may be limited presence or absent sampling of their respective characteristic features (curvilinear vessels of myxofibrosarcoma and lipoblasts of pleomorphic liposarcoma; **Fig. 11**). Immunohistochemistry is useful in excluding other entities, including

DDLPS. Most are signed out descriptively (eg, "high-grade pleomorphic sarcoma") which is sufficient for patient management; patients undergo surgical resection often with neoadjuvant therapy. The surgical resection specimen must be thoroughly sampled and examined to identify characteristic histologic features. After exclusion of myxofibrosarcoma and pleomorphic liposarcoma and all other diagnostic entities, some cases are ultimately classified as undifferentiated pleomorphic sarcoma (UPS). UPS is a diagnosis of exclusion, and classification on cytology specimens is not possible apart from established patients with recurrent or metastatic disease.

PRECISION MEDICINE: RELEVANT IMPLICATIONS FOR CYTOPATHOLOGISTS

Most sarcomas are treated with one-size-fits-all chemotherapy approach, with established treatment regiments for only a small number of tumor types (eg, Ewing sarcoma). However, there is an

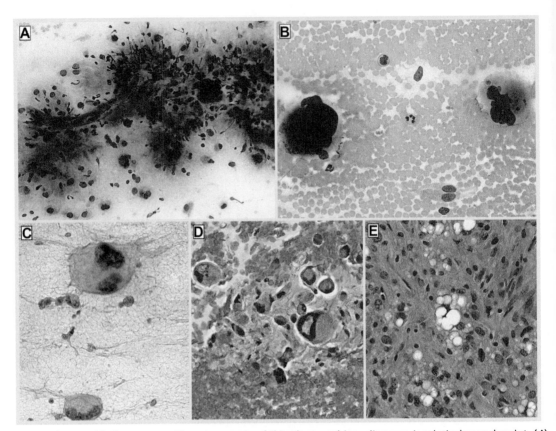

Fig. 11. Pleomorphic liposarcoma. The appearance of this pleomorphic malignancy is relatively nondescript. (*A*) The presence of myxoid stroma can resemble myxofibrosarcoma (Romanowsky stain). (*B*) Multinucleated giant tumor cells can be seen, but are nonspecific (Romanowsky stain). FNAs can sample the pleomorphic tumor cell component with limited or no sampling of diagnostic features (*C*, Papanicolaou stain; *D*, cell block). (*E*) On resection, the final diagnosis is confirmed by the presence of the diagnostic pleomorphic lipoblasts.

expanding role for "precision medicine" as therapeutic and prognostic molecular targets are characterized in soft tissue tumors. Currently, there are only a few Food and Drug Administration (FDA)-approved targeted treatments relative to the large number of soft tissue neoplasms, most of which are used in patients with advanced sarcomas. Far more agents are currently in research and clinical development, and the list of targeted therapies is undoubtedly expanding. In this context, cytopathologists will have important roles in the treatment of these patients with the need for biopsies to confirm recurrent or metastatic disease. Selected examples of FDA-approved targeted agents are mentioned here.

Tyrosine kinase inhibitor (TKI) therapy for GIST is a well-established targeted treatment paradigm, based on the presence of activating *KIT* mutations. Imatinib is the first line in patients with complex or unresectable tumors, while several other TKIs are approved for resistant cases.[126,127] The NCCN guidelines recommend mutational testing whenever TKIs are indicated, since specific mutations confer different sensitivities to these agents and *KIT* secondary mutations are a mechanism of resistance in TKI-refractory GIST.[128,129] *KIT* exon 11 mutations are most common (75%) and importantly render responsivity to imatinib, while *KIT* exon 9 mutations are associated with lower response rates.[128,129] While most tumors with *PDGFRA* mutations respond to imatinib, those with *PDGFRA* D842V are insensitive and are treated with avapritinib.

Targeting kinase mutations has been successful in other tumor types. Crizotinib inhibits c-met, ALK, and ROS1 and shows activity in advanced stage *ALK*-rearranged IMT.[126,127,130] Pexidartinib has selective activity against colony-stimulating factor 1 receptor and is approved for treatment of debilitating tenosynovial giant cell tumor, which overexpresses CSF1 secondary to *CSF1* fusions.[131] Pazopanib, which targets the vascular endothelial growth factor receptor (VEGFR), has shown noninferiority when compared to anthracycline-based therapies and is used as an alternative first-line therapy for advanced/metastatic disease for several sarcoma types.[132] Advanced SFTs show responses to TKIs that have antiangiogenic activity, such as pazopanib, sunitinib, and sorafenib.[133,134]

PEComas are associated with frequent *TSC1/2* alterations, and the loss of TSC function gives rise to activation of the mTOR pathway. The mTOR inhibitor nab-sirolimus shows responses in locally advanced or metastatic malignant PEComa, with durable disease control and survival, as well as better benefit for patients with *TSC1/2* mutations.[135]

Epigenetic mechanisms of carcinogenesis can also be targeted. ES is characterized by *SMARCB1* inactivation, leading to loss of function of the encoded INI1 subunit of the chromatin remodeling complex SWI/SNF, leading to constituent activation of the methyltransferase EZH2. Tazemetostat is a selective EZH2 inhibitor that has been approved for patients with ES.[136]

Histology-agnostic treatments targeting specific molecular alterations are now available, with relevant applications for some sarcomas. Larotrectinib and entrectinib are approved for solid tumors harboring *NTRK* fusions which are seen in several soft tissue neoplasms; responses are seen in patients with metastatic or locally aggressive infantile fibrosarcoma (which have *NTRK1/2/3* fusions).[137] Dabrafenib and trametinib are approved for solid tumors with *BRAF* V600 E mutations,[138] which include rare *BRAF*-mutant GISTs.

Data are still limited regarding the efficacy of immune checkpoint inhibitor (ICI) in sarcomas, and promising responses have only been seen in a small number of selected tumor types. The ICI pembrolizumab is used for subsequent treatment in patients with high tumor mutational burden, microsatellite instability-high, or DNA mismatch repair-deficient tumors, regardless of histology.[10] Currently, it is only used for a small number of sarcomas in advanced stages, mostly myxofibrosarcoma, UPS, and cutaneous angiosarcoma. Mismatch repair deficiency is very rare (1%) in sarcomas (mostly in high-grade and undifferentiated sarcomas)[139,140] and predictive markers (if any) for responsivity to ICI therapy in sarcomas remain to be elucidated.

SUMMARY

The goals of soft tissue FNA are to provide accurate diagnoses when possible or to triage lesions based on grade even when a definitive diagnosis is not possible, ultimately to ensure appropriate clinical management. There are many reliable ancillary tests that enable the cytologic diagnosis of many soft tissue tumors, even very rare entities. Immunohistochemistry is practical and efficient in the workup of soft tissue FNAs, and there are now many reliable markers that can serve as surrogates of underlying molecular alterations. A pattern-based framework is recommended for guiding the formulation of differentials, ensuring that immunohistochemical and molecular tests are judiciously selected based on clinical and morphologic features. There are benefits for the incorporation of routine NGS in sarcoma diagnostics, but morphologic evaluation remains key. In this era of precision medicine, an expansion of targeted therapies for sarcomas is expected, underscoring the importance of accurate classification by cytopathologists.

DISCLOSURE

The authors have no disclosures.

REFERENCES

1. Chambers M, O'Hern K, Kerr DA. Fine-needle aspiration biopsy for the diagnosis of bone and soft tissue lesions: a systematic review and meta-analysis. J Am Soc Cytopathol 2020;9(5):429–41.
2. von Mehren M, Kane JM, Agulnik M, et al. Soft Tissue Sarcoma, Version 2.2022, NCCN Clinical Practice Guidelines in Oncology. J Natl Compr Canc Netw 2022;20(7):815–33.
3. Roy-Chowdhuri S, Chen H, Singh RR, et al. Concurrent fine needle aspirations and core needle biopsies: a comparative study of substrates for next-generation sequencing in solid organ malignancies. Mod Pathol 2017;30(4):499–508.
4. Lam SW, Cleton-Jansen AM, Cleven AHG, et al. Molecular Analysis of Gene Fusions in Bone and Soft Tissue Tumors by Anchored Multiplex PCR-Based Targeted Next-Generation Sequencing. J Mol Diagn 2018;20(5):653–63.
5. Mantilla JG, Ricciotti RW, Chen E, et al. Detecting disease-defining gene fusions in unclassified round cell sarcomas using anchored multiplex PCR/targeted RNA next-generation sequencing-Molecular and clinicopathological characterization of 16 cases. Genes, chromosomes & cancer. 2019;58(10):713–22.
6. Chebib I, Taylor MS, Nardi V, et al. Clinical Utility of Anchored Multiplex Solid Fusion Assay for Diagnosis of Bone and Soft Tissue Tumors. Am J Surg Pathol 2021;45(8):1127–37.
7. Dermawan JK, Cheng YW, Tu ZJ, et al. Diagnostic Utility of a Custom 34-Gene Anchored Multiplex PCR-Based Next-Generation Sequencing Fusion Panel for the Diagnosis of Bone and Soft Tissue Neoplasms With Identification of Novel USP6

Fusion Partners in Aneurysmal Bone Cysts. Arch Pathol Lab Med 2021;145(7):851–63.

8. Walaas L, Kindblom LG. Lipomatous tumors: a correlative cytologic and histologic study of 27 tumors examined by fine needle aspiration cytology. Hum Pathol 1985;16(1):6–18.

9. Dey P. Fine needle aspiration cytology of well-differentiated liposarcoma. A report of two cases. Acta Cytol 2000;44(3):459–62.

10. Kapila K, Ghosal N, Gill SS, et al. Cytomorphology of lipomatous tumors of soft tissue. Acta Cytol 2003;47(4):555–62.

11. Klijanienko J, Caillaud JM, Lagace R. Fine-needle aspiration in liposarcoma: cytohistologic correlative study including well-differentiated, myxoid, and pleomorphic variants. Diagn Cytopathol 2004; 30(5):307–12.

12. Binh MB, Sastre-Garau X, Guillou L, et al. MDM2 and CDK4 immunostainings are useful adjuncts in diagnosing well-differentiated and dedifferentiated liposarcoma subtypes: a comparative analysis of 559 soft tissue neoplasms with genetic data. Am J Surg Pathol 2005;29(10):1340–7.

13. Lemos MM, Kindblom LG, Meis-Kindblom JM, et al. Fine-needle aspiration characteristics of hibernoma. Cancer. 2001;93(3):206–10.

14. Marino-Enriquez A, Hornick JL, Dal Cin P, et al. Dedifferentiated liposarcoma and pleomorphic liposarcoma: a comparative study of cytomorphology and MDM2/CDK4 expression on fine-needle aspiration. Cancer cytopathology 2014;122(2):128–37.

15. Wakely PE Jr, Wangsiricharoen S, Ali SZ. Pleomorphic liposarcoma: A clinicopathologic study of 20 FNA cases. Cancer Cytopathol 2022;130(9):705–13.

16. Marino-Enriquez A, Fletcher CD, Dal Cin P, et al. Dedifferentiated liposarcoma with "homologous" lipoblastic (pleomorphic liposarcoma-like) differentiation: clinicopathologic and molecular analysis of a series suggesting revised diagnostic criteria. Am J Surg Pathol 2010;34(8):1122–31.

17. Wakely PE Jr, Jin M. Myxoid liposarcoma: Fine-needle aspiration cytopathology in the molecular era. A report of 24 cases. J Am Soc Cytopathol 2016;5(3):162–9.

18. Scapa JV, Cloutier JM, Raghavan SS, et al. DDIT3 Immunohistochemistry Is a Useful Tool for the Diagnosis of Myxoid Liposarcoma. Am J Surg Pathol 2021;45(2):230–9.

19. Baranov E, Black MA, Fletcher CDM, et al. Nuclear expression of DDIT3 distinguishes high-grade myxoid liposarcoma from other round cell sarcomas. Mod Pathol 2021;34(7):1367–72.

20. Domanski HA, Carlen B, Jonsson K, et al. Distinct cytologic features of spindle cell lipoma. A cytologic-histologic study with clinical, radiologic,

electron microscopic, and cytogenetic correlations. Cancer 2001;93(6):381–9.

21. Lopez-Rios F, Alberti N, Perez-Barrios A, et al. Fine-needle aspiration of pleomorphic lipoma. Diagn Cytopathol 2001;24(4):296–7.

22. Chen BJ, Marino-Enriquez A, Fletcher CD, et al. Loss of retinoblastoma protein expression in spindle cell/pleomorphic lipomas and cytogenetically related tumors: an immunohistochemical study with diagnostic implications. Am J Surg Pathol 2012;36(8):1119–28.

23. Wakely PE Jr. Atypical spindle cell/pleomorphic lipomatous tumour (ASPLT): A report of three FNA cases and comparison with spindle cell/pleomorphic lipoma cytopathology. Cytopathology 2023; 34(4):346–52.

24. Creytens D, van Gorp J, Savola S, et al. Atypical spindle cell lipoma: a clinicopathologic, immunohistochemical, and molecular study emphasizing its relationship to classical spindle cell lipoma. Virchows Arch : an international journal of pathology 2014;465(1):97–108.

25. Marino-Enriquez A, Nascimento AF, Ligon AH, et al. Atypical Spindle Cell Lipomatous Tumor: Clinicopathologic Characterization of 232 Cases Demonstrating a Morphologic Spectrum. Am J Surg Pathol 2017;41(2):234–44.

26. Anderson WJ, Fletcher CDM, Jo VY. Atypical Pleomorphic Lipomatous Tumor: Expanding Our Current Understanding in a Clinicopathologic Analysis of 64 Cases. Am J Surg Pathol 2021; 45(9):1282–92.

27. Wakely Jr PE, Bos GD, Mayerson J. The cytopathology of soft tissue mxyomas: ganglia, juxta-articular myxoid lesions, and intramuscular myxoma. Am J Clin Pathol 2005;123(6):858–65.

28. Domanski HA, Mertens F, Panagopoulos I, et al. Low-grade fibromyxoid sarcoma is difficult to diagnose by fine needle aspiration cytology: a cytomorphological study of eight cases. Cytopathology : official journal of the British Society for Clinical Cytology. 2009;20(5):304–14.

29. Yang EJ, Hornick JL, Qian X. Fine-needle aspiration of soft tissue perineurioma: A comparative analysis of cytomorphology and immunohistochemistry with benign and malignant mimics. Cancer cytopathology 2016;124(9):651–8.

30. Mustafa S, VandenBussche CJ, Ali SZ, et al. Cytomorphologic findings of low-grade fibromyxoid sarcoma. J Am Soc Cytopathol 2020;9(3):191–201.

31. Doyle LA, Moller E, Dal Cin P, et al. MUC4 is a highly sensitive and specific marker for low-grade fibromyxoid sarcoma. Am J Surg Pathol 2011;35(5):733–41.

32. Kilpatrick SE, Ward WG. Myxofibrosarcoma of soft tissues: cytomorphologic analysis of a series. Diagn Cytopathol 1999;20(1):6–9.

33. Wakely PE Jr. Cytopathology of myxofibrosarcoma: a study of 66 cases and literature review. J Am Soc Cytopathol 2021;10(3):300–9.

34. Machado I, Lopez-Soto MV, Rubio L, et al. Soft tissue myoepithelial carcinoma with rhabdoid-like features and EWSR1 rearrangement: Fine needle aspiration cytology with histologic correlation. Diagn Cytopathol 2015;43(5):421–6.

35. Wang G, Tucker T, Ng TL, et al. Fine-needle aspiration of soft tissue myoepithelioma. Diagn Cytopathol 2016;44(2):152–5.

36. Wakely PE Jr, Siddiqui MT. Fine-needle aspiration cytopathology of soft tissue myoepithelioma: an analysis of seven cases. J Am Soc Cytopathol 2022;11(1):31–9.

37. Wang L, Yee-Chang M, Sun W, et al. Myoepithelial carcinoma of soft tissue is a diagnostic challenge on fine-needle aspiration: Case report and review of literature. Diagn Cytopathol 2022;50(7):E203–9.

38. Bahrami A, Dalton JD, Krane JF, et al. A subset of cutaneous and soft tissue mixed tumors are genetically linked to their salivary gland counterpart. Genes, chromosomes & cancer. 2012;51(2):140–8.

39. Antonescu CR, Zhang L, Chang NE, et al. EWSR1-POU5F1 fusion in soft tissue myoepithelial tumors. A molecular analysis of sixty-six cases, including soft tissue, bone, and visceral lesions, showing common involvement of the EWSR1 gene. Genes Chromosomes Cancer 2010;49(12):1114–24.

40. Le Loarer F, Zhang L, Fletcher CD, et al. Consistent SMARCB1 homozygous deletions in epithelioid sarcoma and in a subset of myoepithelial carcinomas can be reliably detected by FISH in archival material. Genes, chromosomes & cancer. 2014;53(6):475–86.

41. Suurmeijer AJH, Dickson BC, Swanson D, et al. A morphologic and molecular reappraisal of myoepithelial tumors of soft tissue, bone, and viscera with EWSR1 and FUS gene rearrangements. Genes Chromosomes Cancer 2020;59(6):348–56.

42. Santos F, Martins C, Lemos MM. Fine-needle aspiration features of extraskeletal myxoid chondrosarcoma: A study of cytological and molecular features. Diagn Cytopathol 2018;46(11):950–7.

43. Wakely PE Jr. Extraskeletal myxoid chondrosarcoma: combining cytopathology with molecular testing to achieve diagnostic accuracy. J Am Soc Cytopathol 2021;10(3):293–9.

44. Mohanty SK, Srinivasan R, Rajwanshi A, et al. Cytologic diagnosis of ossifying fibromyxoid tumor of soft tissue: a case report. Diagn Cytopathol 2004; 30(1):41–5.

45. Kumari N, Anthony ML, Durgapal P, et al. Ossifying fibromyxoid tumor: Fine-needle aspiration cytology findings of a rare soft tissue neoplasm. Diagn Cytopathol 2020;48(4):396–400.

46. Graham RP, Weiss SW, Sukov WR, et al. PHF1 rearrangements in ossifying fibromyxoid tumors of soft parts: A fluorescence in situ hybridization study of 41 cases with emphasis on the malignant variant. Am J Surg Pathol 2013;37(11):1751–5.

47. Kao YC, Sung YS, Zhang L, et al. Expanding the molecular signature of ossifying fibromyxoid tumors with two novel gene fusions: CREBBP-BCORL1 and KDM2A-WWTR1. Genes, chromosomes & cancer. 2017;56(1):42–50.

48. Kao YC, Sung YS, Argani P, et al. NTRK3 overexpression in undifferentiated sarcomas with YWHAE and BCOR genetic alterations. Mod Pathol 2020; 33(7):1341–9.

49. Chebib I, Hornicek FJ, Nielsen GP, et al. Cytomorphologic features that distinguish schwannoma from other low-grade spindle cell lesions. Cancer cytopathology 2015;123(3):171–9.

50. Wakely PE Jr. Benign peripheral nerve tumors: Analysis of 89 FNA cases emphasizing diagnostic accuracy and their morphologic spectrum. Cancer Cytopathol 2023;131(5):300–12.

51. Tao LC, Davidson DD. Aspiration biopsy cytology of smooth muscle tumors. A cytologic approach to the differentiation between leiomyosarcoma and leiomyoma. Acta Cytol 1993;37(3):300–8.

52. Wieczorek TJ, Faquin WC, Rubin BP, et al. Cytologic diagnosis of gastrointestinal stromal tumor with emphasis on the differential diagnosis with leiomyosarcoma. Cancer. 2001;93(4):276–87.

53. Stelow EB, Stanley MW, Mallery S, et al. Endoscopic ultrasound-guided fine-needle aspiration findings of gastrointestinal leiomyomas and gastrointestinal stromal tumors. Am J Clin Pathol 2003; 119(5):703–8.

54. West RB, Corless CL, Chen X, et al. The novel marker, DOG1, is expressed ubiquitously in gastrointestinal stromal tumors irrespective of KIT or PDGFRA mutation status. Am J Pathol 2004; 165(1):107–13.

55. Hwang DG, Qian X, Hornick JL. DOG1 antibody is a highly sensitive and specific marker for gastrointestinal stromal tumors in cytology cell blocks. Am J Clin Pathol 2011;135(3):448–53.

56. Dalen BP, Meis-Kindblom JM, Sumathi VP, et al. Fine-needle aspiration cytology and core needle biopsy in the preoperative diagnosis of desmoid tumors. Acta Orthop 2006;77(6):926–31.

57. Owens CL, Sharma R, Ali SZ. Deep fibromatosis (desmoid tumor): cytopathologic characteristics, clinicoradiologic features, and immunohistochemical findings on fine-needle aspiration. Cancer 2007;111(3):166–72.

58. Rege TA, Madan R, Qian X. Long fascicular tissue fragments in desmoid fibromatosis by fine needle aspiration: a new cytologic feature. Diagn Cytopathol 2012;40(1):45–7.

59. Erickson-Johnson MR, Chou MM, Evers BR, et al. Nodular fasciitis: a novel model of transient

neoplasia induced by MYH9-USP6 gene fusion. Lab Invest 2011;91(10):1427–33.

60. Allison DB, Wakely PE Jr, Siddiqui MT, et al. Nodular fasciitis: A frequent diagnostic pitfall on fine-needle aspiration. Cancer Cytopathol 2017; 125(1):20–9.

61. Stoll LM, Li QK. Cytology of fine-needle aspiration of inflammatory myofibroblastic tumor. Diagn Cytopathol 2011;39(9):663–72.

62. Sharma S, Gupta N, Rajwanshi A, et al. Inflammatory myofibroblastic tumour: a diagnostic challenge on fine needle aspiration cytology. Cytopathology 2016;27(6):512–6.

63. Coffin CM, Hornick JL, Fletcher CD. Inflammatory myofibroblastic tumor: comparison of clinicopathologic, histologic, and immunohistochemical features including ALK expression in atypical and aggressive cases. Am J Surg Pathol 2007;31(4): 509–20.

64. Cheah AL, Zou Y, Lanigan C, et al. ALK Expression in Angiomatoid Fibrous Histiocytoma: A Potential Diagnostic Pitfall. Am J Surg Pathol 2019;43(1): 93–101.

65. Wakely PE Jr, Rekhi B. Cytopathology of solitary fibrous tumor: a series of 34 cases. J Am Soc Cytopathol 2021;10(4):382–90.

66. Tani E, Wejde J, Astrom K, et al. FNA cytology of solitary fibrous tumors and the diagnostic value of STAT6 immunocytochemistry. Cancer 2018;126(1): 36–43.

67. Kao YC, Lin PC, Yen SL, et al. Clinicopathological and genetic heterogeneity of the head and neck solitary fibrous tumours: a comparative histological, immunohistochemical and molecular study of 36 cases. Histopathology 2016;68(4): 492–501.

68. Mohajeri A, Tayebwa J, Collin A, et al. Comprehensive genetic analysis identifies a pathognomonic NAB2/STAT6 fusion gene, nonrandom secondary genomic imbalances, and a characteristic gene expression profile in solitary fibrous tumor. Genes, chromosomes & cancer. 2013;52(10):873–86.

69. Kilpatrick SE, Teot LA, Stanley MW, et al. Fine-needle aspiration biopsy of synovial sarcoma. A cytomorphologic analysis of primary, recurrent, and metastatic tumors. Am J Clin Pathol 1996;106(6): 769–75.

70. Akerman M, Ryd W, Skytting B, et al. Fine-needle aspiration of synovial sarcoma: criteria for diagnosis: retrospective reexamination of 37 cases, including ancillary diagnostics. A Scandinavian Sarcoma Group study. Diagn Cytopathol 2003; 28(5):232–8.

71. Wakely PE Jr, Saoud C, Ali SZ. Synovial sarcoma: cytopathology of 51 cases highlighting the application of ancillary molecular testing. J Am Soc Cytopathol 2023;12(4):284–95.

72. Baranov E, McBride MJ, Bellizzi AM, et al. A Novel SS18-SSX Fusion-specific Antibody for the Diagnosis of Synovial Sarcoma. Am J Surg Pathol 2020;44(7):922–33.

73. Zaborowski M, Vargas AC, Pulvers J, et al. When used together SS18-SSX fusion-specific and SSX C-terminus immunohistochemistry are highly specific and sensitive for the diagnosis of synovial sarcoma and can replace FISH or molecular testing in most cases. Histopathology 2020;77(4):588–600.

74. Klijanienko J, Caillaud JM, Lagace R, et al. Cytohistologic correlations of 24 malignant peripheral nerve sheath tumor (MPNST) in 17 patients: the Institut Curie experience. Diagn Cytopathol 2002; 27(2):103–8.

75. Wakely PE Jr, Ali SZ, Bishop JA. The cytopathology of malignant peripheral nerve sheath tumor: a report of 55 fine-needle aspiration cases. Cancer cytopathology 2012;120(5):334–41.

76. Lee W, Teckie S, Wiesner T, et al. PRC2 is recurrently inactivated through EED or SUZ12 loss in malignant peripheral nerve sheath tumors. Nat Genet 2014;46(11):1227–32.

77. Cleven AH, Sannaa GA, Briaire-de Bruijn I, et al. Loss of H3K27 tri-methylation is a diagnostic marker for malignant peripheral nerve sheath tumors and an indicator for an inferior survival. Mod Pathol : an official journal of the United States and Canadian Academy of Pathology, Inc. 2016;29(6): 582–90.

78. Schaefer IM, Fletcher CD, Hornick JL. Loss of H3K27 trimethylation distinguishes malignant peripheral nerve sheath tumors from histologic mimics. Mod Pathol 2016;29(1):4–13.

79. Mito JK, Qian X, Doyle LA, et al. Role of Histone H3K27 Trimethylation Loss as a Marker for Malignant Peripheral Nerve Sheath Tumor in Fine-Needle Aspiration and Small Biopsy Specimens. Am J Clin Pathol 2017;148(2):179–89.

80. Hornick JL, Nielsen GP. Beyond "Triton": Malignant Peripheral Nerve Sheath Tumors With Complete Heterologous Rhabdomyoblastic Differentiation Mimicking Spindle Cell Rhabdomyosarcoma. Am J Surg Pathol 2019;43(10):1323–30.

81. Domanski HA, Akerman M, Rissler P, et al. Fine-needle aspiration of soft tissue leiomyosarcoma: an analysis of the most common cytologic findings and the value of ancillary techniques. Diagn Cytopathol 2006;34(9):597–604.

82. Klijanienko J, Couturier J, Bourdeaut F, et al. Fine-needle aspiration as a diagnostic technique in 50 cases of primary Ewing sarcoma/peripheral neuroectodermal tumor. Institut Curie's experience. Diagn Cytopathol 2012;40(1):19–25.

83. Hung YP, Fletcher CD, Hornick JL. Evaluation of NKX2-2 expression in round cell sarcomas and other tumors with EWSR1 rearrangement: imperfect

specificity for Ewing sarcoma. Mod Pathol : an official journal of the United States and Canadian Academy of Pathology, Inc. 2016;29(4):370–80.

84. Russell-Goldman E, Hornick JL, Qian X, et al. NKX2.2 immunohistochemistry in the distinction of Ewing sarcoma from cytomorphologic mimics: Diagnostic utility and pitfalls. Cancer Cytopathol 2018;126(11):942–9.

85. Chebib I, Jo VY. Round cell sarcoma with CIC-DUX4 gene fusion: Discussion of the distinctive cytomorphologic, immunohistochemical, and molecular features in the differential diagnosis of round cell tumors. Cancer cytopathology 2016; 124(5):350–61.

86. Tang S, Dodd LG. CIC-DUX4 sarcoma diagnosed by fine-needle aspiration cytology: A case report. Diagn Cytopathol 2018;46(11):958–63.

87. Specht K, Sung YS, Zhang L, et al. Distinct transcriptional signature and immunoprofile of CIC-DUX4 fusion-positive round cell tumors compared to EWSR1-rearranged Ewing sarcomas: further evidence toward distinct pathologic entities. Genes, chromosomes & cancer. 2014;53(7):622–33.

88. Italiano A, Sung YS, Zhang L, et al. High prevalence of CIC fusion with double-homeobox (DUX4) transcription factors in EWSR1-negative undifferentiated small blue round cell sarcomas. Genes, chromosomes & cancer. 2012;51(3): 207–18.

89. Choi EY, Thomas DG, McHugh JB, et al. Undifferentiated small round cell sarcoma with t(4;19)(q35;q13.1) CIC-DUX4 fusion: a novel highly aggressive soft tissue tumor with distinctive histopathology. Am J Surg Pathol 2013;37(9):1379–86.

90. Sugita S, Arai Y, Tonooka A, et al. A novel CIC-FOXO4 gene fusion in undifferentiated small round cell sarcoma: a genetically distinct variant of Ewing-like sarcoma. Am J Surg Pathol 2014; 38(11):1571–6.

91. Connolly EA, Bhadri VA, Wake J, et al. Systemic treatments and outcomes in CIC-rearranged Sarcoma: A national multi-centre clinicopathological series and literature review. Cancer Med 2022; 11(8):1805–16.

92. Specht K, Zhang L, Sung YS, et al. Novel BCOR-MAML3 and ZC3H7B-BCOR Gene Fusions in Undifferentiated Small Blue Round Cell Sarcomas. Am J Surg Pathol 2016;40(4):433–42.

93. Kao YC, Sung YS, Zhang L, et al. Recurrent BCOR Internal Tandem Duplication and YWHAE-NUTM2B Fusions in Soft Tissue Undifferentiated Round Cell Sarcoma of Infancy: Overlapping Genetic Features With Clear Cell Sarcoma of Kidney. Am J Surg Pathol 2016;40(8):1009–20.

94. Kao YC, Owosho AA, Sung YS, et al. BCOR-CCNB3 Fusion Positive Sarcomas: A Clinicopathologic and Molecular Analysis of 36 Cases With Comparison to Morphologic Spectrum and Clinical Behavior of Other Round Cell Sarcomas. Am J Surg Pathol 2018;42(5):604–15.

95. Gajdzis P, Laé M, Pierron G, et al. Fine-Needle Aspiration Features of BCOR-CCNB3 Sarcoma. Am J Clin Pathol 2020;153(3):315–21.

96. Cohen-Gogo S, Cellier C, Coindre JM, et al. Ewing-like sarcomas with BCOR-CCNB3 fusion transcript: a clinical, radiological and pathological retrospective study from the Societe Francaise des Cancers de L'Enfant. Pediatr Blood Cancer 2014;61(12): 2191–8.

97. Akhtar M, Ali MA, Bakry M, et al. Fine-needle aspiration biopsy diagnosis of rhabdomyosarcoma: cytologic, histologic, and ultrastructural correlations. Diagn Cytopathol 1992;8(5):465–74.

98. Pohar-Marinsek Z, Bracko M. Rhabdomyosarcoma. Cytomorphology, subtyping and differential diagnostic dilemmas. Acta Cytol 2000;44(4):524–32.

99. Dias P, Chen B, Dilday B, et al. Strong immunostaining for myogenin in rhabdomyosarcoma is significantly associated with tumors of the alveolar subclass. Am J Pathol 2000;156(2):399–408.

100. Rutland CD, Gedallovich J, Wang A, et al. Diagnostic utility of FOXO1 immunohistochemistry for rhabdomyosarcoma classification. Histopathology 2023;83(1):49–56.

101. Leca LB, Vieira J, Teixeira MR, et al. Desmoplastic small round cell tumor: diagnosis by fine-needle aspiration cytology. Acta Cytol 2012;56(5):576–80.

102. Klijanienko J, Colin P, Couturier J, et al. Fine-needle aspiration in desmoplastic small round cell tumor: a report of 10 new tumors in 8 patients with clinicopathological and molecular correlations with review of the literature. Cancer cytopathology 2014; 122(5):386–93.

103. Tsuda Y, Zhang L, Meyers P, et al. The clinical heterogeneity of round cell sarcomas with EWSR1/FUS gene fusions: Impact of gene fusion type on clinical features and outcome. Genes Chromosomes Cancer 2020;59(9):525–34.

104. Gonzalez-Peramato P, Jimenez-Heffernan JA, Cuevas J. Fine-needle aspiration cytology of "proximal-type" epithelioid sarcoma. Diagn Cytopathol 2001;25(2):122–5.

105. Lemos MM, Chaves P, Mendonca ME. Is preoperative cytologic diagnosis of epithelioid sarcoma possible? Diagn Cytopathol 2008;36(11):780–6.

106. Hornick JL, Dal Cin P, Fletcher CD. Loss of INI1 expression is characteristic of both conventional and proximal-type epithelioid sarcoma. Am J Surg Pathol 2009;33(4):542–50.

107. Murali R, Zarka MA, Ocal IT, et al. Cytologic features of epithelioid hemangioendothelioma. Am J Clin Pathol 2011;136(5):739–46.

108. VandenBussche CJ, Wakely PE Jr, Siddiqui MT, et al. Cytopathologic characteristics of epithelioid

vascular malignancies. Acta Cytol 2014;58(4): 356–66.

109. Tanas MR, Sboner A, Oliveira AM, et al. Identification of a disease-defining gene fusion in epithelioid hemangioendothelioma. Sci Transl Med 2011; 3(98):98ra82.

110. Doyle LA, Fletcher CD, Hornick JL. Nuclear Expression of CAMTA1 Distinguishes Epithelioid Hemangioendothelioma From Histologic Mimics. Am J Surg Pathol 2016;40(1):94–102.

111. Antonescu CR, Le Loarer F, Mosquera JM, et al. Novel YAP1-TFE3 fusion defines a distinct subset of epithelioid hemangioendothelioma. Genes Chromosomes Cancer 2013;52(8):775–84.

112. Anderson WJ, Fletcher CDM, Hornick JL. Loss of expression of YAP1 C-terminus as an ancillary marker for epithelioid hemangioendothelioma variant with YAP1-TFE3 fusion and other YAP1-related vascular neoplasms. Mod Pathol 2021; 34(11):2036–42.

113. Rao V, Rekhi B. Cytomorphological spectrum, including immunohistochemical results of 16 cases of clear cell sarcoma of soft tissue, along with positive EWSR1 gene rearrangement result in two cases. Cytopathology 2020;31(4):280–7.

114. Wangsiricharoen S, Larman TC, Wakely PE Jr, et al. Cytopathology of extra-renal perivascular epithelioid cell tumor (PEComa): a series of 7 cases and review of the literature. J Am Soc Cytopathol 2021;10(2):175–86.

115. Argani P, Aulmann S, Illei PB, et al. A distinctive subset of PEComas harbors TFE3 gene fusions. Am J Surg Pathol 2010;34(10):1395–406.

116. Lopez-Ferrer P, Jimenez-Heffernan JA, Vicandi B, et al. Cytologic features of alveolar soft part sarcoma: report of three cases. Diagn Cytopathol 2002;27(2):115–9.

117. Wakely PE Jr, McDermott JE, Ali SZ. Cytopathology of alveolar soft part sarcoma: a report of 10 cases. Cancer 2009;117(6):500–7.

118. Schoolmeester JK, Lastra RR. Granular cell tumors overexpress TFE3 without corollary gene rearrangement. Hum Pathol 2015;46(8):1242–3.

119. Janeway KA, Kim SY, Lodish M, et al. Defects in succinate dehydrogenase in gastrointestinal stromal tumors lacking KIT and PDGFRA mutations. Proceedings of the National Academy of Sciences of the United States of America 2011;108(1):314–8.

120. Doyle LA, Nelson D, Heinrich MC, et al. Loss of succinate dehydrogenase subunit B (SDHB) expression is limited to a distinctive subset of gastric wild-type gastrointestinal stromal tumours: a comprehensive genotype-phenotype correlation study. Histopathology 2012;61(5):801–9.

121. Wagner AJ, Remillard SP, Zhang YX, et al. Loss of expression of SDHA predicts SDHA mutations in gastrointestinal stromal tumors. Mod Pathol : an official journal of the United States and Canadian Academy of Pathology, Inc. 2013;26(2):289–94.

122. Mason EF, Hornick JL. Conventional Risk Stratification Fails to Predict Progression of Succinate Dehydrogenase-deficient Gastrointestinal Stromal Tumors: A Clinicopathologic Study of 76 Cases. Am J Surg Pathol 2016;40(12):1616–21.

123. Marino-Enriquez A, Wang WL, Roy A, et al. Epithelioid inflammatory myofibroblastic sarcoma: An aggressive intra-abdominal variant of inflammatory myofibroblastic tumor with nuclear membrane or perinuclear ALK. Am J Surg Pathol 2011;35(1):135–44.

124. Lee JC, Wu JM, Liau JY, et al. Cytopathologic features of epithelioid inflammatory myofibroblastic sarcoma with correlation of histopathology, immunohistochemistry, and molecular cytogenetic analysis. Cancer cytopathology 2015;123(8): 495–504.

125. Gronchi A, Collini P, Miceli R, et al. Myogenic differentiation and histologic grading are major prognostic determinants in retroperitoneal liposarcoma. Am J Surg Pathol 2015;39(3):383–93.

126. Butrynski JE, D'Adamo DR, Hornick JL, et al. Crizotinib in ALK-rearranged inflammatory myofibroblastic tumor. N Engl J Med 2010;363(18): 1727–33.

127. Schöffski P, Sufliarsky J, Gelderblom H, et al. Crizotinib in patients with advanced, inoperable inflammatory myofibroblastic tumours with and without anaplastic lymphoma kinase gene alterations (European Organisation for Research and Treatment of Cancer 90101 CREATE): a multicentre, single-drug, prospective, non-randomised phase 2 trial. Lancet Respir Med 2018;6(6):431–41.

128. Group GSTM-A. Comparison of Two Doses of Imatinib for the Treatment of Unresectable or Metastatic Gastrointestinal Stromal Tumors: A Meta-Analysis of 1,640 Patients. J Clin Oncol 2010; 28(7):1247–53.

129. National Comprehensive Cancer Network. NCCN Clinical Practice Guidelines in Oncology: Gastrointestinal Stromal Tumors. In. Version 1.2023 ed2023.

130. Comandini D, Catalano F, Grassi M, et al. Outstanding Response in a Patient With ROS1-Rearranged Inflammatory Myofibroblastic Tumor of Soft Tissues Treated With Crizotinib: Case Report. Front Oncol 2021;11:658327.

131. Gelderblom H, Wagner AJ, Tap WD, et al. Long-term outcomes of pexidartinib in tenosynovial giant cell tumors. Cancer 2021;127(6):884–93.

132. Grünwald V, Karch A, Schuler M, et al. Randomized Comparison of Pazopanib and Doxorubicin as First-Line Treatment in Patients With Metastatic Soft Tissue Sarcoma Age 60 Years or Older: Results of a German Intergroup Study. J Clin Oncol 2020;38(30):3555–64.

133. Stacchiotti S, Negri T, Libertini M, et al. Sunitinib malate in solitary fibrous tumor (SFT). Ann Oncol 2012;23(12):3171–9.

134. Valentin T, Fournier C, Penel N, et al. Sorafenib in patients with progressive malignant solitary fibrous tumors: a subgroup analysis from a phase II study of the French Sarcoma Group (GSF/GETO). Invest New Drugs 2013;31(6):1626–7.

135. Wagner AJ, Ravi V, Riedel RF, et al. Phase II Trial of nab-Sirolimus in Patients With Advanced Malignant Perivascular Epithelioid Cell Tumors (AMPECT): Long-Term Efficacy and Safety Update. J Clin Oncol 2024Jco2302266. https://doi.org/10.1200/JCO.23.02266.

136. Gounder M, Schöffski P, Jones RL, et al. Tazemetostat in advanced epithelioid sarcoma with loss of INI1/SMARCB1: an international, open-label, phase 2 basket study. Lancet Oncol 2020;21(11):1423–32.

137. Shulman DS, DuBois SG. The Evolving Diagnostic and Treatment Landscape of NTRK-Fusion-Driven Pediatric Cancers. Paediatr Drugs 2020;22(2):189–97.

138. Hanrahan AJ, Chen Z, Rosen N, et al. BRAF - a tumour-agnostic drug target with lineage-specific dependencies. Nat Rev Clin Oncol 2024;21(3):224–47.

139. Doyle LA, Nowak JA, Nathenson MJ, et al. Characteristics of mismatch repair deficiency in sarcomas. Mod Pathol 2019;32(7):977–87.

140. Lam SW, Kostine M, de Miranda N, et al. Mismatch repair deficiency is rare in bone and soft tissue tumors. Histopathology 2021;79(4):509–20.

The Current and Future Impact of Lymph Node Fine-Needle Aspiration Cytology on Patient Care

Elisabetta Maffei, MD[a], Angela D'Ardia, BS[a],
Valeria Ciliberti, MD[b], Bianca Serio, MD[c],
Francesco Sabbatino, MD[d], Pio Zeppa, MD, PhD[a],*,
Alessandro Caputo, MD[a]

KEYWORDS

- Lymph node • FNAC • Triage • ROSE • Ancillary techniques • Core-needle biopsy
- Molecular testing • Classification

Key points

- Lymph node fine-needle aspiration cytology (LN-FNAC) has a triaging role in the identification of benign, suspicious, and malignant lymphadenopathies. LN-FNAC can indicate the surveillance for reactive cases and core-needle biopsy (CNB) or surgical biopsy for suspicious or primary malignant lymphadenopathies. Combined FNAC and CNB in one setting enhances the advantages of both the techniques producing definitive and actionable diagnoses.

- Rapid on-site evaluation enhances the efficiency of LN-FNAC through the immediate repetition of inadequate cases, indications in management of diagnostic material, and the choice of appropriate ancillary tests to perform.

- Molecular testing on lymph node metastases is routinely used on cytologic samples and next generation sequencing (NGS) technology has further increased their application. LN-FNAC allows molecular assessment of LN metastases to obtain information for treatment and other predictive purposes.

ABSTRACT

Lymph node (LN) fine-needle aspiration cytology (FNAC) is a common diagnostic procedure for lymphadenopathies. Despite the qualities and potentialities of LN-FNAC, the number of possible pathologies and the variety of clinical contexts represent a challenge and require a continuous upgrading of the procedure according to the emerging clinical requests and new technologies. This study presents an overview of the current and future impact of LN-FNAC on the care of patients with lymphadenopathy.

OVERVIEW

Since the pioneering studies of the last century,[1,2] lymph node (LN) fine-needle aspiration cytology (FNAC) has been routinely used to diagnose lymphadenopathies caused by different pathologies, in different clinical contexts. In fact, the applications of LN-FNAC span from infectious to neoplastic processes and from palpable up to deep-seated LNs, approached by palpation, US or EUS/EBUS guide. Hundreds of studies have assessed that LN-FNAC is an accurate, safe, effective, cheap, and well-tolerated diagnostic procedure for the diagnosis

[a] Pathology Department, University Hospital "San Giovanni di Dio e Ruggi d'Aragona", Salerno, Italy; [b] Department of Advanced Biomedical Sciences, Pathology Unit, University of Naples Federico II, Naples, Italy; [c] Haematology Department, University Hospital "San Giovanni di Dio e Ruggi d'Aragona", Salerno, Italy; [d] Oncology Department, University Hospital "San Giovanni di Dio e Ruggi d'Aragona", Salerno, Italy
* Corresponding author. Department of Pathology, University Hospital "San Giovanni di Dio e Ruggi d'Aragona", Largo città d'Ippocrate n.1, Salerno 84100, Italy.
E-mail address: pzeppa@unisa.it

Surgical Pathology 17 (2024) 509–519
https://doi.org/10.1016/j.path.2024.04.010
1875-9181/24/© 2024 Elsevier Inc. All rights are reserved, including those for text and data mining, AI training, and similar technologies.

- LN-FNAC guidelines, classification, and reporting: the Sydney System and the near to be published World Health Organization (WHO) System for Reporting Lymph Node Cytopathology classify LN-FNAC into 5 basic categories: inadequate/insufficient, benign, atypical, suspicious, and malignant providing a standardized and useful report system.

- High-throughput sequencing will probably utilized in the diagnosis of NHL. LN-FNAC may have a role in this procedure through the harvest of up to 40 ng of high-quality DNA suitable for whole exome or genome sequencing.

- Digital cytology promises to be conveniently utilized on LN-FNAC. Furthermore, telecytology will allow quick, cheap, and safe circulation of slides worldwide, including LN-FNAC slides.

of reactive processes, lymphoma, and metastases.[3–11] Moreover, LN-FNAC provides samples that are suitable for different ancillary techniques, especially for molecular testing.[11,12] Above all, LN-FNAC, due to its flexibility, speed of execution, and integration with different clinical contexts, represents a bridge between clinic and pathology, as foreseen by the first studies that defined FNAC as "clinical cytology," including LN-FNAC.[2] In this review, an overview of the current and future impact of LN-FNAC on patient care is reported.

THE CURRENT IMPACT OF LYMPH NODE FINE-NEEDLE ASPIRATION CYTOLOGY ON PATIENT CARE

TRIAGING ROLE

Lymph nodes may become enlarged for different reasons in extremely variable clinical presentations. In much of the cases, the link between clinical evidence of benign conditions and corresponding lymphadenopathies is straightforward and does not require a direct diagnosis on the enlarged LN; in other cases, mainly in adults and elderly patients, the causes of LN enlargements may be not clear or unique hence their direct evaluation may be necessary. Lymph node excision and histologic control are the gold standard for this purpose, followed by core-needle biopsy (CNB) when available and feasible. However, these procedures are longer and more expensive than LN-FNAC and more demanding for the patients; moreover, LN excision may result in oversized reactive processes. In this perspective, LN-FNAC is often used for triaging lymphadenopathies, distinguishing with high sensitivity and specificity reactive lymphadenopathies to be followed up clinically from neoplastic lymphadenopathies to be further diagnosed by CNB or excision.[13–15]

RAPID ON-SITE EVALUATION

Rapid on-site evaluation (ROSE) can be performed on air-dried smears, immediately stained with Diff-Quik and observed microscopically[8,11,12,16–18]

(Fig. 1). The whole procedure takes a few minutes from the smearing to the microscopic evaluation and represents the fastest, most effective, and easiest microscopic diagnostic procedure. ROSE can avoid a final diagnosis of inadequate by allowing immediate repetition of inadequate passes[8,11]; ROSE is also the first step for the management of residual diagnostic material and ancillary techniques.[3,8,11] Advantages of ROSE have been conveniently exploited on touch imprints of surgical samples and biopsies requested for frozen sections.[19] The main disadvantage of ROSE is its cost in terms of time and the lack of rewarding in many institutions.[8,11]

ANCILLARY TESTING AND MANAGEMENT OF CYTOLOGIC MATERIAL

Differently from other organs investigated by FNAC, LN-FNAC needs ancillary techniques more frequently for accurate diagnoses. To achieve accurate diagnoses, mainly in cases of lymphoma but also in hyperplasia to be differentiated from non-Hodgkin lymphoma (NHL) and metastases to assess their origin, ancillary techniques are necessary and effective in most cases. The most common procedures are flow-cytometry (FC), immunocytochemistry (ICC), and molecular testing including clonality testing and fluorescent in-situ hybridization (FISH).[3,6,8–11,15–18,20–26] However, these techniques are differently effective depending on the different pathologic processes (reactive, Hodgkin lymphoma, NHL, and metastases) and are performed on different technical supports ranging from additional smears, suspension of vital cells in buffered solutions, cell-blocks, or other supports. Therefore, the management of LN-FNAC material and the choice of the ancillary technique that fits with specific diagnostic requests is crucial (see Fig. 1).

COMBINED FINE-NEEDLE ASPIRATION CYTOLOGY AND CORE-NEEDLE BIOPSY IN ONE SETTING

Despite its association with ROSE and ancillary techniques, LN-FNAC may be insufficient to reach an actionable diagnosis in many pathologies, especially those which require large ICC panels or those in which the study of histologic/architectural features is mandatory. CNB may provide tissue architectural details and sufficient material for ancillary studies. CNB is generally performed by radiologists and clinicians, lacking in this way information obtained by FNAC and ROSE. Performing LN-FNAC, ROSE, and CNB in the same setting may overcome these limitations (see **Fig. 1**; **Fig. 2**).[13,14,27–29] Patients eligible for CNB are selected according to specific requests from clinicians or cytopathologists after FNAC and ROSE. Criteria for CNB selection are LN diameter of 20 mm or greater; lesion being accessible by palpation or by US guide; distance from large vessels of 10 mm or greater; and absence of evidence of hemorrhage or necrosis at ROSE. CNB procedures are generally performed using needles of different gauges after disinfection and local anesthesia.[13,14,27–29] CNB samples are fixed in formalin and embedded in paraffin according to standard techniques.[8,12,13,29,30] The combined LN-FNAC/CNB approach may represent an alternative to surgical excision for reaching a definitive diagnosis[13,27–30] because this method produces a formal histologic report with indication of the specific pathologic process in most cases. An accurate classification of NHL has been reported up to 81% of cases[3,13,28–30] (see **Figs. 1** and **2**), being equally effective for both initial diagnoses and relapses.

MOLECULAR TESTING ON LYMPH NODE METASTASES

Molecular tests are routinely used on cytologic samples,[3,5,16,17,20,21,24,25,31] and the introduction of NGS technology has further increased their application.[3,16,22,24,26,32] Although CNB has decreased the use of FNAC in specific organs such as the breast, lung, and liver, FNAC is still widely used as it allows to sample small or multiple lesions and harvest tumoral cells with minimal contamination of stroma and other tissues when compared to CNB.[3] From a clinical point of view, advanced-stage patients can tolerate neither invasive biopsies nor prolonged times for target therapies therefore these cases benefit from the qualities of FNAC. Moreover, FNAC has been simultaneously utilized on primary tumor and concomitant metastasis to compare the possible differences in molecular profile.[20] Molecular testing has been mainly performed on thyroid, pancreas, lung tumors, and melanoma.[17,22,24,26,32] However, since LNs are frequent sites of metastases, molecular testing on LN-FNAC is used in early or advanced neoplasms. LN-FNAC coupled with molecular techniques is an ideal technique also for longitudinal tracking of tumors and their molecular profile, including drug resistance and other molecular features useful for predictive purposes (**Fig. 3**). Regarding sample adequacy, 1 or 2 LN-FNACs can easily harvest 40 ng or greater of DNA, which is sufficient for a complete molecular profiling.[7]

THE FUTURE IMPACT OF LYMPH NODE FINE-NEEDLE ASPIRATION CYTOLOGY ON PATIENT CARE

LYMPH NODE FINE-NEEDLE ASPIRATION CYTOLOGY GUIDELINES, CLASSIFICATION, AND REPORTING

Despite high values of sensitivity, specificity, and accuracy, LN-FNAC is not uniformly accepted by

Fig. 1. Proposed flowchart for LN-FNAC, rapid on-site evaluation, ancillary techniques, and CNB in one setting.

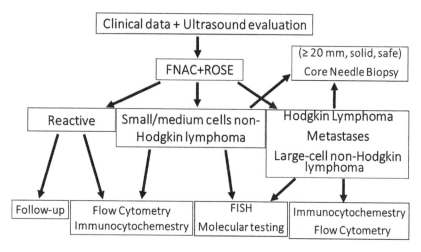

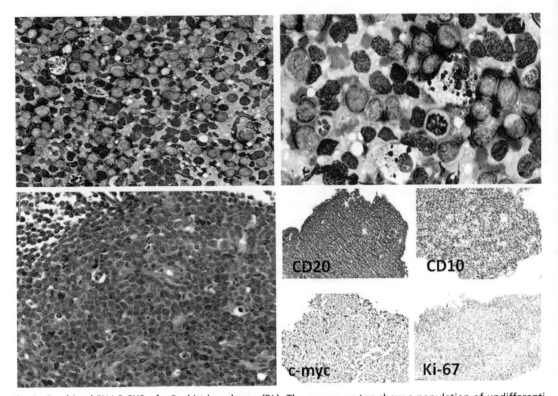

Fig. 2. Combined FNAC-CNB of a Burkitt lymphoma (BL). The smears on top show a population of undifferentiated, monomorphous, medium size cells with dense, coarse chromatin and inconspicuous nucleoli. Numerous mitoses are present (*upper left*) and scattered macrophages confer a starry sky appearance. The CNB histologic features, on the bottom, show the same undifferentiated cells with scattered macrophages. The IHC demonstrates diffuse positivity for CD20, C10, c-myc, and a high proliferative rate (Ki67 >90% of the cells).

clinicians and pathologists.[30] This was mainly due to the lack of shared and accepted guidelines and a cytopathological classification that directly relates to the management of corresponding lymphadenopathies. In 2020, a system for performance, classification, and reporting for LN-FNAC was proposed and termed the Sydney system.[30] This system provides indications for essential clinical data evaluation, LN-FNAC, technical procedures, and ancillary techniques with specific recommendations. The Sydney system then proposes to report LN-FNAC on 2 diagnostic levels. The first level includes 5 categories: inadequate/insufficient, benign, atypical, suspicious, and malignant; for each category, specific recommendations are provided. The second diagnostic level, when achievable, indicates the specific benign or malignant entity responsible for the lymphadenopathy. The Sydney system will be merged in the near to be published World Health Organization (WHO) Reporting System for Lymph Node, Spleen, and Thymus Cytopathology, which classifies LN-FNAC in the same basic 5 diagnostic categories plus a second diagnostic level when possible. Classification and recommendations for LN-

FNAC are summarized in **Table 1**. The risk of malignancy for each diagnostic category has been retrospectively evaluated in different studies[5]; a relatively high ROM for the inadequate category and a very high ROM for atypical, suspicious, and malignant categories have also been reported. However, the number of atypical and suspicious, in the evaluated series, was largely influenced by the application or the lack of ancillary techniques. Further studies with application of guidelines and diagnostic criteria are needed to homogenize the results of different laboratory tests. The LN-FNAC classification system may lead to a greater acceptance and utilization of LN-FNAC and to a better interdisciplinary communication and understanding of corresponding results.

MOLECULAR CYTOPATHOLOGY FOR LYMPHOMAS

The diagnosis of lymphoma by LN-FNAC represents the most controversial issue of LN-FNAC.[11,30] The ever-expanding complexity of NHL classification, ROSE indispensability but not

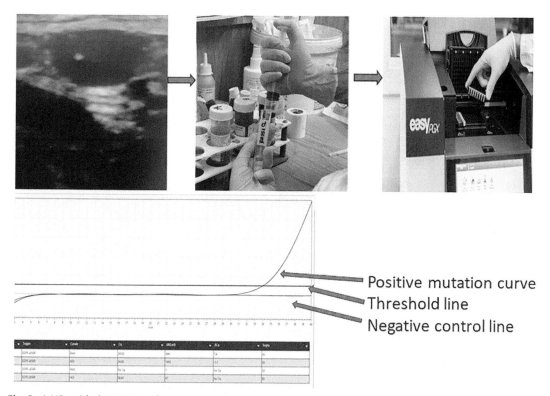

Fig. 3. A US-guided LN-FNAC of a metastasis from lung adenocarcinoma was utilized for DNA extraction and for the detection of gene mutations. A real-time PCR was processed and a point mutation of epidermal growth factor receptor (EGFR), namely p.L8R8R was identified (*arrows*).

always reliable, the necessity of standardized ancillary techniques and the loss of archival material for research are the main impediments to LN-FNAC as first-line or sole approach to NHL (and some reactive) diagnoses.[11,30] Traditionally, FISH and polymerase chain reaction (PCR)-based techniques are utilized to assess the clonality of lymphoproliferative processes and chromosomal alterations (translocations and deletions) that are specific to some NHLs; FISH and PCR are successfully utilized on LN-FNAC samples too.[3,9,33,34] Moreover, through the application of high-throughput sequencing (HTS) to LN pathology many improvements are foreseeable in the understanding, diagnosis, and treatment of NHL.[35–39] It is predictable that, applying HTS to LN-FNAC samples, the efficacy and accuracy of the procedure will increase and even the role of LN-FNAC in the management of NHL might change. In fact, chromosomal alterations, single nucleotide variants, and immunoglobulin (IG) / T-cell receptor (TR) clonality, which are traditionally evaluated by single tests, and are hardly performed in sequence on cytologic samples, can be evaluated in a single test. For instance, chromosomal alterations, detected by cytogenetics, may be useful or indispensable to identify certain NHL, and FISH is

most often used to detect chromosomal translocations and deletions. FISH can be successfully used on cytologic samples, but it is performed one test per sample, and an analysis spanning on all the possible chromosomal abnormalities, mainly on limited samples like LN-FNAC is almost impossible. Clonality assessment of IG and TR loci rearrangements is a basic information mainly obtained by PCR-based analyses, but they are single tests, which require their own technology and material that are not always performable in combination with other tests on LN-FNAC samples.[33,34] Single nucleotide variants detected by HTS mainly produce prognostic and predictive information on specific pathologic entities also useful for diagnosis and about the cell origin of lymphomas. For instance, TP53 mutations are unfavorable prognostic occurrence in chronic lymphocytic leukemia/small lymphocytic lymphoma (CLL/SLL) or enhancer of zeste homolog 2 (EZH2) mutation that occurs in 15% to 30% of follicular lymphomas has a prognostic value and is predictive of response to EZH2 inhibitors. Regarding the potential contribution of HTS to the diagnosis of NHL, there are mutations that are indicative of few NHLs or specific for single entities such as proto-oncogene B-Raf (BRAF) V600 E mutation for hairy

Table 1
Lymph node fine-needle aspiration cytology classification according to the Sydney system and the World Health Organization system for reporting lymph node cytopathology

Diagnostic Classes and 1° Diagnostic Level (Clinic, US, Cytology Ancillary Techniques)	Description	2° Diagnostic Level (Clinic, US, Cytology Ancillary Techniques)	Recommendations
L1 Inadequate/insufficient	Cases that cannot be diagnosed due to scant cellularity, extensive necrosis, or technical limitations	—	Repeat LN-FNAC with immunophenotyping, preferably by FC, required
L2 Negative hyperplasia, suppurative, granulomatous	Heterogeneous lymphoid cells, small lymphocytes, germinal center cells, dendritic cells, tingible body macrophages. Process diagnosable as reactive with or without FC or ICC. Suppurative, granulomatous	Etiology, specific processes (mononucleosis, TBC, and so forth)	Repeat FNAC, preferably with FC and cytogenetics, or CNB or excisional biopsy regardless of clinical and US findings
L3 Atypical Atypical lymphoid (cells) of uncertain significance/atypical (cells) undetermined of significance (ALUS/AUS)	ALUS: heterogeneous lymphoid population whose features suggest a reactive process, but an NHL cannot be excluded, AUS: presence of atypical cells that may be not lymphoid	—	Repeat FNAC, preferably with FC and cytogenetics, or CNB or excisional biopsy is required regardless of clinical and US findings
L4 Suspicious	Small or medium-sized, atypical lymphoid cells suspicious of NHL, but the cytomorphology alone is not sufficient for diagnosis; or the presence of rare Hodgkin-like or Reed-Sternberg-like cells not sufficient for diagnosis; or atypical cells suspicious for metastasis are present but are too scant to be diagnostic	—	Repeating FNAC or CNB or excisional biopsy
L5 Malignant (lymphoma, metastasis)	—	Specific entities (SLL/CLL, FL, MCL, DLBCL, BL, PTCL, and so forth)	Histologic confirmation for primary NHL and metastases NOS, actionable diagnoses in cases of NHL relapses and identified primary tumors

High throughpout sequencing of 125 genes panel for lymphomas and oncohematological diseases

AICDA	CBFB	CREBBP **X**	FGFR1	LZTS1	NRAS	RANBP1	
AKT3	CCDC50	CTLA4	FOXP1	MAL	P2RY8	RHOA	
ALK	CCND1	CYB5R2	FUT8	MALT1	PAICS	S1PR2	
ASB13	CCND2	DEK	IDH1	MAML3	PDCD1	SERPINA9	
BATF3	CCND3	DENND3	IDH2	MKL1	PDCD1LG2	SF3B1	
BAX	CD274	DLEU1	IL16	MLF1	PDGFRA	SH3BP5	
BCL2 **X**	CD44	DNMT3A	IRF4	MLLT10	PIM1	STAT3	
BCL2A1	CD79B	DNMT3B	IRF8 **X**	MME	PIM2	STAT5B	
BCL3	CDC25A	DNTT	ITPKB	MUC1	PLCG1	STAT6 **X**	
BCL6 **X**	CDK6	DUSP22	JAK1	MYBL1	PLCG2	STIL	
BCR	CDKN2A	E2F2	JAK2	MYC **X**	PPAT	STRBP	
BIRC3	CDKN2B	EIF4A1	JAK3	MYD88 **X**	PRDM16	TCF3	
BLNK	CEBPD	ENTPD1	KIAA0101	NEK6	PRKAR2B	TNFRSF13B **X**	
BMF	CEBPE	ETV6	KMT2A	NFKB1	PTPN1	TNFSF4	
BMP7	CEBPG	EXOC2	KRAS	NFKB2	PYCR1	TP63 **X**	
BRAF **X**	CHIC2	EZH2 **X**	LIMD1	NME1	RAB29	WT1	
BTK	CIITA	FAM216A	LMO2	NOTCH1	RAG1	XPO1	
CARD11 **X**	CREB3L2	FBXW7	LRMP	NOTCH2 **X**	RAG2		

MCL KLF2, NOTCH2, PTPRD, CARD11, IRF8. **FL** CREBBP, EZH2, TNFRSF13, STAT6.
HCL **BRAF.** **CLL/SLL** TP53, TP63. **LPL** MYD88. **DLBCL** MYC, BCL2, BCL6.

Legend
- ◆ SNV or indel
- ▢ Expression
- ● Fusion, splicing or exon skipping

Fig. 4. High throughput sequencing of 125 genes panel for lymphomas and oncohematological diseases is herein reported. The rearrangements and point mutations, commonly observed in specific entities, are marked by X; BRAF and MYD88 are exclusive for HCL and LPL, respectively (X reported in *bold*). CLL/SLL, chronic lymphocytic leukemia/small lymphocytic lymphoma; DLBCL, diffuse, large, B-cell lymphoma; FL, follicular lymphoma; HCL, hairy cell leukemia; LPL, lymphoplasmacytic lymphoma; MCL, mantle cell lymphoma.

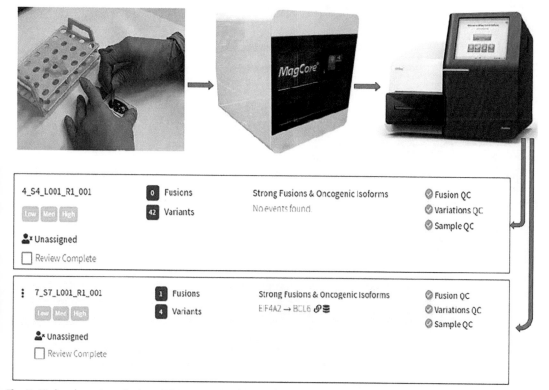

Fig. 5. Molecular cytopathology RNA extraction from Diff-Quik stained LN-FNAC. A sequencing of 125 genes was processed using NGS Illumina (Miseq) (5200 Illumina Way, San Diego, CA 92122 U.S.A.). Two analyses are reported on the bottom: no variations emerged from the analysis of the first sample; the second one showed BCL6 gene fusion with an uncommon partner.

cell leukemia or myeloid differentiation primary response 88 (MYD88)-L265 mutation for lymphoplasmacytic lymphoma (**Fig. 4**). While phenotyping by ICC or FC allows an accurate classification of most small-cell NHLs, there is a definite percentage of cases in which NHL cells do not express specific antigens or those suitable for classification are not expressed. For instance, CD5-negative, CD10-negative, BCL2-negative small B-cell NHL may represent marginal lymphoma (MZL), or BCL2–negative follicular lymphoma (FL), or even hairy cell leukemia. In these cases, BCL6 rearrangement or 1p36 deletion favor FL. Mutations of KLF2, NOTCH2, PTPRD, CARD11, and IRF8 favor MZL[36,40]; CREB binding protein (CREBBP), EZH2, TNF receptor superfamily member 13B (TNFRSF13), and signal transducer and activator of transcription 6 (STAT6) mutation favor BCL2–negative FL[37] (**Fig. 5**). In peripheral T-cell lymphoma (PTCL), mutations and small indels in genes are often found[38,39]; HTS demonstration of

genomic alterations may be useful to assess clonality and support the diagnosis. The classification of diffuse, large B-cell lymphoma (DLBCL) according to the cell of origin (between activated B-cell–like and germinal center B-cell–like subtypes) can be performed either by gene expression profiling or by surrogate immunohistochemistry (IHC), but it is predictable that target therapies for DLBCL will require the incorporation of genetic profiling by whole exome sequencing (WES) or whole genome sequencing (WGS) analysis of MYC proto-oncogene (MYC), BCL2, and BCL6 rearrangements. Therefore, HTS will be an integral part in the diagnosis and genetic profiling of NHL through the evaluation of up to 200 to 250 genes, and LN-FNAC may have a role starting from 1 or 2 passes that may contain up to 40 ng of high-quality DNA suitable for WES/WGS. The limitation of molecular tests in lymphomas is the high cost of the method; in our laboratory, it is estimated that a single complete profiling costs approximately 600

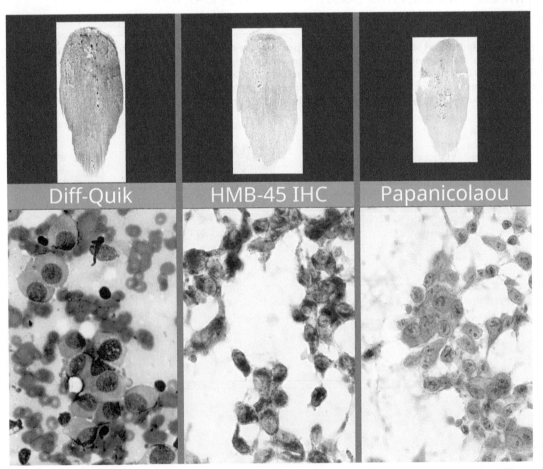

Fig. 6. A virtual slide tray composed of 3 WSIs depicting smears from a LN-FNAC showing metastatic malignant melanoma. These slides can be shared worldwide immediately and without the risks and costs associated with moving slides or pathologists. Left: Diff-Quik, middle: HMB-45 diaminobenzidine immunohistochemistry, and right: Papanicolaou. Magnifications: × 1 (*top*) and × 400 (*bottom*).

euros, even if it is foreseeable that the costs will decrease with time.

DIGITAL CYTOLOGY

Telepathology and digital pathology have shown their promise in histology and are here to stay[41]; nonetheless, technical issues have slowed down their application to cytologic preparations.[42] Nowadays, slide scanners are capable of producing diagnostic whole-slide images (WSIs) of cytologic preparations[4] and cytology is rapidly adopting these innovations. Telecytology, for example, allows the remote examination of a slide. This has far-reaching implications: ROSE can be performed off-site, saving precious pathologist time,[43] and cytology slides can be circulated worldwide without costs, risks, or delay (Fig. 6).[4,44] In parallel, WSIs are the optimal substrate for artificial intelligence-based techniques, allowing computer-aided diagnosis. Cytology, more than histology, was the first discipline to seek computer assistance to alleviate the heavy screening workloads.[42,45] Today, numerous tools are available to lessen the workload on histopathologists, for instance by automatically detecting LN (micro)metastases, detecting and grading prostate cancer,[46] counting mitoses,[47] and detecting *Helicobacter pylori*.[41,48,49] Several tasks in the routine practice of cytology can benefit from computer-aided diagnosis tools, making the cytologist both faster and more accurate. Urine cytology, for example, can be screened by algorithms that highlight, and optionally extract, suspicious cells for review by a pathologist.[50] Similar tools can be used for other use-cases, such as cervicovaginal[51] and thyroid[52] cytology.

CLINICS CARE POINTS

- Accurate diagnosis of specific entities.
- Molecular assessment for target therapies.

DISCLOSURE

The authors have not to disclose.

REFERENCES

1. Meatheringhm RE, Ackerman LV. Aspiration biopsy of lymph nodes; a critical review of the results of 300 aspirations. Surg Gynecol Obstet 1947;84(6): 1071–1076.11.
2. Zajicek J. 1 Introduction to aspiration biopsy. Monogr Clin Cytol 1974;4(0):1–211.
3. Krishnamurthy S. Applications of molecular techniques to fine-needle aspiration biopsy. Cancer 2007;111(2):106–22.
4. Caputo A, Fraggetta F, Cretella P, et al. Digital Examination of LYmph node CYtopathology Using the Sydney system (DELYCYUS). An international, multi-institutional study. Cancer Cytopathol 2023. https://doi.org/10.1002/cncy.22741.
5. Caputo A, Ciliberti V, D'Antonio A, et al. Real-world experience with the Sydney System on 1458 cases of lymph node fine needle aspiration cytology. Cytopathology 2022;33(2):166–75.
6. Cozzolino I, Vitagliano G, Caputo A, et al. CD15, CD30, and PAX5 evaluation in Hodgkin's lymphoma on fine-needle aspiration cytology samples. Diagn Cytopathol 2020;48(3):211–6.
7. Cozzolino I, Giudice V, Mignogna C, et al. Lymph node fine-needle cytology in the era of personalised medicine. Is there a role? Cytopathology 2019;30(4):348–62.
8. Da Cunha Santos G, Saieg MA, Troncone G, et al. Cytological preparations for molecular analysis: A review of technical procedures, advantages and limitations for referring samples for testing. Cytopathology 2018;29(2):125–32.
9. Peluso AL, Cozzolino I, Bottiglieri A, et al. Immunoglobulin heavy and light chains and T-cell receptor beta and gamma chains PCR assessment on cytological samples. A study comparing FTA cards and cryopreserved lymph node fine-needle cytology. Cytopathology 2017;28(3):203–15.
10. Cozzolino I, Varone V, Picardi M, et al. CD10, BCL6, and MUM1 expression in diffuse large B-cell lymphoma on FNA samples. Cancer Cytopathol 2016; 124(2):135–43.
11. Barroca H, Bode-Lesniewska B, Cozzolino I, et al. Management of cytologic material, preanalytic procedures and biobanking in lymph node cytopathology. Cytopathology 2019;30(1):17–30.
12. Da Cunha Santos G, Ko HM, Saieg MA, et al. "The petals and thorns" of ROSE (rapid on-site evaluation). Cancer Cytopathol 2013;121(1):4–8.
13. Shyu S, Rajgariah A, Saoud C, et al. Image-guided lymph node fine-needle aspiration: the Johns Hopkins Hospital experience. J Am Soc Cytopathol 2021;10(6):543–57.
14. Joudeh AA, Shareef SQ, Al-Abbadi MA. Fine-needle aspiration followed by core-needle biopsy in the same setting: Modifying our approach. Acta Cytol 2016;60(1):1–13.
15. Shah A, Ross C, Sur M. An approach to small lymph node biopsies: Pearls and pitfalls of reporting in the real world. Journal of the American Society of Cytopathology 2021;10(3):328–37.
16. Bailey GE, Maleki Z. Supraclavicular lymph nodes: An easily accessible site for diagnosis and molecular profiling of malignancies in the era of precision medicine. Diagn Cytopathol 2023;51(11):689–97.

17. D'Ardia A, Caputo A, Fumo R, et al. Advanced non-small cell lung cancer: Rapid evaluation of EGFR status on fine-needle cytology samples using Idylla. Pathol Res Pract 2021 Aug;224:153547.

18. Peluso AL, Ieni A, Mignogna C, et al. Lymph Node Fine-Needle Cytology: Beyond Flow Cytometry. Acta Cytol 2016;60(4):372–84.

19. Bharath S, Sharma D, Yadav SK, et al. A Systematic Review and Meta-analysis of Touch Imprint Cytology and Frozen Section Biopsy and Their Comparison for Evaluation of Sentinel Lymph Node in Breast Cancer. World J Surg 2023;47(2):478–88.

20. Li R, Hao J, Zhu Z, et al. Correlation between US-FNAC withBRAF V600E Mutation Analysis and Central Neck Lymph Node Metastasis in cN0 Papillary Thyroid Cancer. BioMed Res Int 2021;2021:9937742.

21. Ronchi A, Montella M, Carraturo E, et al. To Get the Most out of the Least: BRAF Molecular Evaluation in Melanoma Metastases on Cell Suspension from Fine Needle Aspiration Cytology Needle Rinses. Acta Cytol 2023;67(4):357–64.

22. Pisapia P, Pepe F, Iaccarino A, et al. Next generation sequencing in cytopathology: focus on non-small cell lung cancer. Front Med 2021 Feb 11;8:633923.

23. Vigliar E, Cozzolino I, Fernandez LV, et al. Fine-needle cytology and flow cytometry assessment of reactive and lymphoproliferative processes of the breast. Acta Cytol 2012;56(2):130–8.

24. Fielding DI, Dalley AJ, Singh M, et al. Evaluating Diff-Quik cytology smears for large-panel mutation testing in lung cancer-Predicting DNA content and success with low-malignant-cellularity samples. Cancer Cytopathol 2023;131(6):373–82.

25. Vigliar E, Pepe F, Migliatico I, et al. Microfluidic chip technology applied to fine-needle aspiration cytology samples for IGH clonality assessment. Diagn Cytopathol 2019;47(8):749–57.

26. Ghabi EM, Habib JR, Shoucair S, et al. Detecting somatic mutations for well-differentiated pancreatic neuroendocrine tumors in endoscopic ultrasound-guided fine needle aspiration with next-generation sequencing. Ann Surg Oncol 2023;30(12):7720–30.

27. Torres Rivas HE, Villar Zarra K, Pérez Pabón LA, et al. Ultrasound-Guided Fine-Needle Aspiration of Superficial Lymphadenopathy Performed by Interventional Pathologists: The Applicability of the Sydney System from 2 Years of Experience and 363 Cases. Acta Cytol 2021;65(6):453–62.

28. Jelloul FZ, Navarro M, Navale P, et al. Diagnosis of lymphoma using fine-needle aspiration biopsy and core-needle biopsy: A single-institution experience. Acta Cytol 2019;63(3):198–205.

29. Ciliberti V, Maffei E, D'Ardia A, et al. Combined fine needle aspiration cytology and core needle biopsy in the same setting: A two-years' experience. Cytopathology 2024;35(1):78–91.

30. Al-Abbadi M, Barroca H, Bode-Lesniewska B, et al. Letter to the Editor: Fine- needle aspiration cytology and core-needle biopsy in the diagnosis of lymphadenopathies: Words of endorsement. Eur J Haematol 2021;107(2):295–6.

31. Caleo A, Vigliar E, Vitale M, et al. Cytological diagnosis of thyroid nodules in Hashimoto thyroiditis in elderly patients. BMC Surg 2013;13(Suppl 2):S41.

32. Zhang C, Kim RY, McGrath CM, et al. The Performance of an Extended Next Generation Sequencing Panel Using Endobronchial Ultrasound-Guided Fine Needle Aspiration Samples in Non-Squamous Non-Small Cell Lung Cancer: A Pragmatic Study. Clin Lung Cancer 2023;24(2):e105–12.

33. Vigliar E, Cozzolino I, Picardi M, et al. Lymph node fine needle cytology in the staging and follow-up of cutaneous lymphomas. BMC Cancer 2014 Jan 6;14:8.

34. Cozzolino I, Vigliar E, Todaro P, et al. Fine needle aspiration cytology of lymphoproliferative lesions of the oral cavity. Cytopathology 2014;25(4):241–9.

35. De Leval L, Alizadeh AA, Bergsagel PL, et al. Genomic profiling for clinical decision making in lymphoid neoplasms. Blood 2022;140(21):2193–227.

36. Rossi D, Bertoni F, Zucca E. Marginal-zone lymphomas. N Engl J Med 2022;386(6):568–81.

37. Nann D, Ramis-Zaldivar JE, Müller I, et al. Follicular lymphoma t(14;18)-negative is genetically a heterogeneous disease. Blood Adv 2020;4(22):5652–65.

38. Vallois D, Dobay MPD, Morin RD, et al. Activating mutations in genes related to TCR signalling in angioimmunoblastic and other follicular helper T-cell–derived lymphomas. Blood 2016;128(11):1490–502.

39. Watatani Y, Sato Y, Miyoshi H, et al. Molecular heterogeneity in peripheral T-cell lymphoma, not otherwise specified revealed by comprehensive genetic profiling. Leukemia 2019;33(12):2867–83.

40. Clipson A, Wang M, de Leval L, et al. KLF2 mutation is the most frequent somatic change in splenic marginal zone lymphoma and identifies a subset with distinct genotype. Leukemia 2015;29(5):1177–85.

41. Meroueh C, Chen ZE. Artificial intelligence in anatomical pathology: building a strong foundation for precision medicine. Hum Pathol 2023;132:31–8.

42. Pantanowitz L. Digital cytology: Look how much has been achieved. Cytopathology 2020;31(5):370–1.

43. Xing J, Monaco SE, Cuda J, et al. Telecytology rapid on-site evaluation: Diagnostic challenges, technical issues and lessons learned. Cytopathology 2020;31(5):402–10.

44. Caputo A, Macrì L, Gibilisco F, et al. Validation of full-remote reporting for cervicovaginal cytology: the Caltagirone-Acireale distributed lab. J Am Soc Cytopathol 2023;12(5):378–85.

45. Lew M, Wilbur DC, Pantanowitz L. Computational cytology: lessons learned from pap test computer-assisted screening. Acta Cytol 2021;65(4):286–300.

46. Eloy C, Marques A, Pinto J, et al. Artificial intelligence-assisted cancer diagnosis improves the efficiency of pathologists in prostatic biopsies. Virchows Arch 2023;482(3):595–604.

47. Flach RN, Fransen NL, Sonnen AFP, et al. Implementation of Artificial Intelligence in Diagnostic Practice as a Next Step after Going Digital: The UMC Utrecht Perspective. Diagnostics 2022; 12(5):1042.

48. Caputo A, D'Antonio A. Digital pathology: the future is now. Indian J Pathol Microbiol 2021; 64(1):6–7.

49. Berbís MA, McClintock DS, Bychkov A, et al. Computational pathology in 2030: a Delphi study forecasting the role of AI in pathology within the next decade. EBioMedicine 2023;88:104427.

50. Sanghvi AB, Allen EZ, Callenberg KM, et al. Performance of an artificial intelligence algorithm for reporting urine cytopathology. Cancer Cytopathol 2019;127(10):658–66.

51. Ikenberg H, Lieder S, Ahr A, et al. Comparison of the hologic genius digital diagnostics system with the thinprep imaging system-a retrospective assessment. Cancer Cytopathol 2023;131(7):424–32.

52. Dov D, Kovalsky SZ, Feng Q, et al. Use of machine learning-based software for the screening of thyroid cytopathology whole slide images. Arch Pathol Lab Med 2022;146(7):872–8.

Artificial Intelligence Applications in Cytopathology
Current State of the Art

Louis J. Vaickus, MD, PhD[a,b,]*, Darcy A. Kerr, MD[a,b],
Jaylou M. Velez Torres, MD[c], Joshua Levy, PhD[a,d]

KEYWORDS

- Cytopathology • Artificial intelligence • Machine learning • Computational pathology
- Deep learning • Artificial neural network • Convolutional neural network

---

Key points

- The initial applications of machine learning in pathology were developed in cytopathology.
- The field of computational pathology is rapidly taking shape.
- Machine learning is an effective tool for automating defined cytopathology tasks, especially the ones a human practitioner finds tedious.
- While many research articles have been published, few have progressed to clinical implementation.
- The most likely form of machine learning algorithms in pathology is semiautonomous diagnostic aids.

ABSTRACT

The practice of cytopathology has been significantly refined in recent years, largely through the creation of consensus rule sets for the diagnosis of particular specimens (Bethesda, Milan, Paris, and so forth). In general, these diagnostic systems have focused on reducing intraobserver variance, removing nebulous/redundant categories, reducing the use of "atypical" diagnoses, and promoting the use of quantitative scoring systems while providing a uniform language to communicate these results. Computational pathology is a natural offshoot of this process in that it promises 100% reproducible diagnoses rendered by quantitative processes that are free from many of the biases of human practitioners.

OVERVIEW

When people think of pathology-related artificial intelligence/machine learning (AIML), they typically consider the latest, flashy articles touting confident diagnostic predictions made on histologic sections. It is unsurprising that current research endeavors focus on these types of specimens.

---

[a] Department of Pathology and Laboratory Medicine, Dartmouth-Hitchcock Medical Center, One Medical Center Drive, Lebanon, NH 03756, USA; [b] Geisel School of Medicine at Dartmouth, Hanover, NH 03750, USA; [c] Department of Pathology and Laboratory Medicine, University of Miami Miller School of Medicine, Miami, FL 33136, USA; [d] Cedars-Sinai Medical Center, 8700 Beverly Boulevard, Los Angeles, CA 90048, USA
* Corresponding author. 1 Medical Center Drive, Lebanon, NH 03756.
E-mail address: Louis.J.Vaickus@hitchcock.org
Twitter: @darcykerrMD (D.A.K.)

Surgical Pathology 17 (2024) 521–531
https://doi.org/10.1016/j.path.2024.04.011
1875-9181/24/© 2024 Elsevier Inc. All rights reserved.

surgpath.theclinics.com

After all, whole tissue slides have the benefit of architecture, where the likelihood of finding a particular feature is directly related to its regional environment (its so-called spatial characteristics). Moreover, tissue resections are often considered to be the "ground truth" with respect to cytology specimens. Cytology preparations, conversely, are amorphous, random dispersions of cellular elements and small tissue fragments, where ratios of components and pure morphology dictate diagnoses.

It is surprising to some, therefore, that the initial applications of AIML in pathology were indeed cytology-related applications. Part of this misconception has to do with the assumption that AIML is a recent development (dating to the 2010s), and exclusively makes use of advanced deep learning algorithms. However, AIML, at its most fundamental level, is simply *a means of predicting an outcome based on rules/information learned from an initial training dataset.* Under this definition, linear regression is a form of AIML, in that the distribution of unseen data-points can be predicted based on the slope and origin of a line fit to a sample of data (training data). An unspoken rule of predictive modeling is to use the simplest algorithm that can adequately accomplish the goal; therefore, if linear regression is adequate, why bother with the complexity of deep learning? Of course, not all problems can be solved with simple models. Distilling a cytopathologist's knowledge of, for example, urine cytology, is a difficult task as that knowledge encompasses unconscious heuristics, consciously applied rules, and associations and alterations to the visual cortex so far below consciousness as to be completely inaccessible.[1,2] For tasks such as these, models must develop a semantic understanding of, for instance, what distinguishes a urothelial cell from a squamous cell. This task is easy and effortless for a trained cytopathologist, but, if one attempts to lay down a set of rules in a computer program, one immediately realizes the staggering scope of the problem; for example, what logical expression can capture the feeling that a cell "looks squamy"? Even prior to the deep learning era (beginning roughly in 2012), many attempts (some successful) were made to automate tasks that were until then the domain of human experts.

Given the earlier definition, the first such application is likely the automated cell counter. A photometric version was first described by Mercandier and colleagues in 1928 as a means of quantitating blood cells in a dilute solution.[3] This was followed by a more robust implementation utilizing electrical impedance in 1953 by Coulter, which would later become the now ubiquitous and eponymous Coulter Counter.[4] These devices take as input variation in electrical current, decode these signals through a model with statistically defined cutoffs for different cell types, and produce an output: a differential of cells present in the blood. While it is debatable whether this is a cytology application, one can at least argue that it is cytology-adjacent, in that cells without architecture are being analyzed.

The first indisputably cytology-related applications of AIML were developed for Pap smears. There were many attempts to develop morphometric algorithms for detecting atypia in these specimens dating back to the 1960s, but all failed for various reasons.[5–7] A new wave of applications was developed in the 1980s, and although the accuracy of these systems was acceptable, none were commercialized due to cost-effectiveness concerns.[8–12] A new crop of algorithms was developed in the late 1980s following the introduction of liquid-based processing (LBP, ThinPrep, Hologic, Marlborough MA) thus providing a much cleaner and more consistent slide for image analysis.[13–15] Following decades of research, technological improvements (especially in computation, digital imaging, LBP, and AIML) and industrial consolidation, the first commercial applications/devices for the semiautomated screening of Pap smears were granted Food and Drug Administration (FDA) approval and entered clinical use: BD FocalPoint (Beckton-Dickinson, Vernon Hills, IL) (formerly AutoPap 300, TriPath) FDA approved in 1996, Hologic ThinPrep (Hologic, Marlborough, MA) Imaging System (formerly Cytyc) FDA approved in 2003.[16,17] These devices quickly entered cytology practice and became indispensable in an age of increased regulatory scrutiny, particularly in regards to primary screener workload restrictions.[18,19]

The next great push for AIML in cytology came after the advent of truly modern deep learning techniques in the form of AlexNet in 2012.[20] The use of convolutional neural networks (CNNs) revolutionized the field and spurred the current explosion in applications we see everywhere from our smartphone's face identification capabilities, to the predictive text in search engines to the large language models (LLM) currently dominating public discussion of AIML.

The following discussion will examine subsequent developments, based on specimen type (gynecological [GYN], non-gynecological [NON-GYN], and fine needle aspiration [FNA]) and source (Pap, urine, cerebrospinal fluid [CSF], solid organ FNA, and so forth). The next section will discuss the scope of AIML in cytology with discussions of the various types of models employed, the levels of supervision (how much manual curation of data was performed), the domain of the data employed, and the goals of the various research groups.

BREAKDOWN OF ARTIFICIAL INTELLIGENCE/ MACHINE LEARNING PUBLICATIONS IN CYTOLOGY

A brief description of the methodology of the literature search follows. Keyword searches (eg, machine learning cytology) were performed in PubMed over all available dates (with the caveat that AIML articles published before the mid-2000s are rare). Multiple keyword searches were performed using different combinations of keywords. Articles were selected based on their relevance to cytology. After a list of anatomic locations was generated from the primary search, a secondary search was performed using these locations in isolation paired with 3 key phrases ("machine learning," "deep learning," and "artificial intelligence"). Finally, anatomic locations that were not identified in the prior search but that are common in cytology (salivary, head and neck, lymph node, liver, and so forth) as well as general terms (cancer, adenocarcinoma, squamous cell carcinoma, and so forth) were searched independently with the earlier mentioned key phrases. Preprints (eg, arXiv) were excluded as were all other nonpeer reviewed sources. Articles concerning coronavirus disease 2019 (COVID-19) were excluded due to the high incidence of low quality and fraudulent articles in this space. Studies using proprietary algorithms with insufficiently detailed methods were excluded. In total, 89 articles were identified.

The breakdown of specimen sources (**Fig. 1**) shows that 26 articles (∼29%) were GYN focused and 64 (∼71%) were NONGYN. The rate of new publications in the cytology AIML space has increased over time, especially in the late 2010s (**Fig. 2**).

The types of machine learning models employed in these studies included 4 main categories: classification, segmentation, segmentation and classification, and dimensionality reduction. These 4 tasks are summarized in **Table 1**.

TYPES OF MODELS

Classification

This was by far the most common task performed in the identified studies. In classification, the goal is to predict whether an item from a dataset (eg, an image of a cell) belongs to a certain group or class, where there are at least 2 classes. For instance, in cervical cytology, if one was to train a cell type classification model, the desired classes might be squamous cell, inflammatory cell, glandular cell, infectious organism, and so forth. The types of classification models included a mixture of binary (2 classes) and multiclass (3 or more classes) implementations.

Segmentation

Whereas classification models aim to provide a class for an image (eg, a whole cell), segmentation models aim to determine a class for every pixel in a given image. For instance, if a researcher wanted to train a model to determine the nuclear to cytoplasmic (NC) ratio of a given cell, the model would first need to know which pixels correspond to nucleus, which correspond to cytoplasm, and which correspond to background. The output of a segmentation model is often referred to as a mask (**Fig. 3**). From this information, a pixel-wise

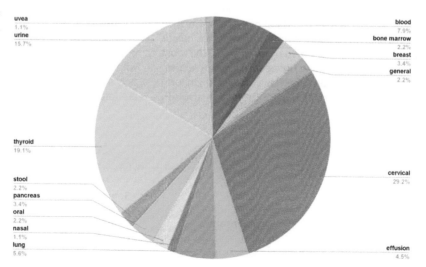

Fig. 1. Breakdown of AIML publication frequency by specimen source.

uvea 1.1%
urine 15.7%
blood 7.9%
bone marrow 2.2%
breast 3.4%
general 2.2%
thyroid 19.1%
cervical 29.2%
stool 2.2%
pancreas 3.4%
oral 2.2%
nasal 1.1%
lung 5.6%
effusion 4.5%

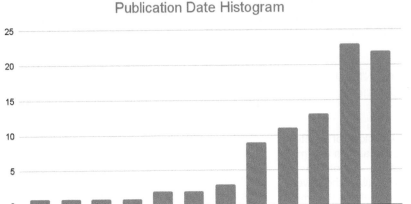

Fig. 2. AIML publication frequency in cytology over time.

calculation could be performed by dividing the number of nucleus pixels by the sum of nucleus and cytoplasm pixels. The complexity of analysis performed in the cited literature ranges from simple (eg, which pixels are part of cells, which are background) to more complicated analyses.

Segmentation and Classification

A subset of articles (~5%) performed both segmentation and classification. In the articles cited, the segmentation model was used to first identify the areas of interest (eg, squamous cells in a Pap smear), which were then served to the classification model for identification (eg, benign squamous cell vs squamous intraepithelial lesion [SIL]). These are slightly more complicated implementations in that the final algorithm is an ensemble of 2 different types of models.

Dimensionality Reduction

This technique takes as input a complex, high-dimensional dataset (eg, a set of cellular statistics containing more than 3 items) and performs calculations to determine which data types are the most salient in distinguishing between different classes. Principal component analysis (PCA) and Uniform Manifold Approximation and Projection (UMAP)

are examples of dimensionality reduction. This technique is often used as a preprocessing step to determine which variables are most important, or after training a model to ensure that the learned features are distinctly separated.

LEVELS OF SUPERVISION

Machine learning models can be trained under multiple different supervision levels. Here, supervision refers to complementary information provided alongside the main training data (eg, images) that define the grouping of the various input objects (eg, squamous cell vs urothelial cell).

Fully Supervised

In fully supervised learning tasks, the model is provided with fully labeled data (eg, a list of images of squamous cells and a list of images of urothelial cells).

Semisupervised

In semisupervised learning, the model is provided with partial or incomplete labels (eg, images where only some of the nuclei are highlighted and the rest are left unlabeled).

Table 1
Frequency of model type employed in cytology artificial intelligence/machine learning research

Classification	Segmentation	Segmentation and Classification	Dimensionality Reduction
79	5	5	1

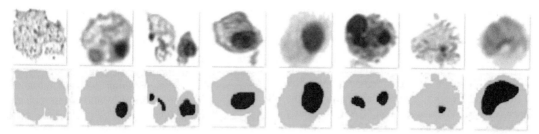

Fig. 3. Output of semantic segmentation model (mask) differentiating nuclear and cytoplasmic compartments as blue and green respectively.

Unsupervised/Self-Supervised

In unsupervised or self-supervised learning, the model is provided with unlabeled data and learns to "cluster" the data into groups that share similar characteristics.

SCOPE OF PREDICTION

Predictions made by machine learning models can be very granular (eg, a type for every cell in an image) or very macro (eg, a single prediction for an entire whole slide image).

Cell Level

Cell level predictions are made at the level of individual cells (eg, highlighting the nuclei of all malignant cells in a slide).

Slide Level

Slide level predictions incorporate information gleaned from the entire slide to apply a single label to the whole slide (eg, taking the average malignancy score of all the regions of a slide to render a final summary of risk).

RESEARCH SUMMARY

GYN

Unsurprisingly, 100% of the GYN-oriented articles focused on cervical cancer screening. A variety of model types were employed with the following breakdown (classification: 80.7%, segmentation: 11.6%, and segmentation and classification: 7.7%). The segmentation models focused on segmenting cells (cell vs background) or cell compartments (nucleus vs cytoplasm),[21–23] while the segmentation and classification models used segmentation as a first step for cell identification followed by classification of the identified cells.[24,25]

The GYN classification tasks ranged in complexity from investigating the effects of image quality on model performance and evaluating a commercial Pap smear algorithm,[26,27] to simpler binary tasks (eg, benign vs atypical squamous

cell, region of interest [ROI] selection),[28,29] to more complex, multiclass cell classification (eg, Benign vs atypical squamous cells of undetermined significance [ASCUS] vs low grade squamous intraepithelial lesion [LSIL] vs high grade squamous intraepithelial lesion [HSIL])[30–44] to prediction of surgical endpoints (eg, inferring cervical intraepithelial neoplasia [CIN] on biopsy from pap smear).[45,46]

A variety of metrics were used to determine the accuracy of these models including raw accuracy, negative predictive value, area under the curve (where high values indicate that the model is very good at differentiating positive and negative inputs), confusion matrix, intersection over union (IoU, essentially how well a predicted pixel assignment for an image overlaps with a ground truth pixel assignment), and DICE (Dice coefficient, similar to IoU but more sensitive to size mismatches of compared images).

Of note, very few of the articles exceeded the complexity of BD FocalPoint and the ThinPrep Imaging system in terms of modeling inputs and outputs. Most are recapitulations of this technology using modern machine learning models. Many of the studies made use of publicly available datasets including Herlev (917 grayscale images of individual cervical cells),[47] ISBI 2015 Cervical Cytology Challenge Data (17 extended depth of field cervical cytology images),[48] and SipakMed (4094 cropped images taken from cervical cytology clusters).[49]

NONGYN

The NONGYN articles covered a variety of specimen types that will be discussed in the order of decreasing frequency.

Thyroid

Investigations of thyroid cytology comprised ~20% of all cytology machine learning articles. All of the reviewed articles trained classification models of varying complexity. Four articles focused on rendering a binary prediction (malignant vs benign) based on overall morphology, nuclear morphology, or morphology plus *BRAF* next generation sequencing (NGS) results.[50–53] Another common theme was correctly predicting a specific malignancy (papillary thyroid carcinoma or medullary thyroid carcinoma [MTC]) or subtyping within multiple carcinoma classes.[54,55,56] Another study used molecular endpoints from FNA specimens to predict MTC prior to surgical resection.[57]

Several articles dealt with more complex modeling scenarios including predicting *BRAF* mutations from images,[58] determining adequacy from images of unstained slides,[59] predicting surgical findings for difficult differential scenarios (Noninvasive follicular thyroid neoplasm with papillary-like nuclear features [NIFTP] vs papillary thyroid carcinoma [PTC],[60] follicular adenoma vs carcinoma,[61,62] benign vs malignant for atypia of undetermined significance [AUS]/ follicular lesion of undetermined significance [FLUS],[63] and prediction of central lymph node metastasis[64]). There was additionally a single article that made use of weakly supervised learning to classify smears as benign or malignant.[65]

Urine

Urine was the next most common specimen utilized for AIML investigations. Several articles made use of segmentation or the combination of segmentation and classification for cluster deconvolution[66] and isolation and classification of cells in voided urine.[67,68] The rest of the articles addressing urine cytology employed classification models for binary malignant versus benign predictions,[69,70] multiclass cell identity prediction,[71,72] risk stratification,[73] slide level diagnosis,[74] and Paris System category prediction.[75,76] Two articles attempted to predict histologic findings from cytology,[77,78] and one article made use of an alternative imaging paradigm (Raman spectroscopy).[79]

Blood and Bone Marrow

While not traditionally considered to be cytology specimens, blood and bone marrow are included in this analysis because of domain similarities (eg, random cellular dispersions lacking architecture). The majority of studies employing blood smears were concerned with cell identification and quantitation.[80–84] More targeted research investigated leukemia lineage prediction[85] and detection of *Plasmodium*-infected red cells.[86]

The marrow aspirate-focused investigations used dimensionality reduction to summarize cell population proportions[87] and deep learning-based classification of marrow cell types.[88]

Lung

The cytology AIML investigations in lung consisted entirely of classification tasks. Four articles focused on binary predictions: malignant vs benign on bronchoscopic/FNA specimens,[89] differentiating between small cell and large cell neuroendocrine carcinoma[90] and non-small cell lung carcinoma typing.[91,92] The final article in this space investigated predicting driver mutations based on cytology alone.[93]

Breast

All of the breast-focused articles involved classification. One article (the earliest article in the entire cohort, published in 1995) utilized handcrafted tabular features derived from examination of cell nuclei and logistic regression to differentiate benign and malignant cells.[94] Another, compared different model architectures for the prediction of benign or malignant cellular features.[95] The final articles dealt with differentiating fibroadenoma from infiltrating carcinoma.[96]

Effusion

All of the effusion-based models concentrated on the binary task of determining whether cellular elements were benign or malignant. One model focused on breast cancer,[97] one focused on adenocarcinoma,[98] and two focused on predicting carcinoma in general.[99,100]

Pancreas

The pancreas-related articles were all binary classification models. Two focused on predicting benign versus malignant cells,[101,102] and one sought to aid in the evaluation of adequacy during Rapid Onsite Assessment.[103]

Oral

Two articles based on oral scrape cytology were identified: one segmentation-based model utilizing multichannel fluorescent images[104] and one model investigating the effect of model hyperparameters (values that affect model performance characteristics during training) on the detection of squamous cells.[105]

Stool

There were 2 articles focused on the detection of parasite eggs in stool smears.[106,107]

Nasal and Ocular

There was a single article in nasal cytology focused on rhinitis classification[108] and one article on predicting uveal melanoma from FNA biopsy.[109]

General

Two articles were classified as general: one sought to classify different types of benign and malignant cells in CSF specimens[110] and the other investigated the effects of LBP technique on the accuracy of cell detection.[111]

FUTURE DIRECTIONS

The number of AIML applications (both research and enterprise) in cytopathology will continue to increase over time. The first few waves of research (represented in the above literature summary) have focused mostly on obvious applications using standard modeling techniques. The next wave will most likely make use of more advanced models, multimodal datasets (eg, incorporating multiple complementary data types, whole slide image (WSI), NGS, fluid chemistry, and so forth), multi-institutional datasets and third party software designed to lower the technical hurdles to performing machine learning research. On the translational research/commercial side, expect continuing clinical validation efforts and new enterprise applications from existing players (Hologic, BD) and newer entrants (Visiopharm, Proscia, AIxMed). As with all new technology, however, the "killer applications" will be unpredictable and may cause significant disruptions to the current status quo. Cytopathologists, cytotechnologists, residents, and fellows must, therefore, cultivate an open mindset and be prepared to incorporate rapidly changing technology in the space.

SUMMARY

AIML promises to fundamentally change the practice of cytopathology from a largely subjective, manual endeavor to a computationally augmented and increasingly quantitative field. Significant progress has already been made in conceiving of and performing initial tests of AIML workflows for various common specimen types. Most of the research is still relatively rudimentary. As researchers and commercial vendors gain more experience in the space, cytology specialists can expect to encounter an increasing array of tools designed to make their practice more efficient, safer, and more quantitative. Cytologists have the advantage of more than a decade of experience with semiautomated Pap smear screening systems and so may be better positioned to adapt to these changes than surgical pathologists.

FUNDING

Grant number: 5 K08 CA267096-03.

DISCLOSURE

Nothing to disclose.

REFERENCES

1. Goldstone, R. L., Schyns, P. G. & Medin, D. L. Perceptual learning. (1997).
2. Rainer G, Lee H, Logothetis NK. The effect of learning on the function of monkey extrastriate visual cortex. PLoS Biol 2004;2:e44.
3. Marcandier M, Bideau L, Dubreuil Y. Applications de la photometrie a la numer- ation des hemities. C R Soc Biol Paris 1928;99:741.
4. Coulter, W. H. Means for counting particles suspended in a fluid. 米国特許第2656508号 (1953).
5. Spencer CC, Bostrom RC. Performance of the cytoanalyzer in recent clinical trials. J Natl Cancer Inst 1962;29:267–76.
6. Spriggs AI, Diamond RA, Meyer EW. Automated screening for cervical smears? Lancet 1968;1: 359–60.
7. Sadakazu W. An automated apparatus for cancer prescreening. CYBEST. Comput Graph Image Process 1974;3:350–8.
8. Zahniser DJ, Oud PS, Raaijmakers MC, et al. Bio-PEPR: a system for the automatic prescreening of cervical smears. J Histochem Cytochem 1979;27: 635–41.
9. Erhardt R, Reinhardt ER, Schlipf W, et al. FAZYTAN: a system for fast automated cell segmentation, cell image analysis and feature extraction based on TV-image pickup and parallel processing. Anal Quant Cytol 1980;2:25–40.
10. Tucker JH, Husain OA. Trials with the cerviscan experimental prescreening device on polylysine-prepared slides. Anal Quant Cytol 1981;3:117–20.
11. Ploem JS. LEYTAS-A cytology screening system using the new modular image analysis computer(-MIAC)from leitz. Clinical Cytometry and Histometry 1987;24–35.
12. Nordin B. The development of an automatic pre-screener for the early detection of cervical cancer: algorithms and implementation. Image Analysis Laboratory 1989.
13. Hutchinson ML, Cassin CM, Ball HG. The efficacy of an automated preparation device for cervical cytology. Am J Clin Pathol 1991;96:300–5.
14. Howell LP, Davis RL, Belk TI, et al. The AUTOCYTE preparation system for gynecologic cytology. Acta Cytol 1998;42:171–7.
15. Bernstein SJ, Sanchez-Ramos L, Ndubisi B. Liquid-based cervical cytologic smear study and conventional Papanicolaou smears: A metaanalysis of prospective studies comparing cytologic diagnosis and sample adequacy. Am J Obstet Gynecol 2001;185:308–17.

16. Autopap(r) 300 QC automatic pap screener/QC system. Available at: https://fda.report/PMA/P950009.

17. Premarket Approval (PMA).

18. Koss LG. The Papanicolaou test for cervical cancer detection. A triumph and a tragedy. JAMA 1989; 261:737–43.

19. CLIA law & regulation. 2022. Available at: https://www.cdc.gov/clia/law-regulations.html.

20. Krizhevsky A, Sutskever I, Hinton GE. ImageNet classification with deep convolutional neural networks. In: Advances in neural information processing systems, 25 2012.

21. Chen J, Zhang B. Segmentation of overlapping cervical cells with mask region convolutional neural network. Comput Math Methods Med 2021;2021.

22. Zhao Y, Fu C, Xu S, et al. LFANet: Lightweight feature attention network for abnormal cell segmentation in cervical cytology images. Comput Biol Med 2022;145.

23. Ji J, Zhang W, Dong Y, et al. Automated cervical cell segmentation using deep ensemble learning. BMC Med Imaging 2023;23.

24. Nambu Y, Mariya T, Shinkai S, et al. A screening assistance system for cervical cytology of squamous cell atypia based on a two-step combined CNN algorithm with label smoothing. Cancer Med 2022;11.

25. Ke J, Shen Y, Lu Y, et al. Quantitative analysis of abnormalities in gynecologic cytopathology with deep learning. Lab Invest 2021;101.

26. Liu W, Li C, Rahaman MM, et al. Is the aspect ratio of cells important in deep learning? A robust comparison of deep learning methods for multi-scale cytopathology cell image classification: From convolutional neural networks to visual transformers. Comput Biol Med 2022;141.

27. Bao H, Sun X, Zhang Y, et al. The artificial intelligence-assisted cytology diagnostic system in large-scale cervical cancer screening: A population-based cohort study of 0.7 million women. Cancer Med 2020;9.

28. Kurita Y, Meguro S, Tsuyama N, et al. Accurate deep learning model using semi-supervised learning and Noisy Student for cervical cancer screening in low magnification images. PLoS One 2023;18.

29. Sornapudi S, Brown GT, Xue Z, et al. Comparing deep learning models for multi-cell classification in liquid- based cervical cytology image. AMIA Annu. Symp. Proc 2020;2019.

30. Hamdi M, Senan EM, Awaji B, et al. Analysis of WSI Images by hybrid systems with fusion features for early diagnosis of cervical cancer. Diagnostics 2023;13.

31. Shinde S, Kalbhor M, Wajire P. DeepCyto: a hybrid framework for cervical cancer classification by using deep feature fusion of cytology images. Math Biosci Eng 2022;19.

32. Zhao S, He Y, Qin J, et al. A semi-supervised deep learning method for cervical cell classification. Anal Cell Pathol 2022;2022.

33. Zhu X, Li X, Ong K, et al. Hybrid AI-assistive diagnostic model permits rapid TBS classification of cervical liquid-based thin-layer cell smears. Nat Commun 2021;12.

34. Hussain E, Mahanta LB, Das CR, et al. A comprehensive study on the multi-class cervical cancer diagnostic prediction on pap smear images using a fusion-based decision from ensemble deep convolutional neural network. Tissue Cell 2020;65.

35. Zhang L, Le L, Nogues I, et al. DeepPap: deep convolutional networks for cervical cell classification. IEEE journal of biomedical and health informatics 2017;21.

36. Aljakouch K, Hilal Z, Daho I, et al. Fast and noninvasive diagnosis of cervical cancer by coherent anti-stokes raman scattering. Anal Chem 2019;91.

37. Kupas D, Harangi B. Classification of Pap-smear cell images using deep convolutional neural network accelerated by hand-crafted features. Conf Proc IEEE Eng Med Biol Soc 2022;2022: 1452–5.

38. Rahaman MM, Li C, Yao Y, et al. DeepCervix: A deep learning-based framework for the classification of cervical cells using hybrid deep feature fusion techniques. Comput Biol Med 2021;136.

39. Sompawong N, Mopan J, Pooprasert P, et al. Automated pap smear cervical cancer screening using deep learning. Conf. Proc. IEEE Eng. Med. Biol. Soc 2019;2019.

40. P BS, Faruqi F, K SH, et al. Deep convolution neural network for malignancy detection and classification in microscopic uterine cervix cell images. Asian Pac J Cancer Prev APJCP 2019;20.

41. Li X, Xu Z, Shen X, et al. Detection of cervical cancer cells in whole slide images using deformable and global context aware faster RCNN-FPN. Curr Oncol 2021;28.

42. Holmström O, Linder N, Kaingu H, et al. Point-of-care digital cytology with artificial intelligence for cervical cancer screening in a resource-limited setting. JAMA Netw Open 2021;4.

43. Lin H, Chen H, Wang X, et al. Dual-path network with synergistic grouping loss and evidence driven risk stratification for whole slide cervical image analysis. Med Image Anal 2021;69.

44. Shi J, Wang R, Zheng Y, et al. Cervical cell classification with graph convolutional network. Comput Methods Progr Biomed 2021;198.

45. Tao X, Zhang H, Zhang H, et al. Scrutinizing high-risk patients from ASC-US cytology via a deep learning model. Cancer Cytopathol 2022;130.

46. Bao H, Bi H, Zhang X, et al. Artificial intelligence-assisted cytology for detection of cervical intraepithelial neoplasia or invasive cancer: A multicenter, clinical-based, observational study. Gynecol Oncol 2020;159.

47. Chowdhury, Y. S. Herlev Dataset. (2022).

48. ISBI 2017. Available at: https://biomedicalimaging.org/2015/program/isbi-challenges/.

49. Cv. Cervical Cancer largest dataset (SipakMed). (2021).

50. Assaad S, Dov D, Davis R, et al. Thyroid Cytopathology Cancer Diagnosis from Smartphone Images Using Machine Learning. Mod Pathol 2023; 36.

51. Gopinath B, Shanthi N. Support Vector Machine based diagnostic system for thyroid cancer using statistical texture features. Asian Pac J Cancer Prev APJCP 2013;14.

52. Fragopoulos C, Pouliakis A, Meristoudis C, et al. Radial basis function artificial neural network for the investigation of thyroid cytological lesions. J Thyroid Res 2020;2020.

53. Dov D. Learning fast screening approach on cytological whole slides for thyroid cancer diagnosis. Cancers 2021;13:3891.

54. Sanyal P, Mukherjee T, Barui S, et al. Artificial intelligence in cytopathology: a neural network to identify papillary carcinoma on thyroid fine-needle aspiration cytology smears. J Pathol Inf 2018;9:43.

55. Lin YJ, Elliott Range D, Cohen J, et al. Deep-learning-based screening and ancillary testing for thyroid cytopathology. Am J Pathol 2023;193:1185–94.

56. Hirokawa M, Niioka H, Suzuki A, et al. Application of deep learning as an ancillary diagnostic tool for thyroid FNA cytology. Cancer Cytopathol 2023;131:217–25.

57. Randolph GW, Sosa JA, Hao Y, et al. Preoperative identification of medullary thyroid carcinoma (mtc): clinical validation of the afirma MTC RNA-sequencing classifier. Thyroid 2022;32:1069–76.

58. Wang CW, Muzakky H, Lee YC, et al. Annotation-free deep learning-based prediction of thyroid molecular cancer biomarker BRAF (V600E) from cytological slides. Int J Mol Sci 2023;24:2521.

59. Jang J, Kim YH, Westgate B, et al. Screening adequacy of unstained thyroid fine needle aspiration samples using a deep learning-based classifier. Sci Rep 2023;13:13525.

60. Maleki S, Zandvakili A, Gera S, et al. Differentiating noninvasive follicular thyroid neoplasm with papillary-like nuclear features from classic papillary thyroid carcinoma: analysis of cytomorphologic descriptions using a novel machine-learning approach. J Pathol Inf 2019;10:29.

61. Alabrak MMA, Megahed M, Alkhouly AA, et al. Artificial intelligence role in subclassifying cytology of thyroid follicular neoplasm. Asian Pac J Cancer Prev APJCP 2023;24:1379–87.

62. Savala R, Dey P, Gupta N. Artificial neural network model to distinguish follicular adenoma from follicular carcinoma on fine needle aspiration of thyroid. Diagn Cytopathol 2018;46:244–9.

63. Saini T, Saikia UN, Dey P. An artificial neural network for the prediction of the risk of malignancy in category III Bethesda thyroid lesions. Cytopathology 2023;34:48–54.

64. Ren W, Zhu Y, Wang Q, et al. Deep learning prediction model for central lymph node metastasis in papillary thyroid microcarcinoma based on cytology. Cancer Sci 2023;114:4114–24.

65. Dov D, Kovalsky SZ, Assaad S, et al. Weakly supervised instance learning for thyroid malignancy prediction from whole slide cytopathology images. Med Image Anal 2021;67.

66. Levy JJ, Liu X, Marotti JD, et al. Uncovering additional predictors of urothelial carcinoma from voided urothelial cell clusters through a deep learning-based image preprocessing technique. Cancer Cytopathol 2023;131.

67. Levy JJ, Chan N, Marotti JD, et al. Examining longitudinal markers of bladder cancer recurrence through a semiautonomous machine learning system for quantifying specimen atypia from urine cytology. Cancer Cytopathol 2023;131.

68. Vaickus LJ, Suriawinata AA, Wei JW, et al. Automating the paris system for urine cytopathology-a hybrid deep-learning and morphometric approach. Cancer Cytopathol 2019;127.

69. Tsuneki M, Abe M, Kanavati F. Deep learning-based screening of urothelial carcinoma in whole slide images of liquid-based cytology urine specimens. Cancers 2022;15.

70. Pantazopoulos D, Karakitsos P, Iokim-Liossi A, et al. Back propagation neural network in the discrimination of benign from malignant lower urinary tract lesions. J Urol 1998;159.

71. Lilli L, Giarnieri E, Scardapane S. A calibrated multiexit neural network for detecting urothelial cancer cells. Comput Math Methods Med 2021;2021.

72. Kaneko M, Tsuji K, Masuda K, et al. Urine cell image recognition using a deep-learning model for an automated slide evaluation system. BJU Int 2022;130.

73. Awan R, Benes K, Azam A, et al. Deep learning based digital cell profiles for risk stratification of urine cytology images. Cytometry 2021;99.

74. Sanghvi AB, Allen EZ, Callenberg KM, et al. Performance of an artificial intelligence algorithm for reporting urine cytopathology. Cancer Cytopathol 2019;127.

75. Ou YC, Tsao TY, Chang MC, et al. Evaluation of an artificial intelligence algorithm for assisting the Paris System in reporting urinary cytology: A pilot study. Cancer Cytopathol 2022;130.

76. Lebret T, Paoletti X, Pignot G, et al. Artificial intelligence to improve cytology performance in urothelial carcinoma diagnosis: results from validation phase of the French, multicenter, prospective VIS-IOCYT1 trial. World J Urol 2023;41.

77. Nojima S, Terayama K, Shimoura S, et al. A deep learning system to diagnose the malignant potential of urothelial carcinoma cells in cytology specimens. Cancer Cytopathol 2021;129.

78. Liu Y, Jin S, Shen Q, et al. A deep learning system to predict the histopathological results from urine cytopathological images. Front Oncol 2022;12.

79. Krauß SD, Roy R, Yosef HK, et al. Hierarchical deep convolutional neural networks combine spectral and spatial information for highly accurate Raman-microscopy-based cytopathology. J Biophot 2018;11.

80. Ma L, Shuai R, Ran X, et al. Combining DC-GAN with ResNet for blood cell image classification. Med Biol Eng Comput 2020;58.

81. Kutlu H, Avci E, Özyurt F. White blood cells detection and classification based on regional convolutional neural networks. Med Hypotheses 2020;135.

82. Wang Q, Bi S, Sun M, et al. Deep learning approach to peripheral leukocyte recognition. PLoS One 2019;14.

83. Shahin AI, Guo Y, Amin KM, et al. White blood cells identification system based on convolutional deep neural learning networks. Comput Methods Progr Biomed 2019;168.

84. Durant TJS, Olson EM, Schulz WL, et al. Very deep convolutional neural networks for morphologic classification of erythrocytes. Clin Chem 2017;63.

85. Boldú L, Merino A, Acevedo A, et al. A deep learning model (ALNet) for the diagnosis of acute leukaemia lineage using peripheral blood cell images. Comput Methods Progr Biomed 2021;202.

86. Fu M, Wu K, Li Y, et al. An intelligent detection method for plasmodium based on self-supervised learning and attention mechanism. Front Med 2023;10.

87. Dehkharghanian T, Mu Y, Ross C, et al. Cell projection plots: A novel visualization of bone marrow aspirate cytology. J Pathol Inf 2023;14.

88. Tayebi RM, Mu Y, Dehkharghanian T, et al. Automated bone marrow cytology using deep learning to generate a histogram of cell types. Commun Med 2022;2.

89. Teramoto A, Tsukamoto T, Yamada A, et al. Deep learning approach to classification of lung cytological images: Two-step training using actual and synthesized images by progressive growing of generative adversarial networks. PLoS One 2020;15.

90. Gonzalez D, Dietz RL, Pantanowitz L. Feasibility of a deep learning algorithm to distinguish large cell neuroendocrine from small cell lung carcinoma in cytology specimens. Cytopathology 2020;31.

91. Tsukamoto T, Teramoto A, Yamada A, et al. Comparison of fine-tuned deep convolutional neural networks for the automated classification of lung cancer cytology images with integration of additional classifiers. Asian Pac J Cancer Prev APJCP 2022;23.

92. Wang D, Ye YK, Zhang Y, et al. [Implementation and application of a digital cytopathological lung cancer diagnosing system]. Zhonghua Wai Ke Za Zhi 2007;45.

93. Ishii S, Takamatsu M, Ninomiya H, et al. Machine learning-based gene alteration prediction model for primary lung cancer using cytologic images. Cancer Cytopathol 2022;130.

94. Wolberg WH, Street WN, Heisey DM, et al. Computer-derived nuclear features distinguish malignant from benign breast cytology. Hum Pathol 1995;26.

95. Saikia AR, Bora K, Mahanta LB, et al. Comparative assessment of CNN architectures for classification of breast FNAC images. Tissue Cell 2019;57.

96. Subbaiah RM, Dey P, Nijhawan R. Artificial neural network in breast lesions from fine-needle aspiration cytology smear. Diagn Cytopathol 2014;42.

97. Park HS, Chong Y, Lee Y, et al. Deep learning-based computational cytopathologic diagnosis of metastatic breast carcinoma in pleural fluid. Cells 2023;12.

98. Sanyal P, Dey P. Using a deep learning neural network for the identification of malignant cells in effusion cytology material. Cytopathology 2023;34.

99. Su F, Sun Y, Hu Y, et al. Development and validation of a deep learning system for ascites cytopathology interpretation. Gastric Cancer 2020;23.

100. Xie X, Fu CC, Lv L, et al. Deep convolutional neural network-based classification of cancer cells on cytological pleural effusion images. Mod Pathol 2022;35:609–14.

101. Sohn A, Miller D, Ribeiro E, et al. A deep learning model to triage and predict adenocarcinoma on pancreas cytology whole slide imaging. Sci Rep 2023;13:16517.

102. Qin X, Zhang M, Zhou C, et al. A deep learning model using hyperspectral image for EUS-FNA cytology diagnosis in pancreatic ductal adenocarcinoma. Cancer Med 2023;12:17005–17.

103. Zhang S, Zhou Y, Tang D, et al. A deep learning-based segmentation system for rapid onsite cytologic pathology evaluation of pancreatic masses: A retrospective, multicenter, diagnostic study. EBioMedicine 2022;80:104022.

104. Sunny SP, Khan AI, Rangarajan M, et al. Oral epithelial cell segmentation from fluorescent multichannel cytology images using deep learning. Comput Methods Progr Biomed 2022;227:107205.

105. Sukegawa S, Tanaka F, Nakano K, et al. Effective deep learning for oral exfoliative cytology classification. Sci Rep 2022;12:13281.

106. Noyan MA, Durdu M, Eskiocak AH. TzanckNet: a convolutional neural network to identify cells in